MYOCARDIAL ISCHEMIA

DEVELOPMENTS IN CARDIOVASCULAR MEDICINE

Perry, H.M., ed.: Lifelong management of hypertension. ISBN 0-89838-582-2.
Jaffe, E.A., ed.: Biology of endothelial cells. ISBN 0-89838-587-3.
Surawicz, B., Reddy, C.P., Prystowsky, E.N., eds.: Tachycardias. 1984. ISBN 0-89838-588-1.
Spencer, M.P., ed.: Cardiac doppler diagnosis. ISBN 0-89838-591-1.
Villareal, H.V., Sambhi, M.P., eds.: Topics in pathophysiology of hypertension. ISBN 0-89838-595-4.
Messerli, F.H., ed.: Cardiovascular disease in the elderly. 1984. ISBN 0-89838-596-2.
Simoons, M.L., Reiber, J.H.C., eds.: Nuclear imaging in clinical cardiology. ISBN 0-89838-599-7.
Ter Keurs, H.E.D.J., Schipperheym, J.J., eds.: Cardiac left ventricular hypertrophy. ISBN 0-89838-612-8.
Sperelakis, N., ed.: Physiology and pathophysiology of the heart. ISBN 0-89838-615-2.
Messerli, F.H., ed.: Kidney in essential hypertension. 1983. ISBN 0-89838-616-0.
Sambhi, M.P., ed.: Fundamental fault in hypertension. ISBN 0-89838-638-1.
Marchesi, D., ed.: Ambulatory monitoring: Cardiovascular system and allied applications. ISBN 0-89838-642-X.
Kupper, W., Macalpin, R.N., Bleifeld, W., eds.: Coronary tone in ischemic heart disease. ISBN 0-89838-646-2.
Sperelakis, N., Caulfield, J.B., eds.: Calcium antagonists: Mechanisms of action on cardiac muscle and vascular smooth muscle. ISBN 0-89838-655-1.
Godfraind, T., Herman, A.S., Wellens, D., eds.: Entry blockers in cardiovascular and cerebral dysfunctions. ISBN 0-89838-658-6.
Morganroth, J., Moore, E.N., eds.: Interventions in the acute phase of myocardial infarction. ISBN 0-89838-659-4.
Abel, F.L., Newman, W.H., eds.: Functional aspects of the normal, hypertrophied, and failing heart. ISBN 0-89838-665-9.
Sideman, S., and Beyar, R., eds.: Simulation and imaging of the cardiac system. ISBN 0-89838-687-X.
van de Wall, E., Lie, K.I., eds.: Recent views on hypertrophic cardiomyopathy. ISBN 0-89838-694-2.
Beamish, R.E., Singal, P.K., Dhalla, N.S., eds.: Stress and heart disease. ISBN 089838-709-4.
Beamish, R.E., Panagia, V., Dhalla, N.S., eds.: Pathogenesis of stress-induced heart disease. ISBN 0-89838-710-8.
Morganroth, J., Moore, E.N., eds., Cardiac arrhythmias: New therapeutic drugs and devices. ISBN 0-89838-716-7.
Mathes, P., ed.: Secondary prevention in coronary artery disease and myocardial infarction. ISBN 0-89838-736-1.
Stone, H. Lowell, Weglicki, W.B., eds., Pathology of cardiovascular injury. ISBN 0-89838-743-4.
Meyer, J., Erbel, R., Rupprecht, H.J., eds., Improvement of myocardial perfusion. ISBN 0-89838-748-5.
Reiber, J.H.C., Serruys, P.W., Slager, C.J.: Quantitative coronary and left ventricular cineangiography. ISBN 0-89838-760-4.
Fagard, R.H., Bekaert, I.E., eds., Sports cardiology. ISBN 0-89838-782-5.
Reiber, J.H.C., Serruys, P.W., eds., State of the art in quantitative coronary arteriography. ISBN 0-89838-804-X.
Roelandt, J., ed.: Color doppler flow imaging. ISBN 0-89838-806-6.
van de Wall, E.E., ed.: Noninvasive imaging of cardiac metabolism. ISBN 0-89838-812-0.
Liebman, J., Plonsey, R., Rudy, Y., eds., Pediatric and fundamental electrocardiography. ISBN 0-89838-815-5.
Higler, H., Hombach, V., eds., Invasive cardiovascular therapy. ISBN 0-89838-818-X.
Serruys, P.W., Meester, G.T., eds., Coronary angioplasty: a controlled model for ischemia. ISBN 0-89838-819-8.
Tooke, J.E., Smaje, L.H., eds.: Clinical investigation of the microcirculation. ISBN 0-89838-833-3.
van Dam, Th., van Oosterom, A., eds.: Electrocardiographic body surface mapping. ISBN 0-89838-834-1.
Spencer, M.P., ed.: Ultrasonic diagnosis of cerebrovascular disease. ISBN 0-89838-836-8.
Legato, M.J., ed.: The stressed heart. ISBN 0-89838-849-X.
Safar, M.E., ed.: Arterial and venous systems in essential hypertension. ISBN 0-89838-857-0.
Roelandt, J., ed.: Digital techniques in echocardiography. ISBN 0-89838-861-9.
Dhalla, N.S., Singal, P.K., Beamish, R.E., eds.: Pathophysiology of heart disease. ISBN 0-89838-864-3.
Dhalla, N.S., Pierce, G.N., Beamish, R.E., eds.: Heart function and metabolism. ISNB 0-89838-865-1.

This book is a volume in the series, "Advances in Myocardiology" (N.S. Dhalla, Series Editor). "Advances in Myocardiology" is a subseries within "Developments in Cardiovascular Medicine".

MYOCARDIAL ISCHEMIA

Proceedings of a Satellite Symposium of the
Thirtieth International Physiological Congress
July 8–11, 1986, Winnipeg, Canada

edited by

Naranjan S. Dhalla
Ian R. Innes
Robert E. Beamish
Youville Research Institute, St. Boniface General
Hospital, and Faculty of Medicine, University of
Manitoba, Winnipeg, Canada

Springer-Science+Business Media, B.V.

Library of Congress Cataloging-in-Publication Data

Myocardial ischemia.

  (Developments in cardiovascular medicine)
  1. Coronary heart disease—Congresses. 2. Ischemia—
Congresses. 3. Physiology, Pathological—Congresses.
I. Dhalla, Naranjan S. II. Innes, Ian R. III. Beamish,
Robert E. IV. International Congress of Physiological
Sciences (30th: 1986: Vancouver, B.C.) V. Series.
[DNLM: 1. Coronary Disease—congresses. W1 DE997VME /
WG 300 M99766 1986]
RC685.C6M959   1986   616.1′23   86-33106
ISBN 978-1-4612-9221-0   ISBN 978-1-4613-2055-5 (eBook)
DOI 10.1007/978-1-4613-2055-5

*This book is dedicated to
Dr. Robert B. Jennings for
his pioneer work in
pathophysiology of
ischemic heart disease*

CONTENTS

Preface   xi
Acknowledgements   xiii

A. MYOCARDIAL CELL DAMAGE AND ARRHYTHMIAS

1. Ultrastructural Abnormalities in Ischemic Heart Disease   3
   J. Schaper

2. Preconditioning with Ischemia: A Means to Delay Cell Death in
   Ischemic Myocardium   11
   C.E. Murry, R.B. Jennings, K.A. Reimer

3. Modification of the Thromboxane/Prostacyclin Balance as an Approach
   to Antiarrhythmic Therapy During Myocardial Ischaemia and
   Reperfusion; The Concept of Endogenous Antiarrhythmic Substances   21
   J.R. Parratt

4. Mechanisms of Coupled Arrhythmias in Guinea Pig Perfused Heart
   and Isolated Ventricular Tissue Models of Ischemia-Reperfusion   37
   G.R. Ferrier, C.M. Guyette

5. The Preventive Effect of Sodium Selenite Against Ischemic Ventricular
   Arrhythmia and Some Clues to its Mechanisms   53
   Y.A. Mei, Y.Q. Xu, H.D. Zhang

B. PATHOPHYSIOLOGIC ASPECTS OF ISCHEMIC INJURY

6. Molecular Events Occurring During Post-Ischaemic Reperfusion   67
   R. Ferrari, C. Ceconi, S. Curello, A. Cargnoni, A. Albertini,
   E.O. Visioli

7. Oxidation of Methionine in Proteins of Isolated Rat Heart Myocytes
   and Tissue Slices by Neutrophil-Generated Oxygen Free Radicals   85
   H. Fliss, G. Docherty

8. Phospholipid Metabolism in Heart Membranes   99
   K.J. Kako, M. Kato

9. Models of Injury of Cardiovascular Membranes by Amphiphiles and
   Free Radicals   113
   W.B. Weglicki, I.T. Mak, B.F. Dickens, J.H. Kramer

10. Inability of Superoxide Dismutase and Catalase to Inhibit Calcium
    Influx on Reoxygenation of Rabbit Myocardium   123
    P.A. Poole-Wilson, M.A. Tones

11. Catecholamine Release in Myocardial Ischemia and its Clinical
    Implications   133
    W. Kubler, R. Dietz, W. Maurer, A. Schomig

12. Coronary Blood Flow in Myocardial Stress with Catecholamine
    Administration in the Dog   145
    R.M. Berne, J.M. Gidday, H.E. Hill, R. Rubio

13. Morphometric Analysis of Regional Myocardial Perfusion in Rats as
Measured by Non-Radioactive Microspheres   149
M. Korpan, K. Rakusan

14. Prostaglandins and Defects in Vascular Function   163
D.B. McNamara, J.A. Bellan, P.R. Mayeux, M.D. Kerstein,
A.L. Hyman, P.J. Kadowitz, D.S. Rush

15. Endothelium Dependent Relaxation and Atherosclerosis   171
N. Sreeharan, R. Jayakody, M. Senaratne, A. Thomson,
T. Kappagoda

C. METABOLIC ASPECTS OF CELL DAMAGE

16. Energy Metabolism in Myocardial Ischemia and Reperfusion   185
R.B. Jennings, K.A. Reimer, C. Steenbergen, C.E. Murry

17. The Role of Beta-Adrenoceptors in Ischemia-Induced Acidosis in the
Isolated Rat Heart: A 31-P NMR Study   199
N. Lavanchy, J. Martin, A. Rossi

18. Protective and Nonprotective Effects of Drugs on Cardia Contractile
Activity and High Energy Phosphates During Anoxia and After
Reoxygenation   213
M. Siess, U. Delabar, K. Stieler, J. Leuchtner, I. Teutsch,
A. Khattab, M.B. El Hawary

19. Myocardial Enzyme Leakage and Succinic Dehydrogenase Activity of
Mitochondria Correlated with the Morphological Changes in the Anoxic
Isolated Perfused Rat Heart   233
J. Yeh-Chih, W. Wen-Hu, H. Yu-Sheng, F. Ling-Xiong

20. Hemodynamic Performance of Isolated Blood-Perfused Working Hearts
of Creatine Depleted Rats in Hypoxemia   243
B. Korecky, Y.A. Brandejs-Barry

21. Phosphorus Nuclear Magnetic Resonance Measurements of Intracellular
pH in Isolated Rabbit Heart During the Calcium Paradox   257
T.J.C. Ruigrok, J.H. Kirkels, C.J.A. Van Echteld, C. Borst,
F.L. Meijler

22. Hypercontracture of Isolated Adult Rat Heart Myocytes: Multiple
Causes and a Common Mechanism   265
R.A. Altschuld, M.R. Lambert, G.P. Brierley

23. Mechanical Restitution and Inotropic Reserve of the Rat Heart
Following Heterothermal Global Ischemia   277
J.S. Juggi, P. Braveny

D. CALCIUM ANTAGONISTS AND MYOCARDIAL ISCHEMIA

24. Calcium Antagonism and the Ischemic Myocardium   285
W.G. Nayler, W.J. Sturrock, S. Panagiotopoulos

25. Biochemical and Ultrastructural Alterations in Cardiac Membranes
During Ischaemia-Reperfusion: Protection by a Calcium Entry Blocker   297
J.M.J. Lamers, C.E. Essed, J.A. Post, A.J. Verkleij, F.J. ten Cate,
W.J. van der Giessen, P.D. Verdouw

26. Effect of Nifedipine and Hyaluronidase Alone and in Combination on Myocardial Preservation in Experimental Myocardial Infarction — A Morphological and Biochemical Profile   311
M.P. Gupta, S.D. Seth, S.C. Manchanda, U. Singh

27. Action of Calcium Antagonists on the Contraction of Isolated Human Coronary Arteries and Myocardium   325
T. Godfraind

28. Inhibitory Effects of Allicin (Diallyl Disulfide-Oxide, A Constituent of Garlic Oil) on Human Platelet and Polymorphonuclear Leukocyte Function   339
P.R. Mayeux, K.C. Agrawal, J-S.H. Tou, B.T. King, A.L. Hyman, P.J. Kadowitz, D.B. McNamara

PREFACE

Whenever the coronary flow is inadequate to provide enough oxygen to meet the energy demands of the tissue, the heart becomes ischemic. Manifestations of myocardial ischemia include depression in contractile activity, changes in metabolic pattern, abnormalities in ultrastructure, and alterations in membrane potential. Ischemic changes during the early phase are reversible but as the period of ischemia is extended, the injury becomes irreversible. The transition from reversible to irreversible ischemic injury is usually associated with some membrane defects. It is worthwhile to consider that the irreversible damage to the ischemic myocardium occurs when the sarcolemmal membrane is altered in such a way that it would promote a net gain of Ca^{2+} in the cardiac cell upon reinstitution of blood flow. Such a lesion could result when mechanisms for the entry as well as removal of Ca^{2+} from the myocardial cell become defective. In this regard, depression of the sarcolemmal Ca^{2+} pump would favour the occurrence of intracellular Ca^{2+} overload. Furthermore, inhibition of the Na^+-K^+ pump would lead to elevation of myoplasmic Na^+ which could then increase the intracellular concentration of Ca^{2+} through the sarcolemmal Na^+-Ca^{2+} exchange mechanism. In fact recent studies have revealed an inhibition of the sarcolemmal Na^+-Ca^{2+} exchange mechanism in the ischemic heart and this change could also contribute towards the occurrence of intracellular Ca^{2+} overload. Another possibility for increased intracellular Ca^{2+} in the ischemic heart upon reperfusion could be an excessive entry of Ca^{2+} through abnormal Ca^{2+} channels in the cardiac cell membrane. Thus membrane defects in the ischemic heart can be conceived to involve different sites for Ca^{2+} movement in the myocardium.

Although the presence of membrane defects in a wide variety of experimental models of ischemic heart disease has now been clearly demonstrated, the exact mechanisms for such a lesion are far from clear. Some of the investigators believe that accumulation of various metabolic intermediates including H^+, long chain fatty acids, acylcarnitine and lysophospholipids is responsible for inducing membrane abnormalities in the ischemic heart. Others are of the view that lowering of the energy state and increasing of the cytoplasmic concentration of Ca^{2+} due to prolonged myocardial ischemia result in membrane abnormalities. Activation of lysosomal enzymes, proteases and phospholipases has been implicated in the development of cell damage in the ischemic heart; however, the role of free radicals in ischemic injury is gaining considerable support. Thus the pathogenesis of the ischemic damage seems to be of a complex nature and accordingly the therapy of myocardial ischemia should be approached from different angles. In this book, several recognized experts have expressed their views on the pathogenesis and therapeutics of ischemic heart disease and have supported their conclusions by experimental findings. For the convenience of our readers we have grouped 28 articles in four sections namely Myocardial Cell Damage and Arrhythmias, Pathophysiologic Aspects of Ischemic Injury, Metabolic Aspects of Cell Damage and Calcium Antagonists and Myocardial Ischemia. We hope the information contained in this book is helpful in further understanding ischemic heart disease and improving its therapy.

Naranjan S. Dhalla, Ph.D.
Ian R. Innes, M.D.
Robert E. Beamish, M.D.

Acknowledgements

We are grateful to the following Agencies and Foundations for their generous financial support of the Symposium, which formed the basis of this book.

A. **Major Contributors:**

1. Manitoba Heart Foundation
2. Sterling-Winthrop Research Institute
3. Squibb Canada, Inc.
4. St. Boniface Hospital Research Foundation
5. Manitoba Medical Service Foundation, Inc.
6. Health Sciences Centre Research Foundation
7. International Society for Heart Research - American Section
8. Knoll Pharmaceuticals Canada Inc.
9. Section of Cardiology - St. Boniface General Hospital
10. Section of Cardiology - Health Sciences Centre
11. Children's Hospital of Winnipeg Research Foundation Inc.
12. Medical Research Council of Canada

B. **Contributors:**

1. Ayerst Laboratories (U.S.A.)
2. Bayer AG/Miles
3. Beckman Instrument, Inc.
4. Boehringer Ingelheim (Canada) Ltd.
5. Canadian Heart Foundation
6. ICI Pharma, Canada
7. Merck Frosst Canada Inc.
8. Merrell Dow Pharmaceutical Ltd. (U.K.)
9. Nordic Laboratories Canada Inc.
10. Rhone-Poulenc Pharma Inc.
11. Sandoz Canada Inc.
12. Schering Corporation (U.S.A.)
13. Smith Kline & French Laboratories (U.S.A.)
14. Syntex International Ltd. (U.S.A.)
15. The Upjohn Company (U.S.A.)
16. Rorer Canada, Inc.

C. **Supporters:**

1. American Critical Care (U.S.A.)
2. Marion Laboratories, Inc. (U.S.A.)

xiv

3. Merck Sharp & Dohme (U.S.A.)
4. Medtronic of Canada Ltd.
5. A.H. Robins Canada Inc.
6. G.D. Searle and Co. (U.S.A.)
7. G.D. Searle and Co. (Canada)
8. NOVOPHARM Ltd., Canada

We are thankful to Mrs. Susie Petrychko and the editorial staff of
Martinus Nijhoff for their valuable assistance in the preparation of this book.
Special thanks are due to the members of the Symposium Organization Committee,
Session Chairmen, participants and all those who helped in so many ways to
make this Symposium an outstanding scientific and social event. We are
indebted to Dr. Arnold Naimark, President, University of Manitoba, Dr. John
Wade, Dean, Faculty of Medicine, and Dr. Henry Friesen, Head, Department of
Physiology for their continued interest and encouragement.

A. MYOCARDIAL CELL DAMAGE AND ARRHYTHMIAS

1

ULTRASTRUCTURAL ABNORMALITIES IN ISCHEMIC HEART DISEASE

JUTTA SCHAPER

Max-Planck-Institut, Abt. Exp. Kardiologie, Benekestraße 2,
6350 Bad Nauheim, FRG

INTRODUCTION

Regional myocardial ischemia is caused by either acute
occlusion of a coronary artery or by slowly occurring stenosis
finally leading to occlusion in a major cardiac vessel. The
effects on the myocardium of either acutely or slowly occurring
vascular occlusion vary widely, from a functional as well as
a metabolic and structural point of view. The present study
is concerned with the histologic and ultrastructural changes
of regional ischemia; it shall describe the effects of acute
ligation of a coronary artery in the canine heart and the
alterations due to chronic ischemia in the human heart.

RESULTS AND DISCUSSION

1. Acute regional ischemia in canine hearts.

In open-chest mongrel dogs the left anterior descending
coronary artery (LAD) was ligated for periods of time varying between 45 minutes up to 24 hours. At the end of the
ischemic period with or without reperfusion needle biopsies
were taken from the center of the area affected by ischemia.

These were investigated by transmission electron microscopy
using a semi quantitative evaluation system (1). Acute ischemia produces reversible injury at early stages, irreversible
injury follows at later time points. Changes include clearing
of mitochondria and nuclei, destruction of sarcomeres as well
as of sarcolemma and occurrence of edema (Figs. 1-3).

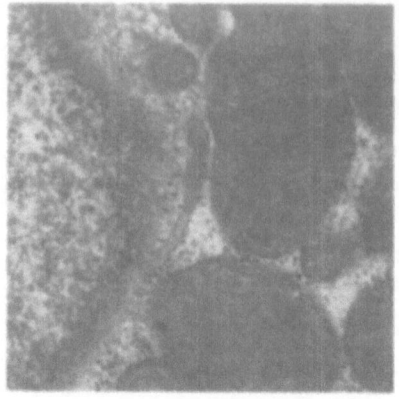

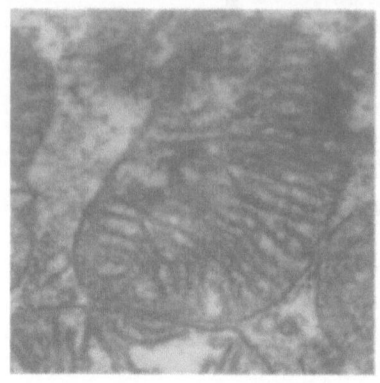

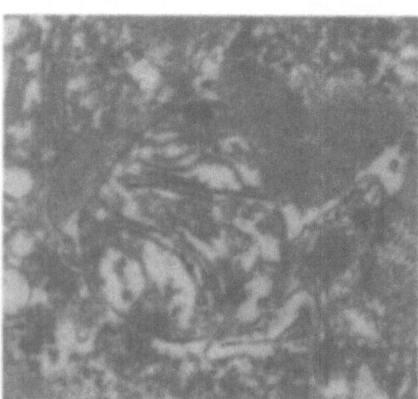

Fig. 1. normal mitochondria
       X 35,100
Fig. 2. reversibly injured
       mitochondria
       X 48,000
Fig. 3. irreversibly injured
       mitochondria
       X 44,000

Acute regional ischemia is characterized by several typical
ultrastructural signs:

- inhomogeneity of the degree of injury of myocardial cells
  at early stages of ischemia
- accumulation of lipid droplets in myocytes
- stickiness and adhesion of neutrophilic leucocytes in capillaries and immigration of these cells into irreversibly
  injured tissue as early as 90 minutes after the onset of
  ischemia
- structural recovery of reversibly injured myocardial cells
  when ischemia is followed by reperfusion

- a more pronounced deterioration of the structural integrity
upon reperfusion of irreversibly injured tissue. The occurrence of contracture bandes is very evident. After periods
of ischemia as long as 180 minutes a hemorrhagic myocardial
infarction develops.

Usually, the degree of ischemic injury is more pronounced in
the subendocardial than in the subepicardial myocardium. A
time dependence of the occurrence of irreversible injury and
hencewith of infarction is existent but it varies between
animals (2) and it varies even more from species to species
depending on the rate of oxygen consumption at the time of
occlusion (3) and of the amount of coronary collateral flow
(4). Generally, it may be stated that reversible injury of a
slight degree occurs as early as 5 minutes after coronary
artery occlusion in the dog heart, and that irreversible injury begins to appear at 45-90 minutes of ischemia. Thus, in
acute regional ischemia following coronary artery ligation a
rapid deterioration of the ultrastructural integrity occurs
followed by cell death, i.e. infarction. The situation is
quite different in slowly developing occlusion of a coronary
vessel as observed in human hearts with coronary heart disease.
2. Chronic ischemia in human hearts.
     Transmural needle biopsies were obtained during open
heart surgery from 40 patients undergoing coronary bypass
surgery. These patients showed a stenosis of the LAD ranging
from 75-98% and they all exhibited hypokinesia of the area
underperfused. Biopsies from patients with ASD who had cli-
nically normal left ventricles served as control. The biopsies
were obtained before induction of intraoperative cardiac
arrest, i.e. from hearts without the influence of global
ischemia. The biopsies were subdivided into subendocardial
and subepicardial samples that were further processed seperate-
ly. Qualitative and quantitative evaluations were carried out
using the light and the electron microscope. By light microscopy, it was evident that the tissue contained an increased
amount of interstitial fibrosis and that cell sizes varied

widely showing the complete range from hypertrophy to atrophy.

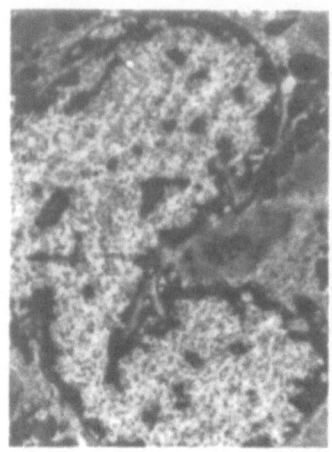

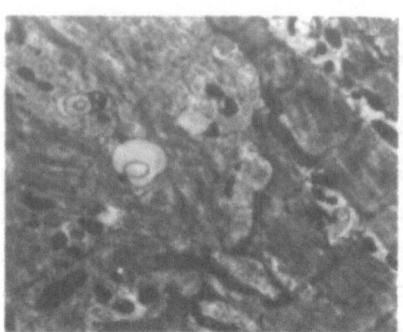

Fig. 4. Enlargement of necleus and clumping of chromatin
X 10,950
Fig. 5. Lack of contractile material and presence of vacuoles
X 8,600

On the ultrastructural level, changes included enlargement of
the nucleus and abnormal chromatin clumping (Fig. 4), lack of
contractile material and occurrence of degenerative vacuoles
(Fig. 5 and 6).

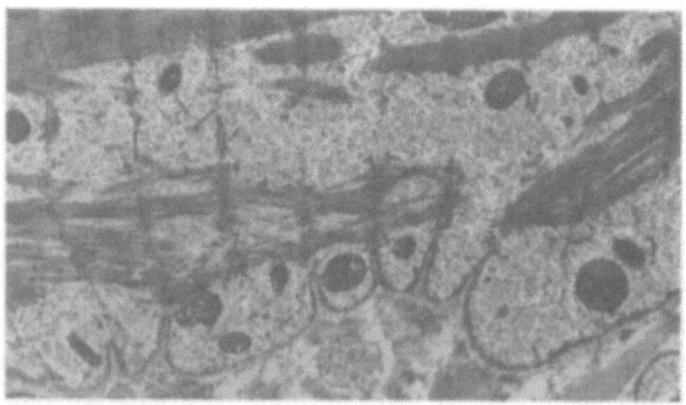

Fig. 6 shows lack of contractile material and cellular debris
in the interstitium
X 21,500

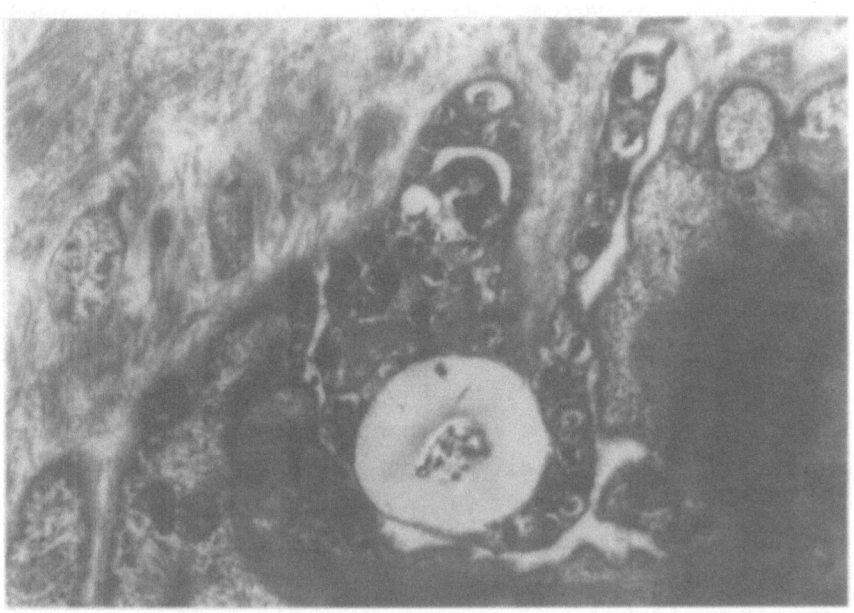

Fig. 7. Pinching-off of a degerated part of a myocardial cell
and myocardial cell particles in the interstitial space
X 21,500

Frequently, degenerating parts of a cell are seen to pinch off
and to occur as isolated particles in the interstitial space
(Fig. 7). This phenonemon might be an explanation for the presence of numerous macrophages and activated proliferation
fibroblasts in the widened interstitial space (Fig. 8).

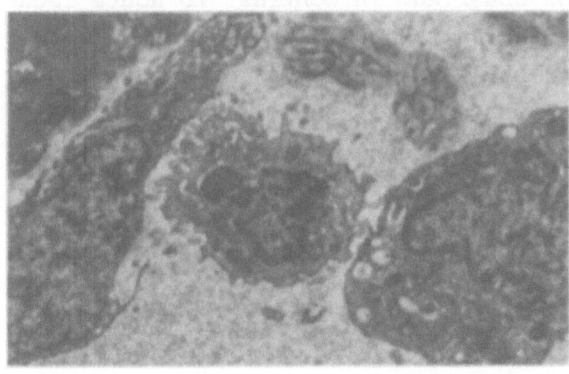

Fig. 8.
Active macrophages
and fibroblasts in
the interstitial
space
X 2,400

The content of fibrosis was measured by light microscopic morphometry and expressed as volume density (V_{vF}). This method is used for the measurement of volume densities of any particular cellular component within a reference volume. These volume densities may be extrapolated to the entire myocardium, and they may be expressed as percentage of the reference volume, which may be either the whole tissue or a total of any cell type within a certain tissue (5). Fibrosis was expressed as percentage of the area distal to the coronary artery stenosis; Table 1 shows the values obtained. When compared with the control group, it is evident that the degree of fibrosis was significantly higher in this group of patients showing hypokinesia of the ischemic left ventricular area. It is also evident that the subendocardial layer contained a higher percentage of fibrosis than the subepicardial layer.

By ultrastructural morphometry the volume densities of mitochondria (V_{vmit}), contractile material (V_{vmyo}), and unspecified cytoplasm (V_{vcyt}) were determined as shown in Table 1. When compared to control, the content of myofibrils was significantly reduced in myocytes from patients with CHD. The amount of cytoplasm was increased whereas the mitochondrial volume density was not different from normal. The reduction of contractile material was more pronounced in the subendocardium than in the subepicardium. Thus, in chronically developing coronary artery stenosis finally leading to occlusion of the vessel, a continuous process of cellular degeneration including all subcellular organelles but mostly the contractile material may be observed. In contrast to acute ischemia as experimentally observed in the canine heart, cell death occurs very slowly, most probably taking months or even years, but the result of this process finally is the same: structural deterioration resulting in disappearance of myocardial cells by slowly occuring necrosis and interstitial phagocytosis of parts of the cells accompanied by replacement with fibrotic material.

In acute ischemia, cell death occurs very early and fast involving the entire cell, and fibrosis=scar formation develops at later times. It may be concluded therefore that regional myocardial ischemia, whether it's effects occur acutely or very slowly in the end produces identical changes: cellular necrosis (total cell or only part of it), accumulation of fibrotic scar tissue and reduction of regional ventricular function, i.e. a decrease in regional wall mobility.

Table 1. Content of fibrosis, mitochondria, contractile material, and cytoplasm in human myocardium.

patients	V_{vF}	V_{vmit}	V_{vmyo}	V_{vcyt}
ASD n=8	11.0	22.8	61.8	15.4
CHD epi n=40	19.8▼	21.5	52.4▼	26.1▼
endo n=40	25.9▼●	23.4	48.3▼●	27.6▼

V_v = volume density, all values in %
n^v = number of patients
▼ = $p < 0.05$ compared to control
● = $P < 0.o5$ epi compared to endo

References:

1. Schaper, J., Mulch, J., Winkler, B., Schaper, W., : Ultrastructural, functional and biochemical criteria for estimation of reversibility of ischemic injury. J.Mol. Cell.Cardiol. 11: 521-41, 1979.
2. Schaper, J., Alpers, P., Gottwik, M., Schaper, W.: Ultrastructural characteristics of regional ischaemia and infarction in the canine heart. Europ.Heart.J. 6: 21-31, 1985.
3. Müller, K.D., Klein, H., Naujocks, S., Schaper, W.: Manipulation der Infarktgröße durch drastische Änderung des kardialen Sauerstoffverbrauchs nach 45' Koronarokklusion, Z. Kardiol. 68: 266, 1979.
4. Schaper, W.: Residual perfusion of acutely ischemic heart muscle. In: The Phathophysiology of Myocardial Perfusion (ed. W. Schaper), Elsevier/North-Holland Biomedical Press, Amsterdam, New York, Oxford, 1979, pp. 345-377.
5. Weibel, E.R., Bolender, R.P.: Stereological techniques for electron microscopic morphometry. In: Principles of Electron microscopy, Biological application (Ed. Hayat), Van Nostrand Reinhold, New York, 1974, pp. 239-299.

2

PRECONDITIONING WITH ISCHEMIA: A MEANS TO DELAY CELL DEATH IN ISCHEMIC MYOCARDIUM

CHARLES E. MURRY, ROBERT B. JENNINGS, KEITH A. REIMER

Department of Pathology, Duke University Medical Center, Durham, NC 27710, USA

ABSTRACT

We have previously shown that a brief episode of ischemia slows the rate of ATP depletion during subsequent ischemic episodes (1). Additionally, intermittent reperfusion washes out ischemic catabolites which may be harmful to the myocardium. Thus, we proposed that brief, repetitive episodes of ischemia might actually protect the heart from a subsequent sustained ischemic insult. To test this hypothesis, two sets of experiments were performed. In the first set, dogs were "preconditioned" with four 5 minute circumflex occlusions, each separated by 5 minutes of reperfusion, following which they received a sustained 40 minute occlusion. The control group received a single 40 minute occlusion. In the second study animals were preconditioned in an identical manner, following which they received a sustained 3 hour occlusion. Control animals received a single 3 hour occlusion. All animals were allowed 4 days of reperfusion to permit histologic infarct sizing. Infarct size was then related to baseline predictors of infarct size, namely the size of the area at risk and collateral blood flow. In the 40 minute study, preconditioning paradoxically limited infarct size to 25% of that seen in control animals (p<.001). Collateral blood flow (microspheres) was not significantly different between the groups. In the 3 hour study, preconditioning had no effect on infarct size. The protective effect in the 40 minute study may have been due to reduced ATP depletion and/or reduced catabolite accumulation during the sustained occlusion. These results suggest that multiple anginal episodes, which often precede myocardial infarction in man, may delay cell death after coronary occlusion, and thereby allow for greater salvage of myocardium by reperfusion therapy.

INTRODUCTION

Recovery of myocardial adenine nucleotides after a brief episode of non-lethal ischemia requires several days (2,3). Additionally, our laboratory has observed a close temporal relationship between severe depletion of tissue ATP stores and irreversible ischemic injury (4,5). Because repletion of ATP is so slow, we postulated that repeated brief episodes of ischemia should cause cumulative loss of ATP. Furthermore, if ATP depletion is a proximate cause of cell death, then repeated brief episodes of ischemia should cause myocyte necrosis. However, results of recent experiments have shown that four consecutive 10 minute episodes of ischemia separated by 20 minutes of reperfusion cause no necrosis and no more ATP depletion than a single 10 minute episode of ischemia (1). This preservation of ATP and viability by intermittent reperfusion was associated with a reduced rate of ATP depletion in subsequent ischemic episodes compared to the first. However, the molecular mechanism underlying the preservation of ATP remains unknown.

Given these beneficial effects of intermittent ischemia and reperfusion, vis-à-vis sustained ischemia, we postulated that multiple brief episodes of ischemia might actually protect the heart from a subsequent sustained ischemic insult. This experiment was designed to answer two basic questions: 1) Will preconditioning myocardium with four 5 minute episodes of ischemia and reperfusion result in smaller infarcts from a sustained 40 minute coronary occlusion, when compared to animals given a single 40 minute occlusion? and 2) If so, will this protective effect extend through a 3 hour period of sustained ischemia? The results of this study, summarized below, have been described in more detail previously (6).

MATERIALS AND METHODS

In general, animal selection and surgical preparation were performed according to the criteria of the multicenter AMPIM study (7). In brief, pentobarbital-anesthetized dogs were subjected to a left thoracotomy and circumflex coronary isolation. Polyethylene catheters were placed in the right femoral artery and vein, and into the left atrium via its appendage. Arterial pressure, atrial pressure and lead II of the EKG were monitored on a Gould recorder throughout the experiment. Any animal which developed ventricular fibrillation was cardioverted, if possible, with an MRL 560 defibrillator using internal paddles. Upon completion of the experiment, surgical wounds were closed and the animals were allowed to survive for 4 days to permit histologic infarct sizing. On the fourth postoperative day the animals were reanesthetized, given 5000 U heparin and their hearts excised for post mortem analysis.

Regional myocardial blood flow was measured at the times indicated in the experimental design section by injecting radiolabeled microspheres through a catheter in the left atrium. Beginning just before injection and continuing for 2.5 minutes, reference blood flow samples were withdrawn from the femoral artery at a rate of 7.75 ml/min. Tissue and blood samples were counted in a gamma counter with corrections made for overlap of isotope spectra. Myocardial blood flow was calculated according to the formula:

Tissue flow = (Tissue counts) (Reference flow)/Reference counts

and is expressed in ml/min·gm wet wt.

Post Mortem Analyses

The primary experimental endpoint was histologic infarct size, which was then related to the major baseline predictors of infarct size: the size of the area at risk and the amount of collateral blood flow to this region. A detailed presentation of the methods used to obtain these parameters has been done previously (7,8). In brief, the size of the area at risk was determined by post mortem simultaneous perfusion of the ischemic and non-ischemic vascular beds with different colored dyes. Collateral blood flow was measured by counting microsphere radioactivity in tissue samples which were carefully cut to avoid admixture of ischemic and non-ischemic vascular beds, and then separated into subendocardial, middle and subepicardial thirds of the ventricular wall. Infarct size was determined from morphometric analysis of histologic slides.

Statistics

All results are expressed as group means, ± SEM. A two-tailed unpaired Student's t-test was used to compare data between groups of animals, and the corresponding paired t-test was used to compare data from the same animals at different times. A p value ≤ 0.05 was considered statistically significant.

Experimental Design

The experimental design is shown in Figure 1. In the 40 minute study the preconditioned group (n=12) received four 5 minute circumflex occlusions, each separated by 5 minutes of reperfusion, followed by a sustained 40 minute occlusion. The control group (n=9) received a single 40 minute occlusion. Myocardial blood flow was measured prior to occlusion and midway through the 40 minute occlusion in both groups. To test for an effect of preconditioning on collateral blood flow, collateral flow was measured 2.5 minutes into the first occlusion of the preconditioning period, and 2.5 minutes into the 40 minute occlusion of the control group.

The 3 hour study followed an identical protocol, except that the preconditioned group (n=13) received a 3 hour sustained occlusion after preconditioning, and the control group (n=9) received a single 3 hour occlusion. Myocardial blood flow was measured prior to and 105 minutes into the 3 hour occlusion in both groups. As before, to test for an effect of preconditioning on collateral flow, flow was measured 2.5 minutes into the first occlusion of preconditioning and 2.5 minutes into the 3 hour occlusion of the control group.

EXPERIMENTAL DESIGN

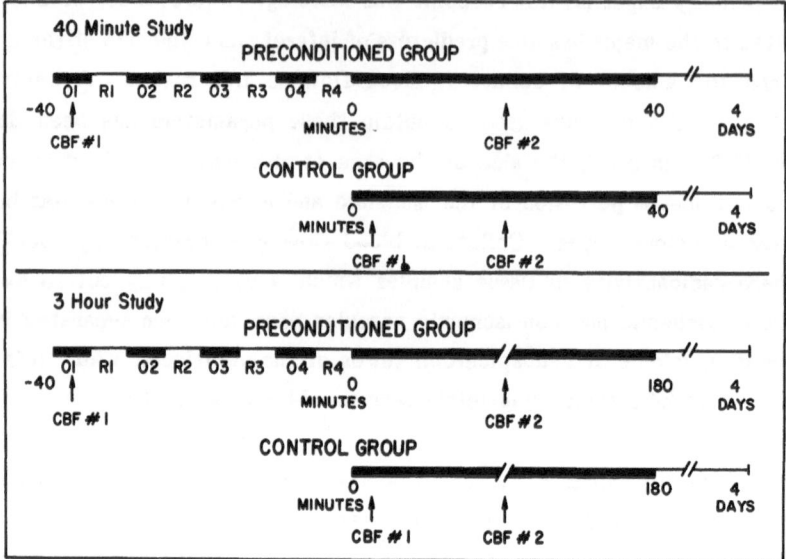

Fig. 1. 40 minute study: Preconditioned animals received four 5 minute circumflex occlusions, each separated by 5 minutes of reperfusion, followed by a sustained 40 minute occlusion. Control animals received a single 40 minute occlusion.
3 hour study: This study followed an identical protocol, except that the preconditioning period was followed by a 3 hour sustained occlusion. The control group received a single 3 hour occlusion.
O = occlusion; R = reperfusion; CBF = collateral blood flow measurement

This and all other figures are reproduced from reference 6 by permission.

RESULTS

Mortality in the study is shown in Table 1. There was no significant difference in overall mortality between the experimental and control groups in either study. None of the groups experienced an increase in collateral blood flow to the subendocardium between the first and second flow measurements. All groups exhibited a modest increase in collateral flow to the subepicardium between the first and second flow measurements (data not shown). Because the flow changes from the first to the fifth occlusion in the preconditioned animals were similar to the flow changes which occurred over time in control animals, we believe that preconditioning did not increase ultimate collateral flow. In any case, we used the later flow measurements for group comparison, thereby eliminating any preconditioning-induced effects on collateral flow.

TABLE 1. Mortality in 40 min and 3 hr studies

Group	No. of dogs enrolled	VF	Defibrillated	Late deaths	Survival (n/%)
40 min study					
Preconditioned	12	5	2	0	9/75
Control	9	2	0	1	6/67
3 hr study					
Preconditioned	12	2	1	1	10/83
Control	9	0	--	2	7/78

Two animals were excluded for technical reasons.
VF = ventricular fibrillation.

Forty Minute Study

Infarct size and collateral blood flow midway through the 40 minute occlusion are shown in Figure 2. Infarct size in control hearts averaged 29.4 ± 4.4% of the area at risk. In sharp contrast, infarct size in preconditioned hearts

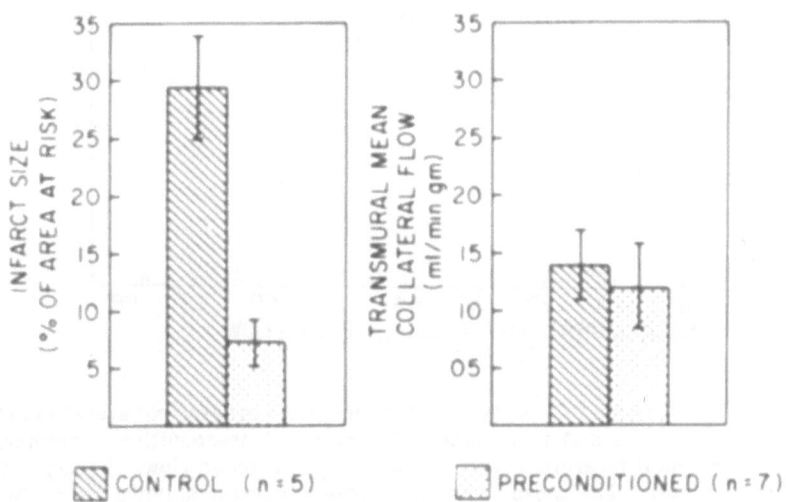

INFARCT SIZE AND COLLATERAL BLOOD FLOW IN
CONTROL AND PRECONDITIONED HEARTS
40 MINUTE STUDY

CONTROL (n=5)   PRECONDITIONED (n=7)

Fig. 2. Infarct size in control animals receiving a single 40 minute occlusion averaged 29.4% of the area at risk. In sharp contrast, in animals which were first preconditioned with four 5 minute episodes of ischemia and then subjected to 40 minutes of sustained ischemia, infarct size averaged only 7.4% of the area at risk (p<.001). Transmural mean collateral blood flows were not significantly different.

averaged only 7.3 ± 2.1% of the area at risk (p<0.001). Collateral blood flows in the subendocardium (zone of infarction) or as a transmural mean were not significantly different between groups. Thus, despite the fact that they received 60 minutes of cumulative ischemia, preconditioned animals had infarcts which were only one fourth the size of their control counterparts receiving 40 minutes of ischemia.

The relationship between infarct size and collateral blood flow in control and preconditioned hearts is shown in Figure 3. For control animals (closed circles and triangles) there was a general inverse relationship, i.e. animals with low collateral flow had large infarcts and vice-versa. However, in preconditioned hearts (open circles) infarcts were small, regardless of collateral flow.

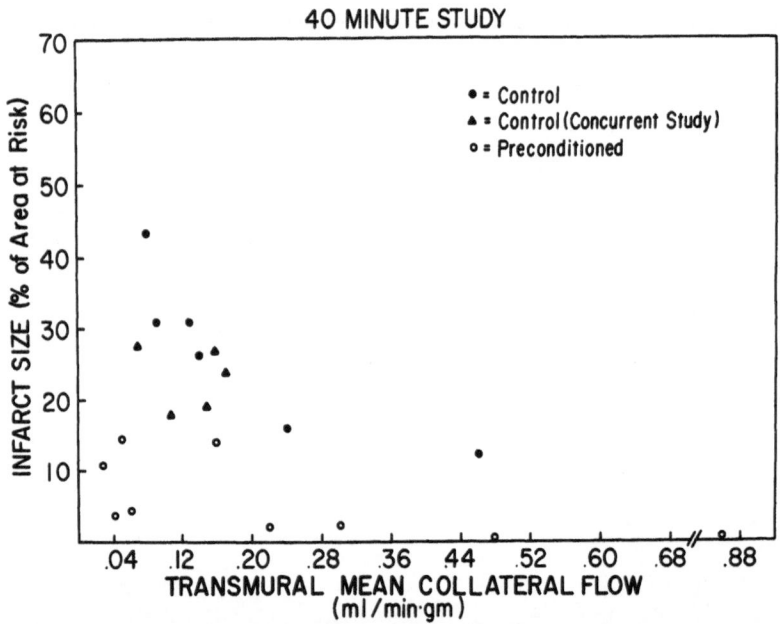

Fig. 3. For control animals (closed symbols), hearts with greater collateral blood flow had smaller infarcts and vice-versa. However, all preconditioned animals (open circles) had small infarcts, regardless of collateral blood flow. Each point represents one animal. The closed circles represent control animals from this study; the closed triangles represent control animals from a concurrent study, included to better define the relationship between necrosis and collateral blood flow.

Three Hour Study

Infarct size and collateral blood flow measured midway through the 3 hour occlusion are shown in Figure 4. Infarct size in control animals averaged 47.9 ± 6.6% of the area at risk. Infarct size in preconditioned animals averaged 47.1 ± 4.8% of the area at risk, not significantly different from controls. Collateral blood flows were not significantly different between the groups.

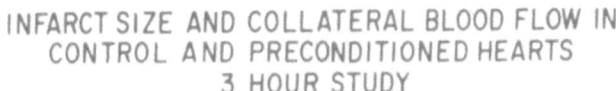

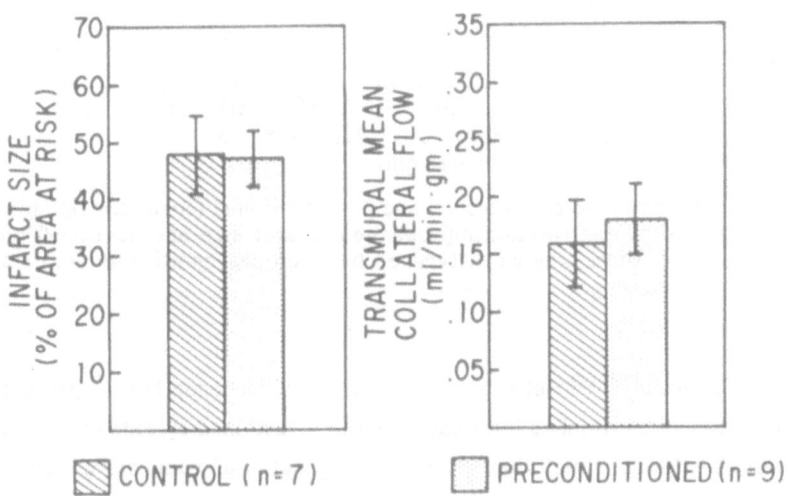

Fig. 4. Infarct size in control animals receiving a single 3 hour circumflex occlusion averaged 47.9% of the area at risk. Infarct size in preconditioned animals averaged 47.1% of the area at risk (p=NS). Transmural mean collateral blood flows were not significantly different between the two groups.

Figure 5 illustrates the relationship between infarct size and collateral blood flow in the 3 hour study. It is apparent in this figure that animals with high collateral flow had small infarcts and vice versa. It is also apparent that there was no difference between preconditioned and control animals in this relationship; the lines are virtually superimposable.

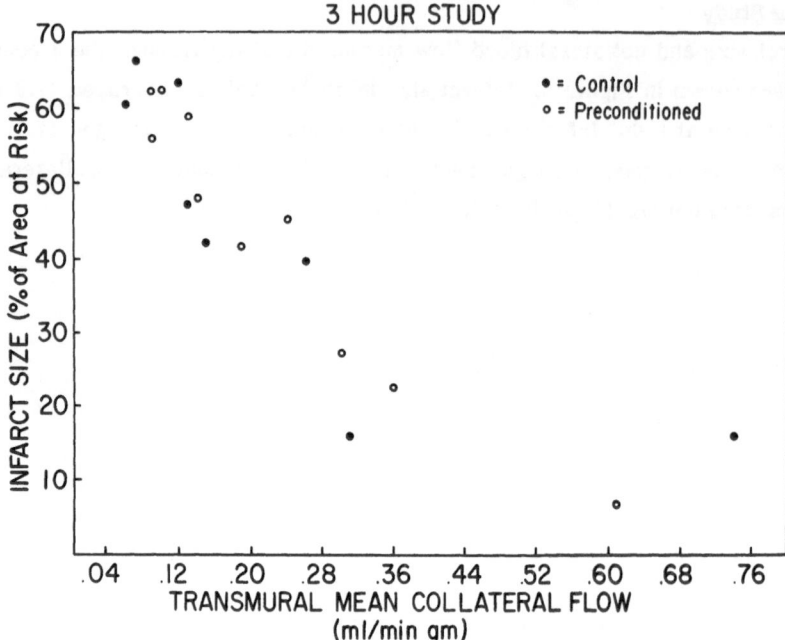

Fig. 5. For both control (closed circles) and preconditioned (open circles) animals there was a close inverse relationship between infarct size and collateral blood flow. Additionally, there was no difference between preconditioned and control groups in the relationship.

DISCUSSION

We have shown that brief repetitive episodes of ischemia have a protective effect on myocardium which is later subjected to a sustained episode of ischemia. Indeed, despite the fact that they received 60 minutes of cumulative ischemia, preconditioned hearts suffered only 25% of the necrosis incurred by the control "virgin" hearts receiving only 40 minutes of sustained ischemia. However, this protective effect could only delay cell death. When the duration of ischemia was extended to 3 hours there was no difference between infarct size in control and preconditioned animals.

Other investigators have studied the effects of multiple coronary occlusions on myocardial metabolism, structure, contractile function and viability. Several groups have shown that repeated ischemic episodes do not cause a cumulative loss of adenine nucleotides (1,9,10). Inasmuch as adenine nucleotide repletion requires days after a single brief episode of ischemia (2,3), the absence of cumulative loss in repeated ischemic episodes indicates a slowed rate of ATP depletion in later vs. the first episode (1). In addition to adenine nucleotides, myocardial ultrastructure, tissue water and electrolyte content are altered by a single 10 minute episode of ischemia but do not show cumulative changes after four 10 minute ischemic episodes (11). Lange et al (12) have demonstrated that three 5 or 15 minute occlusions produce no greater impairment of regional contractile function than a single occlusion.

With respect to cell death, Geft et al (13) have reported that 18 brief periods of ischemia caused small subendocardial infarcts in a minority of dogs studied, while we have shown (1) that four 10 minute circumflex occlusions caused virtually no necrosis. The reason for this difference may be the greater number of occlusions used in the former study. In any case, intermittent reperfusion appears to prevent or greatly attenuate the cumulative effects of brief repeated ischemic episodes.

At present we do not know the mechanism by which preconditioning serves to protect the heart during a sustained episode of ischemia. Although we have not investigated the mechanism in this study, one or both of two general mechanisms seem likely to be involved: 1) a reduced rate of ATP depletion and 2) a reduced rate of catabolite accumulation. Up to the present time we have not been able to distinguish between these possibilities.

The failure of preconditioning to limit infarct size after 3 hours of sustained ischemia has two facets:

1) The previously protected subendocardial region failed to survive the 3 hour occlusion. Thus it appears that preconditioning can only delay cell death; the additional 140 minutes of ischemia overwhelmed the protective effect.

2) Preconditioning with four 5 minute occlusions and reperfusions failed to protect the mid- and subepicardial myocardium from its normal time course of cell death. The failure to delay cell death in these layers must result from a difference in the effect of preconditioning on these regions, or from differences in the mechanism of ischemic cell death in the inner vs. the outer layers of the myocardial wall. It seems likely that the outer layers of myocardium, by virtue of having greater collateral flow and a lower metabolic rate (14), and therefore less severe ischemia, would not be as well preconditioned as the inner layers. If so, it might be possible to protect the mid- and subepicardial region by using longer occlusions in the preconditioning period. Additionally, if reduced catabolite accumulation plays a role in protecting the subendocardial region, one might expect that the mid- and subepicardial regions would not be as dramatically protected, since greater collateral flow to these regions naturally limits their catabolite accumulation.

Clinical Relevance

Although one must always use caution when extrapolating from animal studies to the clinical setting, myocardial infarction in man is frequently preceded by multiple episodes of angina pectoris. It is possible, therefore, that patients who experience repeated anginal episodes may similarly precondition their myocardium, and thereby slow the transmural progression of cell death after a sustained coronary occlusion. A slower progression of cell death implies a longer window of time in which myocardium could be salvaged by reperfusion therapy, e.g. with thrombolysis or coronary angioplasty.

ACKNOWLEDGEMENTS

The authors are grateful for the technical assistance of Jean A. Wakefield in animal surgery, blood flow measurements and infarct sizing.

REFERENCES

1. Reimer, K.A., Murry, C.E., Yamasawa, I., Hill, M.L. and Jennings, R.B. Am. J. Physiol., in press, December 1986.
2. Reimer, K.A., Hill, M.L. and Jennings, R.B. J. Mol. Cell. Cardiol. 13:229-239, 1981.
3. Swain, J.L., Sabina, R.L., McHale, P.A., Greenfield, J.C., Jr. and Holmes, E.W. Am. J. Physiol. 242:H818-H826, 1982.
4. Jennings, R.B., Hawkins, H.K., Lowe, J.E., Hill, M.L., Klotman, S. and Reimer, K.A. Am. J. Pathol. 92:187-214, 1978.
5. Reimer, K.A., Jennings, R.B. and Hill, M.L. Circ. Res. 49:901-911, 1981.
6. Murry, C.E., Jennings, R.B. and Reimer, K.A. Circulation 74: In Press, November 1986.
7. Reimer, K.A., Jennings, R.B., Cobb, F.R., Murdock, R.H., Greenfield, J.C. Jr., Becker, L.C., Bulkley, B.H., Hutchins, G.M., Schwartz, R.P. Jr., Bailey, K.R. and Passamani, E.R. Circ. Res. 56:651-665, 1985.
8. Reimer, K.A. and Jennings, R.B.. Circulation 71:1069-1075, 1985.
9. Swain, J.L., Sabina, R.L., Hines, J.J., Greenfield, J.C., Jr. and Holmes, E.W. Cardiovasc. Res. 18:264-269, 1984.
10. Lange, R., Ingwall, J.S., Hale, S.L., Alker, K.J. and Kloner, R.A. Bas. Res. Cardiol. 79:469-478, 1984.
11. Basuk, W.L., Reimer, K.A. and Jennings, R.B. J. Am. Coll. Cardiol. 8:33A-41A, 1986.
12. Lange, R., Ware, J. and Kloner, R.A. Circulation 69:400-408, 1984.
13. Geft, I.L., Fishbein, M.C., Ninomiya, K., Hashida, J., Chaux, E., Yano, J., Y.-Rit J., Genov, T., Shell, W. and Ganz, W. Circulation 66:1150-1153, 1982.
14. Murry, C.E., Reimer, K.A., Hill, M.L., Yamasawa, I. and Jennings, R.B. Fed. Proc. 44:823, 1985 (abstr.).

3

MODIFICATION OF THE THROMBOXANE/PROSTACYCLIN BALANCE AS AN APPROACH TO ANTIARRHYTHMIC THERAPY DURING MYOCARDIAL ISCHAEMIA AND REPERFUSION; THE CONCEPT OF ENDOGENOUS ANTIARRHYTHMIC SUBSTANCES

James R. Parratt

Department of Physiology & Pharmacology, University of Strathclyde, Glasgow, G1 1XW, Scotland, UK.

INTRODUCTION

Most of the standard approaches to antiarrhythmic therapy in myocardial ischaemia are covered elsewhere in this symposium. They include administration of drugs with various mechanisms of action that have been classified mainly on the basis of direct effects on ion channels. There are however, less direct, ways of reducing the severity of the different arrhythmias that arise during myocardial ischaemia and reperfusion that depend on either preventing the release (or effects at cellular level) of endogenous arrhythmogenic substances or that promote the release (or effects at cellular level) of other endogenous substances that reduce the severity of arrhythmias. A well established example of the first approach is the use of β-adrenoceptor blocking drugs to prevent the arrhythmogenic effects of adrenaline and noradrenaline released in myocardial ischaemia but there are other, less well appreciated, possibilities which are suggested by the ability of certain 5-HT and opioid receptor antagonists to reduce ischaemic arrhythmias in experimental animals (1,2,3). Even less attention has been paid to the possibility that the myocardium might elaborate 'endogenous antiarrhythmic substances' during ischaemia as a protective mechanism. This concept was, I think, first enunciated by Werner Förster (4). He suggested, partly on the basis of the efficacy of various prostaglandins (and prostacyclin) in protecting against chemically-induced arrhythmias in experimental animals, that endogenous prostaglandins might have a functional role in protecting the myocardium. It was this concept that acted as the stimulus for our own studies in this field and the purpose of this brief review is to attempt to summarise the possible role of products derived from arachidonic acid in the genesis and severity of those ischaemia and reperfused-induced ventricular arrhythmias that, in the clinical situation, are responsible for sudden cardiac death.

However, in concentrating on this particular group of substances we should
not ignore the possibility that other endogenous antiarrhythmic agents
are released during ischaemia. Thus, we have recently drawn attention
to the fact that adenosine, administered in amounts similar to those produced by the myocardium under conditions of reduced coronary blood flow,
reduces the severity of the ventricular arrhythmias which arise soon
after coronary artery occlusion as well as decreasing the incidence of
ventricular fibrillation following reperfusion (5,6). On the basis of
such results we have suggested that adenosine might act as a protective
endogenous 'antiarrhythmic' agent (6).

EVIDENCE FOR ACTIVATION OF THE ARACHIDONIC ACID CASCADE BY MYOCARDIAL
ISCHAEMIA AND ITS INVOLVEMENT IN PARTLY DETERMINING THE SEVERITY OF
ISCHAEMIC AND REPERFUSION-INDUCED ARRHYTHMIAS
Evidence for release of products derived from arachidonic acid in
myocardial ischaemia

Although there were earlier reports of the appearance of prostaglandins (and prostaglandin (PG)-like substances) in coronary sinus
blood following coronary artery occlusion (7,8) the first indication of
myocardial thromboxane release following coronary blood flow reduction
came from local coronary venous sampling studies in dogs following
mechanical obstruction of a coronary vessel (9). Levels of the major
metabolite of thromboxane $(Tx)A_2$, the more stable thromboxane B_2, were
elevated in venous blood sampled from the ischaemic region within one
minute of coronary artery occlusion; only later were coronary sinus
blood levels also elevated (9). Increased coronary sinus blood TxA_2
levels have also been found in patients with ischaemic heart disease
(10,11,12) and during coronary occlusion following unsuccessful
percutaneous transluminal coronary angioplasty (13).

During ischaemia prostacyclin (PGI_2) is also released from cellular
elements in the myocardium, as determined by increased coronary sinus
(or local coronary venous) levels of 6-keto $PGF_{1\alpha}$ (9,11). This release
can be substantially increased by antithrombotic drugs such as
nafazatrom (14) and the polydeoxyribonucleotide defibrotide (15). Although
there is evidence that calcium antagonists such as diltiazem can
potentiate prostacyclin release from human vascular tissue in vitro (16)
there is no evidence that such a release occurs from the myocardium

following nifedipine administration in doses that suppress ischaemia-
induced arrhythmias (17).

Relation of prostanoid release to the severity of early ischaemia-induced
arrhythmias and the effects of administered thromboxanemimetics and
prostacyclin-like substances

The early increase in local coronary venous levels of TxA_2 and PGI_2
appears to be related to the number of ventricular ectopic beats (VEB's)
that had occurred up to the time of blood sampling (9). This is
illustrated in Fig. 1 from a series of greyhound dogs where the number of

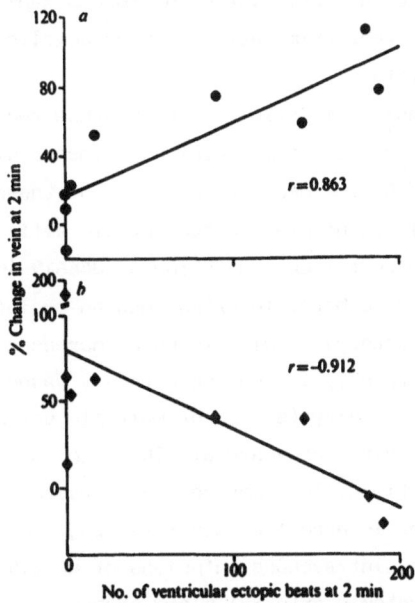

Fig. 1. The relationship between changes in the levels of the major
metabolites of thromboxane A_2 (thromboxane B_2; a) of prostacyclin
(6-keto $PGF_{1\alpha}$; b) and the number of ventricular ectopic beats that had
occurred at the time of the first local coronary venous sampling (2 min)
in dogs subjected to coronary artery occlusion. Note that higher levels
of TxB_2 in blood draining the ischaemic region at this time were
associated with a greater number of ventricular ectopic beats and that
higher levels of 6-keto $PGF_{1\alpha}$ in these samples were associated with
fewer ventricular ectopic beats (data from ref. 9).

VEB's during the initial 2 minutes of ischaemia varied from 0-195. Those
dogs which had the greater number of VEB's by 2 minutes were those that

also had the highest levels of TxA_2 in local coronary venous blood draining the ischaemic myocardial region and/or the lowest levels of PGI_2.
There are two possible explanations for this observation. One is that
ventricular ectopic activity during the period just after the coronary
blood flow reduction may in some way induce TxA_2 release (e.g. from
platelets). The alternative, and more likely, explanation is that the
severity of this early ventricular ectopic activity results from a
change in the TxA_2/PGI_2 balance. The changes could of course be unrelated
to each other and might merely reflect the severity of the blood flow
reduction. The possibility that the TxA_2/PGI_2 balance is important in
determining the severity of early ischaemic (phase 1a) arrhythmias is
supported by evidence that stimulation of thromboxane receptors induces
ectopic activity and that stimulation of prostacyclin receptors
decreases such activity.

The evidence that stimulation of thromboxane receptors results in
ventricular ectopic activity comes from experiments with the
thromboxanemimetic U46619. However, only one of these studies relates
to spontaneous, early ischaemia-induced ectopic activity. Thus, in
greyhound dogs the direct local injection of U46619 into the ischaemic
myocardium (through a catheter inserted into an occluded left anterior
descending coronary artery) results in both increases in peripheral
coronary pressure (probably indicating coronary vasoconstriction) and
ventricular ectopic activity (single or multiple ectopic beats and,
occasionally, ventricular tachycardia; 18). In this respect U46619 is
considerably (10-50 times) less active than noradrenaline. There is also
evidence from studies in anaesthetised rats subjected to coronary artery
occlusion. In these, intravenous infusions of U46619, in doses which do
not affect either systemic arterial blood pressure or heart rate, increase
the severity of early ischaemia-induced ventricular arrhythmias; both
the number of VEB's and the duration of VT are significantly increased
in animals receiving U46619 compared to control, coronary artery ligated,
rats (19). The incidence and duration of VF are also increased.

There is considerable evidence that prostacyclin, and related more
stable analogs, reduce chemically-induced arrhythmias as well as arrhythmias
induced by ischaemia and reperfusion. The indication, in some reports
(20,21), including our own (22), that prostacyclin increases rather
than decreases the severity of ischaemia-induced arrhythmias can

probably be attributed to peripheral vasodilation with a resultant reflex
increase in cardiac sympathetic activity (22). The beneficial antiarrhythmic effects of prostacyclin (and more stable analogs such as
iloprost) in ischaemia (20,22,23,24,25) have been variably explained by
direct actions on cardiac muscle action potentials (26), by systemic
hypotension (24,27) and by a reduction in the severity of ischaemia as a
result of coronary vasodilation and de-aggregation of platelets.

Fig. 2 (taken from ref. 22) demonstrates the difference between the
systemic and local (intracoronary) administration of prostacyclin and
iloprost on ischaemia and reperfusion-induced arrhythmias. The doses of
PGI_2 used resulted in similar levels of 6-keto $PGF_{1\alpha}$ (up to 2000 pg/ml)
in coronary venous blood. Systemic administration resulted in marked
hypotension, tachycardia and (with iloprost) a reduction in left
ventricular filling pressure; the incidence of ventricular fibrillation
on occluding the left anterior descending coronary artery was significantly increased (Fig. 2). The most pronounced effect of the

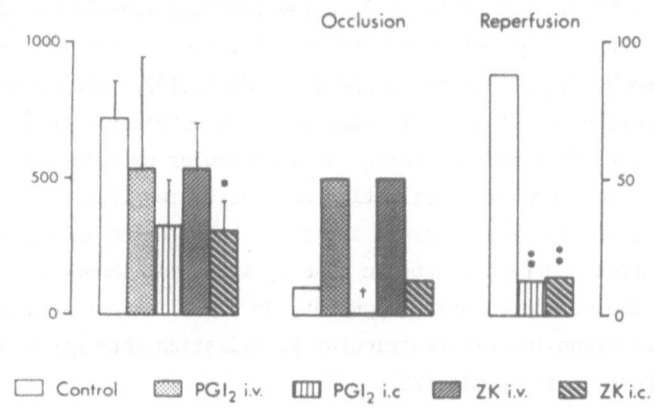

Fig. 2. A comparison of the effects of systemically (intravenous) and
local (intra-coronary) administration of prostacyclin (PGI_2) and iloprost
(ZK 36374) on the number of ventricular ectopic beats (left) and the
percentage incidence of ventricular fibrillation (middle) during coronary
artery occlusion in anaesthetised greyhound dogs. On the right is shown
the effect of locally administered PGI_2 or iloprost on the incidence of
reperfusion-induced ventricular fibrillation. The local (but not
systemic) administration of these agents reduced the severity of
ischaemic and (especially) reperfusion-induced arrhythmias. *P< 0.05;
**P< 0.01 (drugs versus controls); +P< 0.05 (local PGI_2 versus iv PGI_2).
(Data from Coker & Parratt (1983); ref. 22).

intracoronary administration of both substances was a greatly reduced
incidence of fibrillation on reperfusion (Fig. 2).

EVIDENCE THAT MODIFICATION OF THE THROMBOXANE/PROSTACYCLIN BALANCE RESULTS
IN CHANGES IN THE INCIDENCE AND SEVERITY OF ISCHAEMIA AND REPERFUSION-
INDUCED ARRHYTHMIAS

If we accept the above hypothesis (9,32) that the incidence and
severity of the life-threatening arrhythmias resulting from ischaemia
and reperfusion depend in part upon the balance between the local myocardial release of thromboxaneA_2 and prostacyclin, then there are
several possible approaches to beneficially modifying the balance
between these two derivatives of arachidonic acid. These approaches
are summarised in Fig. 3.

Antagonism of the effects of thromboxane

There are now several drugs that prevent the effects of thromboxane
A_2 (and/or the cyclic endoperoxides PGG_2 and PGH_2) on platelets and on
coronary vascular smooth muscle. Released thromboxane (Fig. 1) from
elements (probably mainly platelets) in the coronary vessels would result
in further platelet aggregation and vasoconstriction. These effects can
be antagonised by drugs such as AH 23848 and BM.13.177. The administration of either of these drugs to dogs prior to coronary artery
occlusion results in a reduced number of ventricular ectopic beats,
and a reduced incidence of fibrillation on reperfusion (28,29) and an
improved survival from the combined ischaemic/reperfusion insult (from
10-11% in control, untreated dogs to 50-67%, Table 1). However, for
reasons that are not immediately apparent, AH 23848 is ineffective in
reducing reperfusion-induced ventricular fibrillation when given during,
rather than before, ischaemia (28).

Selective inhibition of thromboxane synthesis

The theoretical advantages of this approach would be the possibility
of diverting (shunting) endoperoxides towards prostacyclin and the
classical prostaglandins. If, as we have seen, prostacyclin production
is helpful in ischaemia then this approach might have advantages over
thromboxane receptor blockade. However, there is also the possibility
of shunting endoperoxides to pro-aggregatory prostaglandins. Measurements

Fig. 3 Possible modification of the thromboxane/prostacyclin balance as an approach to antiarrhythmic therapy.

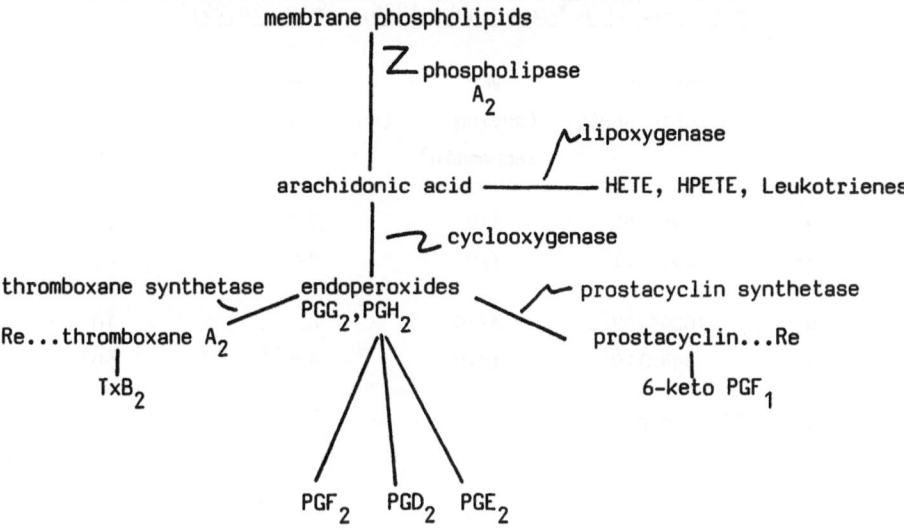

Sites of action:

1. thromboxane receptor blocking drugs (AH 23848; BM.13.177; LC 636,499; SQ 29,548 refs. 28,29,30) (really TxA_2/endoperoxide antagonists)

2. thromboxane synthetase inhibitors (dazoxiben, dazmegrel, CGS-13080 refs. 31-34)

3. 'prostacyclin promotors' (nafazatrom, defibrotide refs. 35-40)

4. cyclooxygenase inhibitors (non-steroidal antiinflammatory drugs e.g. aspirin, indomethacin; refs. 41-46)

5. lipoxygenase inhibitors (e.g. BW 755C, but also inhibits 4; nafazatrom)

6. leukotriene antagonists (e.g. FPL 55712; FPL 57231)

7. inhibitors of phospholipase A_2 (e.g. mepacrine)

Table 1.　Effects of thromboxane receptor antagonists on arrhythmias resulting from myocardial ischaemia and reperfusion in anaesthetised greyhound dogs (Data from Coker & Parratt, 1985;　Parratt & Wainwright, 1986;　Refs. 28,29)

	Ventricular ectopic beats	VF (during ischaemia)	VF (on reperfusion)	Survival (%)
Controls	736 ± 155	1/9	7/8	11
AH 23848*	$339 \pm 111^{+}$	1/9	$2/8^{+}$	67^{+}
Controls	1084 ± 159	3/10	6/7	10
BM 13.177**	$544 \pm 179^{+}$	1/10	$4/9^{++}$	50^{+}

$^{+}P < 0.05$　　$^{++}P < 0.07$

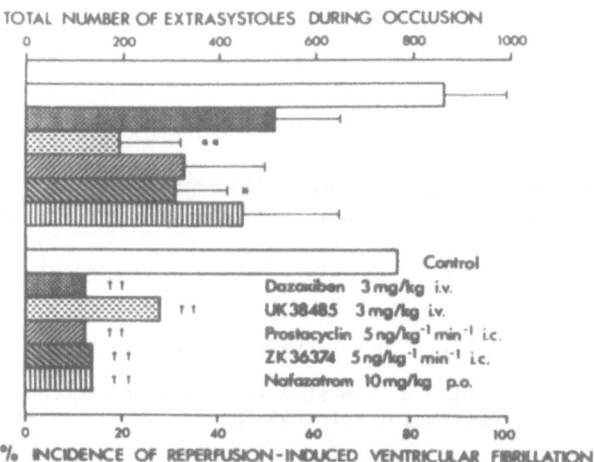

Fig. 4.　A summary of the effect of various procedures relating to the local balance between thromboxane and prostacyclin, on the number of ventricular ectopic beats occurring within the first 30 min of coronary artery occlusion in anaesthetised greyhounds and the incidence of ventricular fibrillation following reperfusion after a 40 min occlusion period.　Procedures that inhibit thromboxane synthesis or which increase the local levels of prostacyclin are especially protective against reperfusion-induced ventricular fibrillation.

of levels of every possible endoperoxide derivative have not been made
following selective thromboxane synthetase inhibition in myocardial
ischaemia but the results thus far obtained (31,32) indicate that there
is no conclusive evidence for a pronounced or significant diversion of
endoperoxides towards prostacyclin during coronary artery occlusion
following administration of these agents.

Inhibition of thromboxane production results in a reduction in the
incidence of ventricular ectopic beats during coronary artery occlusion
(32,34; Fig. 4) and a very significant reduction in the incidence of
fibrillation following reperfusion (31-33; Table 2). Survival from the
combined ischaemic/reperfusion insult is therefore again significantly
increased (from 12-20% up to 71-88%; Table 2).

Table 2. Effects of selective inhibition of thromboxane synthesis on
arrhythmias resulting from myocardial ischaemia and reperfusion in anaesthetised greyhound dogs (Data from Coker & Parratt,
1983*; Coker, 1984**; and Coker et al, 1982*; Refs. 31,32,33)

	Ventricular ectopic beats	VF (on reperfusion)	Survival %
Controls	875±264	7/8	12.5
Dazoxiben*	511±141	1/8[+]	88[+]
Controls	832±158	7/9	20
Dazmegrel**	193±126[+]	2/7[+]	71[+]

[+]$P < 0.01$

'Promotion' of prostacyclin levels during ischaemia

Both nafazatrom and defibrotide are recently developed
antithrombotic agents that stimulate prostacyclin release from vessel
walls and perhaps also inhibit the prostacyclin-degrading enzyme (36).
When given to dogs nafazatrom results in a two-fold increase in
prostacyclin release into coronary venous blood (draining the ischaemic
region) and these increased prostacyclin levels also lead to a reduction
in thromboxane release (Fig. 5) probably because of a prostacyclin-
induced inhibition of platelet aggregation. Nafazatrom also inhibits
lipoxygenase but the relevance of this to the beneficial effects of this
drug early in ischaemia are unclear since leukotrienes do not induce
ventricular arrhythmias when administered locally into the ischaemic

region except in very large doses (18).

Nafazatrom reduces both the incidence and severity of ischaemia and reperfusion-induced arrhythmias (35-38). This is illustrated from some of our own studies in Fig. 4.

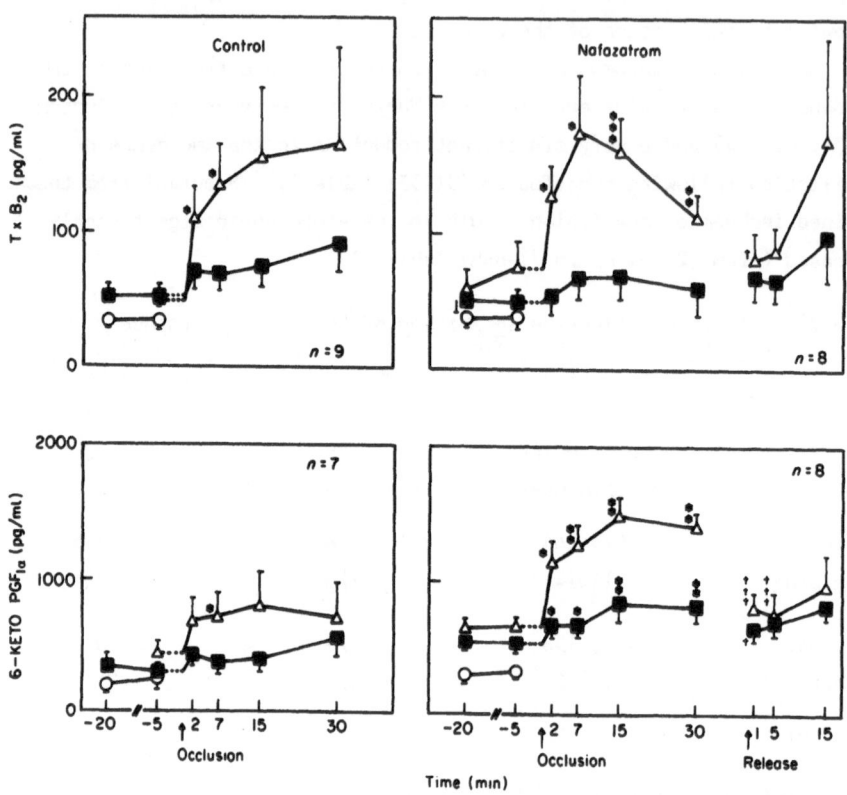

Fig. 5. Plasma concentrations of the major metabolites of thromboxane A_2 (TxB$_2$) and of prostacyclin (6-keto PGF$_{1\alpha}$) in aorta (o), coronary sinus (■) and the local coronary vein (Δ ; which after coronary artery occlusion drains from the ischaemic region) in control dogs (left) and in dogs pretreated with nafazatrom (right). Nafazatrom pretreatment resulted in higher concentrations of 6-keto PGF$_{1\alpha}$ (i.e. increased local generation of prostacyclin during ischaemia. *$P < 0.05$; **$P < 0.01$; ***$P < 0.001$ (post versus 5 min pre-occlusion values). +$P < 0.05$; +++$P < 0.001$ (post-reflow versus 30 min post-occlusion values). Data from Coker & Parratt, 1984 (ref. 35).

Inhibition of cyclooxygenase

Although there have been several conflicting studies on the effects of non-steroidal antiinflammatory drugs on the severity of myocardial

ischaemic damage, much less attention has been paid to the effects of
these drugs on early ischaemia and reperfusion-induced ventricular
arrhythmias. Most of the available evidence comes from studies with
aspirin (41-46) almost all of which demonstrates a protective effect
both during ischaemia (41-46) and during reperfusion (45,46). However,
we should not assume that this protective effect is due solely to
cyclooxygenase inhibition since it is possible that, in the doses used
in some of these studies, aspirin might have direct effects on cardiac
muscle action potentials. The results from some of our own studies are
summarised in Table 3. When given immediately before, or soon after,
coronary artery occlusion aspirin is antiarrhythmic in doses (1-4 mg/kg)
that appear to selectively inhibit thromboxane synthetase without
altering prostacyclin production (43,45), presumably because of a higher
affinity of the drug for platelet cyclooxygenase. The effects of total
inhibition of cyclooxygenase (platelet and vessel wall) on these
arrhythmias have not as yet been sufficiently well examined. There is
some evidence that in dogs this results in loss of aspirin-induced
protection (Table 3 and ref. 46) but in conscious rats (44) indomethacin
(given in a dose likely to completely inhibit cyclooxygenase) is
certainly protective. Whether this is entirely due to effects on the
arachidonic acid cascade is unclear; it would be important to determine
what effect cyclooxygenase inhibition in platelets and vessel walls
has in the early stages of ischaemia and reperfusion.

Rather little work has been done on the role of lipoxygenase
inhibition, leukotriene antagonism and phospholipase A_2 inhibition in
the genesis and severity of ischaemic arrhythmias. It is clear that
although there is accumulating evidence in favour of the 'thromboxane/
prostacyclin balance' hypothesis, there remains the possibility of using
drug combinations that might well be more effective than selectively
inhibiting one particular pathway.

Table 3. The effects of aspirin, given intravenously at different times
before and after coronary artery occlusion, on the arrhythmias
resulting from myocardial ischaemia and reperfusion in anaesthetised greyhound dogs (Data from Coker & Parratt, 1984; 1985;
Refs. 45,46)

	Ventricular ectopic beats	VF (on reperfusion)	Survival (%)
Controls	888 ± 168	88%	10
Aspirin (4 mg kg^{-1} iv; 24h pre-occlusion)	861 ± 345	75%	20
Aspirin (4 mg kg^{-1} iv; 5 min post-occlusion)	282 ± 127*	17%*	83*
Aspirin (1 mg kg^{-1} iv; 5 min post-occlusion)	771 ± 242	50%	50

*$P < 0.005$

Summary

The hypothesis has been reviewed that one major contributory factor
to arrhythmogenesis in myocardial ischaemia and reperfusion is the balance
between the local generation (by platelets, leucocytes and the blood vessel
wall) of thromboxane A_2 (arrhythmogenic) and prostacyclin (an 'endogenous
antiarrhythmic agent'). The ways in which drugs can modify these arrhythmias
by altering the balance between the availability of these two substances to
their receptors is described.

Acknowledgements

The research of the author's own research group is supported by the
Scottish Home and Health Department. This, and the excellent and enthusiastic
work of Drs. Susan Coker and Cherry Wainwright is gratefully acknowledged.

References

1. Fagbemi, O., Leprán, I., Parratt, J.R. and Szekeres, L. Br. J.
    Pharmac., 76: 504-506, 1982.

2. Parratt, J.R. and Sitsapesan, R. Br. J. Pharmac., 87: 21-622, 1986.

3. Coker, S.J., Dean, H.G., Kane, K.A. and Parratt, J.R. Europ. J.
    Pharmac., in press.

4. Forster, W. Acta biol. med. germ. 35: 1101-1112, 1976.

5. Parratt, J.R. and Wainwright, C.L. Br. J. Pharmac., 85: 228P, 1985.

6. Parratt, J.R. and Wainwright, C.L. Br. J. Pharmac., in press.

7. Berger, H.J., Zaret, B.L., Speroff, L., Cohen, L.S. and Wolfson, S. Circulation Res., 38: 566-571, 1976.

8. Kraemer, R.J., Phernetton, T.M. and Folts, J.D. J. Pharmac. exp. Therap., 199: 611-619, 1976.

9. Coker, S.J., Parratt, J.R., Ledingham, I. McA. and Zeitlin, I.J. Nature, 291: 323-324, 1981.

10. Tada, M., Kuzuya, T., Inoue, M., Kodama, K., Mishima, M., Yamada, M., Inui, M. and Abe, H. Circulation, 64: 1107-1115, 1981.

11. Hirsh, P.D., Hills, L.D., Campbell, W.B., Firth, B.G. and Willerson, J.T. N. Eng. J. Med., 304: 685-691, 1981.

12. Tada, M., Hoshida, S., Kuzuya, T., Inoue, M., Minamino, T. and Abe, H. Int. J. Cardiol., 8: 301-312, 1985.

13. Peterson, M.B., Machaj, V., Block, P.C., Palacios, T., Philbin, D. and Watkins, W.D. Am. Heart J., 111: 1-6, 1986.

14. Coker, S.J. and Parratt, J.R. J. Molec. Cell. Cardiol., 16: 43-52, 1984.

15. Thiemermann, C., Lobel, P. and Schror, K. Am. J. Cardiol., 56: 978-982, 1985.

16. Mehta, J., Mehta, P. and Ostrowski, N. Am. J. Med. Sci., 29: 20-24, 1986.

17. Coker, S.J. and Parratt, J.R. J. Cardiovasc. Pharmacol., 5: 406-417,1983.

18. Parratt, J.R. and Wainwright, C.L. Br. J. Pharmac., 88: 397P, 1986.

19. Parratt, J.R., Coker, S.J. and Wainwright, C.L. J. Molec. Cell. Cardiol., in press.

20. Au, T.L.S., Collins, G.A., Harvie, C.J. and Walker, M.J.A. Prostaglandins, 18: 707-720, 1979.

21. Dix, R.K., Kelliher, G.J., Jurkiewicz, N. and Lawrence, T. Prostglandins Med.,3: 173-184, 1979.

22. Coker, S.J. and Parratt, J.R. J. Cardiovasc. Pharmacol., 5: 557-567, 1983.

23. Starnes, V.A., Primm, R.K., Woosley, R.L., Oates, J.A. and Hammon, J.W. J. Cardiovasc. Pharmacol. 4: 765-769, 1982.

24. Jouve, R., Puddu, P-E., Langlet, F., Guillen, J-C., Gautier, T., Cano, J-P. and Serradimigni, A. J. Pharmacol. (Paris), 16: 139-157, 1985.

25. Coker, S.J. and Parratt, J.R. Br. J. Pharmac., 74: 155-159, 1981.

26. Kecskemeti, V., Kelemen, K., and Knoll, J. In: Prostanoids (ed. V. Kecskemeti) Academiai Kiado and Pergamon, Budapest, 1980, pp. 89-93.

27. Kowey, P.R., Verrier, R.L. and Lown, B. Europ. J. Pharmacol., 80: 83-92, 1982.

28. Coker, S.J. and Parratt, J.R. Br. J. Pharmac, 86: 259-264, 1985.

29. Parratt, J.R. and Wainwright, C.L. Br. J. Pharmac., 88: 291P, 1986.

30. Fitzgerald, D.J., Doran, J., Jackson, E. and Fitzgerald, G.A. J. Clin. Invest., 77: 496-502, 1986.

31. Coker, S.J. and Parratt, J.R. Br. J. Clin Pharmac. 15: 87S-95S, 1983.

32. Coker, S.J., Parratt, J.R., Ledingham, I.McA. and Zeitlin, I.J. J. Molec. Cell., Cardiol. 14: 483-485, 1982.

33. Coker, S.J. J. Molec. Cell. Cardiol., 16: 633-641, 1984.

34. O'Connor, K.M., Friehling, T.D., Kelliher, G.J., MacNab, M.W., Wetstein, L. and Kowey, P.R. Am. Heart J. 111: 683-688, 1986.

35. Coker, S.J. and Parratt, J.R. J. Molec. Cell. Cardiol. 16: 43-52, 1984.

36. Fiedler, V.B. Europ. J. Pharmac., 88: 263-267, 1983.

37. Fiedler, V.B. Europ. J. Pharmac., 114: 189-195, 1985.

38. Fiedler, V.B., Mardin, M., Perzborn, E. and Grutzmann, R. Arch. Pharmac., 331: 267-274, 1985.

39. Lobel, P. and Schror, K. Arch. Pharmacol., 331: 125-130, 1985.

40. Thiemermann, C., Lobel, P. and Schror, K. Am. J. Cardiol., 56: 978-982, 1985.

41. Moschos, C.B., Haider, B., de la Cruz, C., Lyons, M.M. and Regan, T.J. Circulation, 57; 681-684, 1978.

42. Moschos, C.B., Haider, B., Escobinas, A.J., Gandhi, A. and Regan, T.J. Am. Heart J., <u>100</u>: 647-652, 1980.

43. Coker, S.J., Ledingham, I.McA., Parratt, J.R. and Zeitlin, I.J. Br. J. Pharmac., <u>72</u>: 593-595, 1981.

44. Lepran, I., Koltai, M. and Szekeres, L. Europ. J. Pharmacol., <u>69</u>: 235-238, 1981.

45. Coker, S.J. and Parratt, J.R. In: Aspirin Symposium, Royal Society of Medicine Symposium Series No. 71, 1984, pp. 71-75.

46. Coker, S.J. and Parratt, J.R. J. Molec. Cell. Cardiol., <u>17</u>: Suppl.3, abs. 109, 1985.

4

MECHANISMS OF COUPLED ARRHYTHMIAS IN GUINEA PIG PERFUSED HEART
AND ISOLATED VENTRICULAR TISSUE MODELS OF ISCHEMIA-REPERFUSION.

GREGORY R. FERRIER AND C. M. GUYETTE

Department of Pharmacology, Dalhousie University, Halifax,
Canada, B3H 4H7

INTRODUCTION

We recently developed an in vitro model of ischemia and
reperfusion in which isolated canine ventricular tissues were
superfused with Tyrode's solutions modified to mimic ischemia and
reperfusion (1,2). Intracellular microelectrode recordings
demonstrated that reperfusion induced a regular orderly sequence
of mechanisms of arrhythmia in Purkinje tissue but not in muscle.
The mechanisms in order of appearance were: oscillatory
afterpotentials (OAP, also known as delayed
afterdepolarizations), conduction block, and depolarization-
induced automaticity (DIA, also known as early
afterdepolarizations). OAP occasionally reached threshold and
induced extrasystoles early in reperfusion (2 min). DIA
regularly induced extrasystolic activity but only after
approximately 20 min of reperfusion. Our superfused tissue model
did not exhibit the characteristic time course of arrhythmic
activity seen in coronary ligation and release (3,4) or perfused
heart models of ischemia and reperfusion (5,6). In these latter
models, ectopic activity frequently appeared as a rapid burst of
activity within the first minute of reperfusion. A valid model
of reperfusion arrhythmias should mimic this characteristic
response. It is possible that "ischemic Tyrode's" mimics the
essential components of ischemia but that slow interstitial
exchange of solutions attenuates the reperfusion response.

The goals of the present study were four fold. First we
wished to determine whether the "ischemic" Tyrode's model would
produce a burst of arrhythmias when adapted to a whole guinea pig
heart preparation perfused through the coronary vasculature. In

doing this we also wished to develop comparable whole heart and isolated tissue models of ischemia/reperfusion arrhythmias using a single species. This would allow one to determine whether arrhythmias in the whole heart exhibited characteristics compatible with cellular mechanisms observed in isolated tissue studies utilizing microelectrode recording techniques. Thirdly, we wished to determine whether mechanisms of arrhythmia similar to those observed in the canine model would be operative in the guinea pig model. And finally, we wished to determine whether the sharp difference in the electrophysiological responses of subendocardial tissues and other regions of myocardium observed in the canine model also occurred in other species.

MATERIALS AND METHODS

Male ginea pigs weighing 500 - 700 g were sacrificed by cervical dislocation. Hearts were quickly excised and placed in room temperature "normal" Tyrode's solution with the following composition in mM: NaCl, 129.0; KCl, 4.0; NaH_2PO_4, 0.9; $NaHCO_3$, 20.0; $CaCl_2$, 2.5; $MgSO_4$, 0.5; and dextrose, 5.5. The solution was gassed with a 95% O_2, 5% CO_2 mixture. Preparations consisted of sections of right or left ventricular free wall 1 cm². In one series of experiments, preparations were pinned endocardial surface up to the bottom of an isolated tissue bath perfused with Tyrode's solution (25 ml/min) at 37° C. In a second series of experiments, the endocardial layer was dissected from left free wall preparations. These preparations were mounted with the epicardial surface up.

Preparations were stimulated with trains of 15 pulses separated by 3 sec pauses via bipolar silver electrodes. Pulses were 1.5 times diastolic threshold and were delivered at a basic cycle length (BCL) of 500 msec. Transmembrane potentials were recorded using standard differential microelectrode techniques. An ECG was recorded by two chlorided silver wires positioned at opposite ends of the tissue bath.

Preparations were equilibrated for 30 min in "normal" oxygenated Tyrode's solution. Tissues were then superfused for

40 min with "ischemic" Tyrode's solution gassed with a 90% N_2, 10% CO_2 mixture, and with the following composition (mM): NaCl, 123.0; KCl, 4.0; NaH_2PO_4, 0.9; $NaHCO_3$, 6.0; $CaCl_2$, 2.5; $MgSO_4$, 0.5; and sodium lactate, 20.0. Reperfusion with control Tyrode's solution was then instituted for an additional 30 min. Our earlier studies demonstrated that elevation of potassium levels during the "ischemic" period did not significantly alter the subsequent response upon reperfusion (2), therefore the concentration of potassium was not elevated in the present study.

In an additional series of experiments whole guinea pig hearts were perfused through the coronary vasculature using a modified Langendorff technique. Stimulation was applied near the base of the left ventricle using close bipolar stainless steel hook electrodes. The stimulation pattern was as above except that hearts were paced at BCL 10% shorter than the spontaneous intervals (180 - 300 msec). Bipolar electrograms were recorded from the apex of the left ventricle using stainless steel hook electrodes. Hearts were perfused with the same solutions and sequence as isolated tissues except that the period of perfusion with "ischemic" Tyrode's solution was shortened to 7.5 min.

RESULTS
Perfused heart experiments.
The effects of perfusion with "ischemic" Tyrode's solution followed by reperfusion with "normal" Tyrode"s solution was studied in 10 hearts. Fig. 1 shows the electrical responses recorded in a representative experiment. Panel A was recorded at the end of the control period. Spontaneous activity was apparent in the pauses in stimulation. Panel B was recorded after 7.5 min of perfusion with "ischemic" Tyrode's solution. Spontaneous activity still occurred in pauses in stimulation but the rate of this activity was slower. Also, postpacing depression, characteristic of normal pacemaker activity, was evident by obvious prolongation of the first spontaneous cycle length. The heart was reperfused immediately following this recording. Heart rate frequently showed an initial biphasic response. Panel C

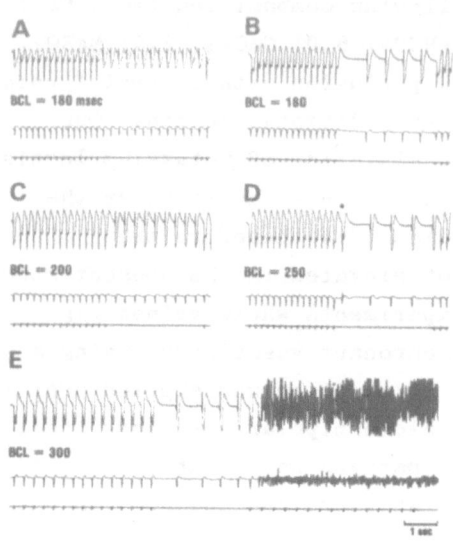

Fig. 1. Effects of "ischemia" and reperfusion on the electrical activity of a perfused guinea pig heart. In each panel the top two records are bipolar electrograms, and the bottom trace is a record of stimulation. Panel A: control; panel B "ischemia"; panels C - E reperfusion. BCL = Basic cycle length.

recorded after 2.0 min of reperfusion shows an increase in spontaneous rate relative to panel B. By 3.0 min (panel D), rate had again slowed. However, spontaneous activity had resolved into activity coupled to the driven beats (marked with a dot in panel C) and slower non-coupled activity. Panel E was recorded after 4 min of reperfusion and demonstrates sudden onset of fibrillation corresponding to the beginning of the second train of stimuli in this panel.

The coupled activity observed upon reperfusion demonstrated postpacing enhancement similar to that characteristic of OAP in other studies (1,7). This is shown in Fig. 2 which shows recordings from the same preparation as Fig. 1 during reperfusion. When the BCL of stimulation was 250 msec, driven activity was followed only by non-coupled spontaneous activity which demonstrated postpacing depression (Fig. 2 A). However, when the BCL was shortened to 180 msec, coupled activity appeared immediately following the train of driven beats (marked with dot). In the experiment illustrated in Fig. 2, coupled activity was limited to single beats following trains. However, periods

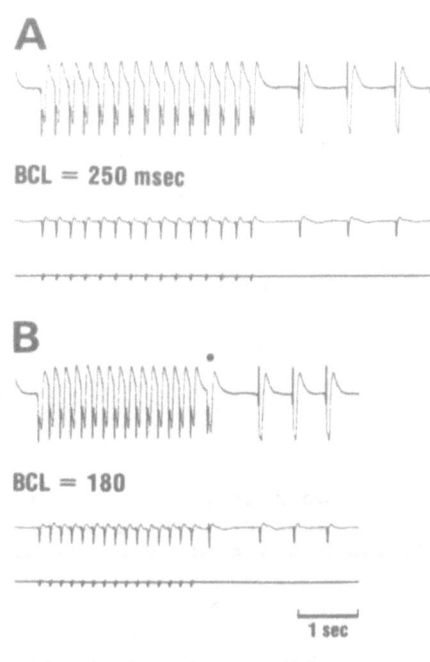

Fig. 2. Postpacing enhancement of coupled spontaneous activity induced by reperfusion in a perfused guinea pig heart. Traces are arranged as in Fig. 1. Coupled activity (marked by dot) appears following train at BCL = 180 msec but not at BCL = 250 msec.

of enhanced spontaneous activity were generated by repetitive coupled activity in several experiments. An example is illustrated in Fig. 3. Panels A and B are continuous and were recorded after 1 min of reperfusion. Panel A shows that, upon reperfusion, slow non-coupled activity gradually slowed and finally disappeared. As shown in panel B, coupled activity first appeared as a single beat following a train of driven beats. With sequential trains, progressively longer series of coupled (triggered) activity appeared until this activity became continuous throughout pauses in stimulation.

Table 1 summarizes the incidence of coupled beats and arrhythmias in hearts perfused with "ischemic" Tyrode's solution followed by "normal" Tyrode's solution. Coupled activity occurred in one preparation before and during perfusion with "ischemic" solution. However, upon reperfusion, coupled activity with characteristics similar to those of OAP occurred in

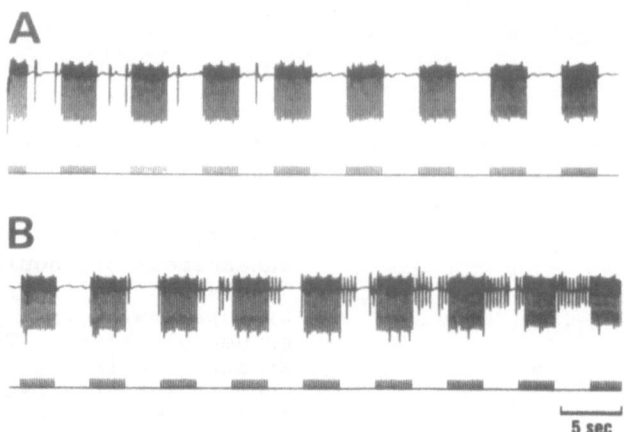

5 sec

Fig. 3. Repetitive coupled activity induced by reperfusion in a perfused guinea pig heart. Top trace: bipolar electrogram; bottom trace: stimulus pattern. Panels A and B are continuous.

Table 1. Incidence of arrhythmias in ischemia and reperfusion. Perfused guinea pig hearts, n = 10.

	Coupled beats	Ventricular tachycardia*	Ventricular fibrillation**
Control	1	0	0
Ischemia	1	1	4
Reperfusion	6	5	7

* Rate > 450/min (BCL < 133 msec)
** Rate > 900/min (mean BCL < 67 msec)

6 of 10 hearts. Neither ventricular tachycardia nor fibrillation occurred during the control period. The incidence of these arrhythmias increased during the ischemic period but was greatest during reperfusion. The arrhythmic response of our whole heart, "ischemic" Tyrode's model is very similar to that reported for underperfusion-reperfusion or ligation and reflow models.

<u>Isolated tissue experiments.</u>

<u>Endocardial preparations.</u> The electrical responses of
isolated tissues to alternate exposure to ischemic conditions and
reperfusion were studied in 9 endocardial preparations. Fig. 4
shows microelectrode and ECG recordings from a representative

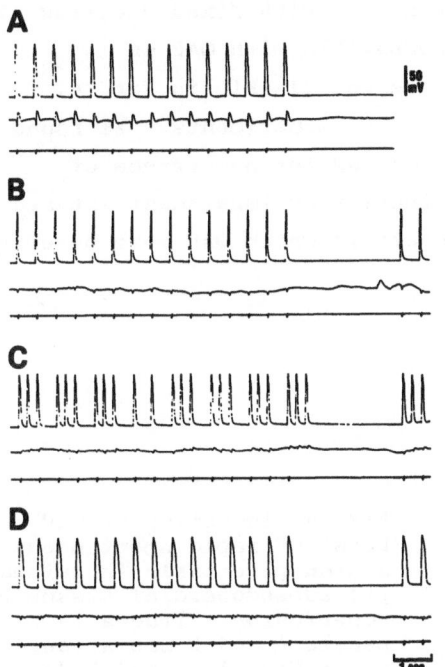

Fig. 4. Effects of
"ischemia" and reperfusion on
electrical activity of
isolated guinea pig
subendocardial tissue. In
each panel the top trace is
an intracellular
microelectrode recording, the
middle trace is an ECG and
the bottom trace is a record
of the stimulus pattern.
Panel A: control; panel B:
"ischemia"; panels C and D:
reperfusion.

experiment. Panel A, illustrates control activity recorded
before this preparation was exposed to ischemic conditions.
Spontaneous activity was absent. Panel B was recorded after 40
min of exposure to ischemic conditions and shows marked
abbreviation of action potential duration plus continued absence
of spontaneous activity. However, within 2 min of reperfusion
with "normal" Tyrode's solution, coupled activity resulted in a
stable trigeminal pattern of arrhythmia (panel C). This
arrhythmia occurred in the continued absence of non-coupled
spontaneous activity as can be seen during the pause in
stimulation. Unlike canine Purkinje preparations, impalements in

isolated guinea pig preparations did not uniformly show evidence of marked depolarization and loss of excitability during reperfusion (1,2). Panel D was recorded after 30 min of reperfusion and shows recovery of the preparation. Recovery was characterized by disappearance of coupled activity and prolongation of action potential duration.

The appearance of a stable trigeminy with fixed coupling at a relatively long cycle length is compatible with OAP as a mechanism (7,8,9). However, OAP are not visible in Fig. 4. Multiple impalements were made in these experiments. We found that OAP could regularly be found during the occurrence of coupled activity, but only at a minority of impalement sites. Fig. 5 shows records from impalements in which OAP were observed.

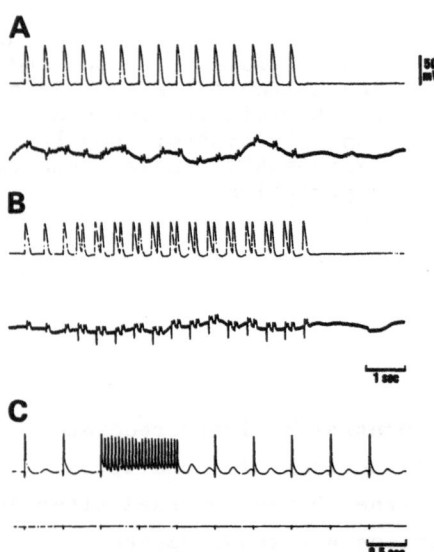

Fig. 5. Induction of OAP and burst of rapid spontaneous action potentials in guinea pig subendocardial tissue by reperfusion. Traces in panels A and B are arranged as in Fig. 4. Panel C does not include an ECG recording.

Panels A and B show sequential trains recorded from a prepartion after 1 min of reperfusion. Small OAP can be seen between driven beats and following the train in the microelectrode recording in panel A. During the train illustrated in panel B, an OAP reached threshold after the third driven beat. This resulted in a

premature beat that occurred in advance of the next stimulus.
Thus the next driven beat was initiated before complete
repolarization of the premature action potential. Subsequently
each driven beat was followed by a premature beat and a stable
bigeminy resulted. The ascending limbs of OAP can be seen
preceding the spontaneous beats. The last driven beat of the
train was followed by one spontaneous coupled beat and then
quiescence.

Panel C in Fig. 5, recorded from a different preparation,
shows large subthreshold OAP coupled to each driven action
potential. This panel also shows a rapid burst of activity
starting before repolarization of the third beat and terminating
abruptly with the fifth stimulus. This activity clearly was
unrelated to the OAP. Bursts of rapid activity occurred only in
one preparation but occurred repetitively. This rapid activity
varied from 1 beat to 3 sec in duration and had a rate equivalent
to 1400/min. All bursts began and ended abruptly with stimuli.
No pacemaker potential was apparent before the upstroke of
individual spikes. Thus this activity may have been reentrant in
origin.

Epicardial preparations. The effects of "ischemia" and
reperfusion were also studied in 6 epicardial preparations.
Recordings from a representative experiment are shown in Fig. 6.
Panel A was recorded at the end of the control period. Panel B
was recorded after 40 min of ischemic conditions. In the
presence of "ischemic" Tyrode's solution, the membrane potential
and action potential decreased. Also, excitability decreased so
that previously effective stimuli were subthreshold. No
arrhythmic activity occurred during the "ischemic" period.
Panels C and D were recorded after 1 and 22 min of reperfusion
respectively. Reperfusion of epicardial preparations was
associated with uneventful recovery of excitability, action
potential duration, and membrane potential. Neither OAP nor
spontaneous beats occurred.

The electrophysiological responses of isolated ventricular
tissues to "ischemia" and reperfusion are summarized in Table 2.

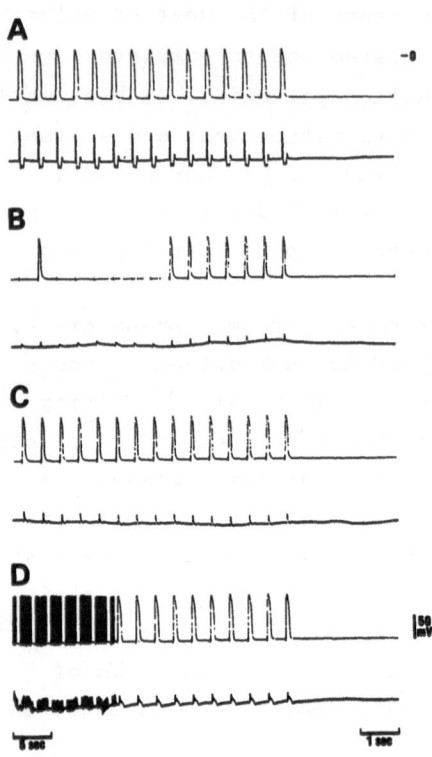

Fig. 6. Electrophysiological response of guinea pig epicardial muscle to "ischemia" and reperfusion. In each panel the top trace is an intracellular microelectrode recording and the lower trace is an ECG. Panel A: control; panel B: "ischemia"; panels C and D: reperfusion.

Table 2. Electrophysiological responses of isolated ventricular tissues to "ischemia" and reperfusion.

	Excit-ability	Spontaneous activity	Coupled beats	V - fib
Endocardium (n=9):				
Control	N/A	1	0	0
Ischemia	- 5	- 1	0	0
Reperfusion	+ 5	++ 8	8	1
Epicardium (n=6):				
Control	N/A	0	0	0
Ischemia	-- 6	0	0	0
Reperfusion	++ 6	0	0	0

+ indicates increase
- indicates decrease

Depression of excitability in endocardial preparations
(designated -) was moderate (drive could be restored by
increasing stimulus voltage 2 fold). Depression of excitability
in epicardial preparations (designated --) was severe (drive
could not be restored by increasing stimulus voltage 2 fold).
Spontaneous activity was present in 1 endocardial preparation
during control conditions. This activity was suppresed by
ischemic conditions. Eight of 9 endocardial preparations
exhibited spontaneous arrhythmic activity upon reperfusion.
Rapid bursts of activity occurred in 1 preparation. This
activity was classified as fibrillation because of its very high
rate. None of 6 epicardial preparations exhibited spontaneous
beats or arrhythmias during either "ischemia" or reperfusion.

DISCUSSION

The present study provides a model of ischemia and
reperfusion that allows comparison of the electrical responses of
whole hearts and isolated tissues. The whole heart preparation
will allow characterization of arrhythmias and comparison of
responses to those seen in underperfusion-reperfusion or
ligation-reflow models in which true ischemia is induced. This
preparation will also allow separate study of various components
of ischemia. The isolated tissue preparation allows the cellular
basis for arrhythmias or antiarrhythmic actions to be studied
within the same species.

In our previous studies utilizing isolated canine tissues, an
immediate burst of arrhythmias was not observed. The present
study shows that the "ischemic" Tyrode's solution model will
induce a burst of arrhythmic activity, including ventricular
fibrillation, when the model is adapted to the Langendorff
perfused heart. It is possible that the different response of
the whole heart reflects the greater mass of surviving transmural
tissue, the greater anatomical complexity of the intact heart, or
the greater rapidity of perfusate changes accomplished in this
model. One of the notable features of the whole heart
experiments is the similarity of the arrhythmic response to that

seen in ligation-reflow experiments. Experiments by others have
provided evidence for both reentry (10) and enhanced automaticity
(11) as mechanisms of reperfusion arrhythmias following ligation
and release of coronary arteries. Kaplinsky et al. (4) noted
that reperfusion arrhythmias occurred in two distinct phases: an
early phase of rapid arrhythmias compatible with a reentrant
mechanism and a later phase of less malignant ectopic activity
compatible with automaticity. Reperfusion - induced automaticity
and digitalis induced OAP share similar responses to adrenergic
influences (12), anoxia (13) and the antiarrhythmic drug,
mexiletine (14). And indeed, we have shown that OAP are induced
by our model of reperfusion in subendocardial tissues both in
canine preparations (1,2) and now in isolated guinea pig tissues.
Furthermore, our experiments in whole hearts perfused with
"ischemic" Tyrode's solution and then reperfused with "normal"
Tyrode's solution exhibit coupled ectopic activity with
characteristics virtually identical to ectopic activity generated
by digitalis induced OAP (7,15).

Our guinea pig tissue and whole heart preparations also
showed rapid arrhythmic activity occurring in response to
reperfusion. In the whole heart preparations this occurred as
ventricular fibrillation which started abruptly with no apparent
causal relationship to the slower coupled activity. In the
isolated tissue experiments only one preparation demonstrated
rapid activity and that occurred in discontinuous bursts. The
mechanism(s) of fibrillatory activity was not apparent in either
preparation. In the isolated tissues this activity was initiated
and terminated by single stimuli and the rapid potentials did not
exhibit prepotentials or pacemaker potentials. Thus rapid
fibrillatory activity may have been reentrant in origin.

Digitalis OAP occur in Purkinje tissue but not in ventricular
muscle in the absence of stretch, depolarization, or very high
drug concentrations (15,16), despite the occurrence of a strong
positive inotropic effect plus prominent aftercontractions in
muscle (17). Similarly, reperfusion - induced OAP were observed
only in Purkinje tissue in our canine tissue experiments (1,2).

In guinea pig preparations the distinction between Purkinje and muscle cells by electrophysiological characteristics is more difficult. However, in the present study we observed OAP only in subendocardial tissues and never in epicardial impalements. In addition, spontaneous activity and arrhythmias only occurred in those preparations with an intact endocardium. Preparations from which the endocardium had been removed did not demonstrate spontaneous activity in response to reperfusion. These observations are in general, although not complete, agreement with observations of others. Ideker et al. (18) noted that the first series of ectopic beats leading to ventricular fibrillation in the dog upon reperfusion did not appear to have an epicardial origin. Janse and coworkers (19,20) showed that early reperfusion ectopy in pig and dog hearts consistently showed activation of Purkinje tissue preceding that of muscle. Destruction of the subendocardial Purkinje system with phenol completely prevented ischemia and reperfusion induced ventricular fibrillation in these same studies. However, other slower reperfusion arrhythmias still occurred. This latter discrepency with our observations might be explained if the phenol treatment did not destroy all of the thicker bundles of Purkinje tissue in the much larger hearts used in these studies, or if damage to underlying myocardium by phenol created an additional new substrate for induction of arrhythmias with yet a different mechanism in these hearts.

The response of guinea pig tissues to "ischemia" and reperfusion was not identical to that of canine tissues. Following appearance of OAP, canine Purkinje tissue exhibited marked depolarization with general inexcitability (1,2). In the present study, marked depolarization and loss of regenerative activity occurred at specific impalements but was not a uniform response of subendocardial tissues. In our studies of canine tissues we found that depolarization only occurred in Purkinje tissue and not in muscle. Furthermore, only Purkinje tissue more than approximately two space constants from muscle exhibited marked depolarization. Action potentials still occurred in thin layers of subendocardial Purkinje tissue when more remote sites were inexcitable. Guinea pig ventricular preparations contain few pure strands of Purkinje tissue extending beyond two space constants from muscle. Thus, strong reperfusion - induced depolarization may be prevented in guinea pig preparations by the electrotonic repolarizing influence of nearby muscle. The specific roles of these different electrophysiological responses to reperfusion in the generation of arrhythmias in hearts of various species including man can only be determined with additional studies.

REFERENCES

1. Ferrier, G.R., Moffat, M.P. and Lukas, A. Circ. Res. **56**: 184 - 194, 1985.
2. Ferrier, G.R., Moffat, M.P., Lukas, A. and Mohabir, R. In: Cardiac Electrophysiology and Arrhythmias (Eds. D.P. Zipes and J. Jalife), Grune and Stratton Inc., New York, N.Y., 1985, pp. 325 - 330.
3. Harris, A.S. and Rojas, A.G. Exp. Med. Surg. **1**. 105 - 122, 1943.
4. Kaplinsky, E., Ogawa, S., Michelson, E.L. and Dreifus, L.S. Circulation **63**: 333 - 340, 1981.
5. Penny, W.J. and Sheridan, D.J. Cardiovasc. Res. **17**: 363 - 372, 1983.
6. Kimura, S., Bassett, A.L., Saoudi, N.C., Cameron, J.S., Kozlovskis, P.L. and Myerburg, R.J. J. Am. Coll. Cardiol. **7**: 833 - 842, 1986.
7. Ferrier, G.R., Saunders, J.H. and Mendez, C. Circ. Res. **32**: 600 - 609, 1973.
8. Zipes, D.P., Arbel, E., Knope,R.F. and Moe, G.K. Am. J. Cardiol. **33**: 248 - 253, 1974.
9. Rosen, M.R., Fisch, C., Hoffman, B.F., Danilo, P., Lovelace, D.E. and Knoebel, S.B. Am. J. Cardiol. **45**: 1272 - 1284, 1980.
10. Murdock, D.K., Loeb, J.M., Euler, D.E. and Randall, W.C. Circulation **61**: 175 - 182, 1980.
11. Penkoske, P.A., Sobel, B.E. and Corr, P.B. Circulation **58**: 1023 - 1035, 1978.
12. Sheridan, D.J., Penkoske, P.A., Sobel, B.E. and Corr, P.B. J. Clin. Invest. **65**: 161 - 171, 1980.
13. Carbonin, P., Di Gennaro, M., Valle, R. and Weisz, A.M. Amer. J. Physiol. **240**: H730 - H737, 1981.
14. Amerini, S., Carbonin, P., Cerbai, E., Giotti, A., Mugelli, A. and Pahor, M. Br. J. Pharmac. **86**: 805 - 815, 1985.
15. Ferrier, G.R. Prog. Cardiovasc. Dis. **19**: 459 - 474, 1977.
16. Ferrier, G.R. Circ. Res. **38**: 156 - 162, 1976.
17. Ferrier, G.R. Circ. Res. **41**: 622 - 629, 1977.

18. Ideker, R.E., Klein, G.J., Harrison, L., Smith, W.M., Kasell, J., Reimer, K.A., Wallace, A.G. and Gallagher, J.J. Circulation 63: 1371 - 1379, 1981.
19. Janse, M.J., Wilms-Schopman, F., Wilensky, R.J. and Tranum-Jensen, J. In: Cardiac Electrophysiology and Arrhythmias (Eds. D.P. Zipes and J. Jalife), Grune and Stratton, New York, N.Y., 1985, pp. 353 - 362.
20. Janse, M.J., Kleber, A.G., Capucci, A., Coronel, R. and Wilms-Schopman, F. J. Mol. Cell. Cardiol. 18: 339 - 355, 1986.

5

THE PREVENTIVE EFFECT OF SODIUM SELENITE AGAINST ISCHEMIC VENTRICULAR
ARRHYTHMIA AND SOME CLUES TO ITS MECHANISMS

Y. A. MEI, Y. Q. XU AND H. D. ZHANG

Department of Physiology, Shanghai Second Medical University, Shanghai,
People's Republic of China

INTRODUCTION

Ventricular arrhythmia is the main cause of sudden deaths of patients
suffering from myocardial infarction. For a long time, workers in the field
have attempted to look for an effective drug in the prevention of ischemic
ventricular arrhythmia and many drugs have been introduced.

Keshan disease is an endemic cardiomyopathy of unknown cause in certain
hilly and mountainuous regions of China. Occurrence of this disease is
found to be invariably associated with a deficiency of selenium in the food
and in the hair of the inhabitants of the involved areas. Oral administration
of sodium selenite is effective in the prevention of this endemic cardiomyopathy (1).

It was also reported that the selenium content of the serum and whole
blood of the patients suffering from coronary heart disease was much lower
than that of healthy persons in Finland (2). Treatment of patients with
coronary heart disease with selenium-Vitamin E can reduce the frequency
of angina pectoris attack (3).

In the present study, the efficacy of sodium selenite in the prevention
of acute ventricular arrhythmia induced by ligation of the anterior descending
coronary artery of the isolated rabbit heart was observed. It could reduce
the rate of development of ischemic ventricular arrhythmia very drastically.
The main electrophysiological effects of sodium selenite on the isolated
cardiac preparations were prolongation of the effective refractory period
and slowing down the conduction velocity of both the fast and slow response
action potentials. All of these effects could be abolished or weakened
by aspirin, an agent which suppresses the endogenous synthesis and release
of the prostanoids including prostacyclin.

MATERIALS AND METHODS

Isolated heart perfusion and the induction of the ischemic ventricular
arrhythmia.

New Zealand rabbits weighing 2-2.5 Kg were stunned by a blow on the
head and the heart was removed immediately. By using the modified Langendorff
perfusion method (De Deckere & Ten Hoor, 1977) (4), the isolated rabbit
heart was perfused with warm Tyrode solution gassed with 95% O_2 and 5% CO_2
at a constant flow rate of 20-25 ml/min. The composition of the Tyrode
solution was as follows (mM): NaCl 137; NaHCO$_3$ 23; KCl 4.5; CaCl$_2$ 1.8; MgCl$_2$
0.5; glucose 11 with pH 7.5. The temperature of the perfusing solution
was kept at 38 ± 0.5 °C.

After the heart was placed in the perfusion apparatus filled with continuously gassed Tyrode solution, the aorta and the pulmonary artery were
each cannulated, the former being the site of inflow of the perfusion fluid
to the coronary arteries, and the latter, the coronary outflow of the perfusion fluid. At the same time, all the veins on both sides of the heart
were ligated so that the perfusion fluid from the cannula in the aorta
entering the coronary system passing through the coronary sinus into the
right atrium and then through the right ventricle to be finally ejected
through the cannula in the pulmonary artery to the outside. However, about
2% of the perfusion fluid was found to be able to leave the coronary vascular
bed and sip through the heart tissues to reach the surface of the heart.
Since the volume of this fluid is small and the concentration of metabolic
products is high, it is more suitable for determination for metabolic product
such as prostacyclin, 6-keto-prostaglandin $F_{1\alpha}$.

The ischemic ventricular arrhythmia was induced by ligation of the
anterior descending coronary artery. By using an electrocardiograph, the
ECG of the isolated perfused heart was recorded by a pair of electrodes
placed separately at the apex and base of the heart.

Intracellular recording of the electrical activities of cardiac muscle cells.

The papillary muscle and trabecular muscle of the right ventricle of
rabbits were isolated. The preparations were superfused in a bath (volume
1.5 ml) with Tyrode solution in a flow speed of 5 ml/min. The composition,
temperature and pH of the Tyrode solution were the same as in the Langendorff
method described above. It was continuously gassed with 95% O_2 and 5% CO_2.

By using a programmatic stimulator designed and manufactured in our
lab, the preparations were stimulated by a bipolar extracellular electrode.

The stimulus parameters were as follows: 1 Hz, 0.5 ms for fast response action potentials and 0.2 Hz, 2-3 ms for slow response action potentials. The strength of the stimulus was 150% of the threshold.

The transmembrane potentials of cardiac muscle cells were recorded by glass microelectrode filled with 3 M KCl having a resistance of 15-20 meg ohms.

After an equilibration period of one hour after penetration of micro-electrode into the cell, the transmembrane potential of cardiac muscles were recorded and displayed via FW-2 type microelectrode amplifier on SBR-1 dual beam oscilloscope. Maximum rate of depolarization during the upstroke of the action potential ($\dot{V}_{max}$) was measured by electrical differentiation and showed at the lower beam of the oscilloscope.

For inducing a slow response action potential, the muscles were depolarized by 22 mM KCl in Tyrode solution, and 0.8 mg/1 isoprenaline was added into the perfusion fluid to increase the calcium inflow.

The effective refractory period (ERP) was measured by an extrasystolic stimulation method. With the basic stimulation frequency mentioned above, the extrasystolic stimulus was given every eight cycles. The coupling interval between the regular stimulus and the extrasystolic stimulus was increased in steps. The shortest coupling interval that an extrasystolic action potential that could be evoked was taken as the duration of the ERP.

The radio-immuno-assay of the endogenous prostacyclin (PGI$_2$).

Since the half life of the prostacyclin is only 2-3 minutes, the stable metabolic end product of prostacyclin, 6-ketoprostaglandin $F_{1\alpha}$ was measured instead of endogenous prostacyclin by using the radio-immuno-assay method introduced by Yilkorkals (1981) (5).

Drugs.

Sodium selenite was synthesized by Beijing Chemical Industrial Company (770428) in a chemical-pure form.

Aspirin was made by Chinese Medical Pharmaceutica Shanghai Branch (831014).

RESULTS

The preventive effect of sodium selenite against acute ischemic ventricular arrhythmia.

In eighteen rabbit hearts, the ligation of the anterior descending coronary artery induced ventricular arrhythmia within 20-30 minutes in 15 of the 18 rabbit hearts. The ventricular arrhythmia included ventricular extrasystoles, ventricular tachycardia and ventricular fibrillation. If the hearts were perfused with 0.05 mM sodium selenite in Tyrode solution for 20 minutes before the ligation, the incidence rate of ventricular arrhythmia was decreased prominently, it only occurred in 2 of 15 rabbit hearts ($p < 0.01$) (Table 1).

The preventive effects of sodium selenite against acute ischemic ventricular arrhythmia could be reversed by aspirin, an inhibitor of endogenous synthesis of prostanoids. If the rabbit hearts were perfused with Tyrode solution containing 0.05 mM sodium selenite plus aspirin 12 mg/1, the preventive effects of sodium selenite disappeared, the ventricular arrhythmia occured in 7 out of 8 hearts ($p < 0.01$, compared with the addition of sodium selenite alone).

Table 1. Effects of sodium selenite and aspirin on the incidence rate of ischemic ventricular arrhythmia

	Number of hearts	Incidence number of ventricular arrhythmia	Incidence rate of arrhythmias (%)
Control	18	15	83 **
Na_2SeO_3 0.05 mM	15	2	13 **
Na_2SeO_3 0.05 mM + aspirin 12 mg/1	8	7	88

** $p < 0.01$

Electrophysiological effects of sodium selenite on the rabbit isolated ventricular muscles.

Effects on fast response action potentials. Sodium selenite in concentrations of 0.05, 0.1 and 0.15 mM had no obvious effect on the resting membrane potential (RP) of the ventricular muscle of rabbits. The amplitude of action potential (APA) and the maximum rate of depolarization during the upstroke of action potential ($\dot{V}_{max}$) were decreased in a dose-dependent manner. The duration of the action potential repolarized to 90% height of APA (APD_{90}) and the ERP were prolonged. Since the prolongation of the ERP was greater than that of the APD, so the ERP/APD_{90} ratio increased (Table 2, Fig. 1).

The above effects of sodium selenite could be partially blocked by aspirin. Aspirin acting alone at concentration of 24 mg/1 had no obvious effect on the parameters of fast response action potential of rabbit ventricular muscles, yet it could block or reverse the prolongation of ERP and APD and the decrease of $\dot{V}_{max}$ induced by sodium selenite (Fig. 2). Fig. 3 shows a typical example of the blocking effect of aspirin against the prolongation effect of sodium selenite on the APD_{90} and the decrease in $\dot{V}_{max}$.

Table 2. Effects of sodium selenite on the parameters of transmembrane potential of ventricular muscle of rabbits (M ± SD, n = 7).

	RP (mV)	APA (mV)	$\dot{V}_{max}$ (V/s)	APD_{90} (ms)	ERP (ms)	ERP/APD_{90} (%)
Control	91 ± 1	120 ± 3	192 ± 21	150 ± 14	137 ± 16	92.0 ± 8
Na_2SeO_3 0.05 mM	91 ± 1 (99.7%)	120 ± 3 (100%)	184 ± 23** (96.3%)	157 ± 14** (104%)	151 ± 17** (110%)	95.7 ± 9* (104%)
Na_2SeO_3 0.10 mM	92 ± 1 (100%)	118 ± 3** (98.3%)	166 ± 23** (86.4%)	172 ± 20** (114%)	166 ± 18** (121%)	96.8 ± 9* (105%)
Na_2SeO_3 0.15 mM	91 ± 1 (99.8%)	116 ± 3** (96.6%)	149 ± 23** (77.6%)	189 ± 21** (126%)	189 ± 25** (137%)	100 ± 9** (108%)

*p < 0.05, **p < 0.01

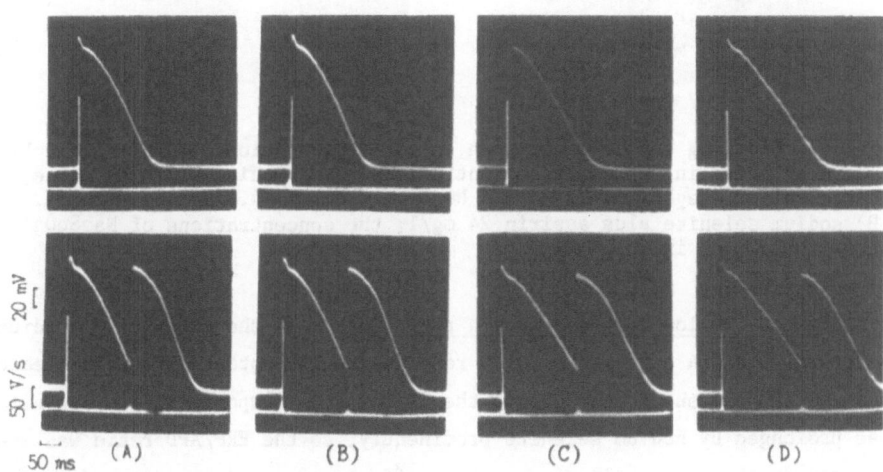

20 mV

50 V/s

50 ms   (A)   (B)   (C)   (D)

Fig. 1. Effects of sodium selenite on the action potential and effective refractory period of the ventricular muscle of rabbits. Upper trace in each panel: action potential; lower trace in each panel: $\dot{V}_{max}$. (A) control; (B) Na_2SeO_3 0.05 mM; (C) Na_2SeO_3 0.10 mM; (D) Na_2SeO_3 0.15 mM.

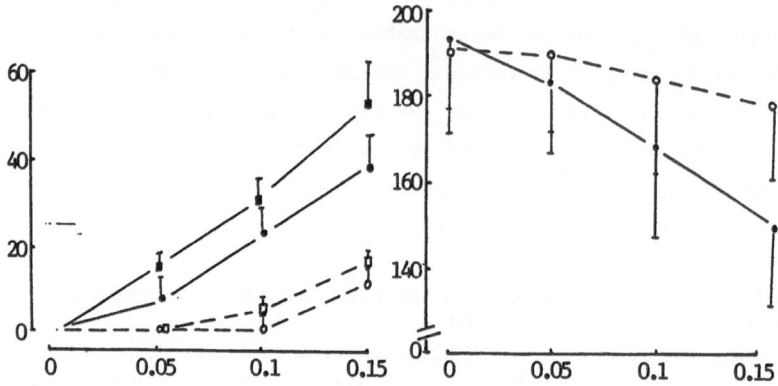

Fig. 2. Blocking effect of aspirin 24 mg/1 on the electrophysiological effects of sodium selenite (n = 7). Left panel: blocking effects on APD and ERP, ordinate: prolongation of ERP and APD in ms, abscissa: Na_2SeO_3 in different concentrations (mM); ■—■ ERP, Na_2SeO_3 alone, □---□ ERP, Na_2SeO_3 plus aspirin, •—• APD, Na_2SeO_3 alone, o---o APD, Na_2SeO_3 plus aspirin. Right panel: blocking effects on $\dot{V}_{max}$, ordinate: $\dot{V}_{max}$ (V/s), abscissa: Na_2SeO_3 in different concentrations (mM); •—• Na_2SeO_3 alone, o---o Na_2SeO_3 plus aspirin.

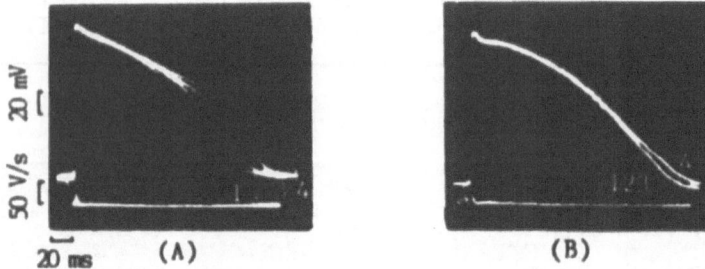

Fig. 3. Blocking effect of aspirin on the prolongation of APD induced by sodium selenite in different concentrations. (A) sodium selenite alone, 1. control; 2. Na_2SeO_3 0.05 mM; 3. Na_2SeO_3 0.10 mM; 4. Na_2SeO_3 0.15 mM. (B) sodium selenite plus aspirin 24 mg/1, the concentrations of Na_2SeO_3 were the same as in (A).

Effect on slow response action potentials. In the presence of sodium selenite, the APA and $\dot{V}_{max}$ of slow response action potential were decreased, and the APD was shortened. Since the ERP of slow response action potential was prolonged by sodium selenite prominently, so the ERP/APD ratio was increased drastically. All of the above effects appeared in a dose-dependent manner (Table 3, Fig. 4).

The effects of sodium selenite on the slow response action potential could also be blocked partially by aspirin 24 mg/1. Aspirin itself had

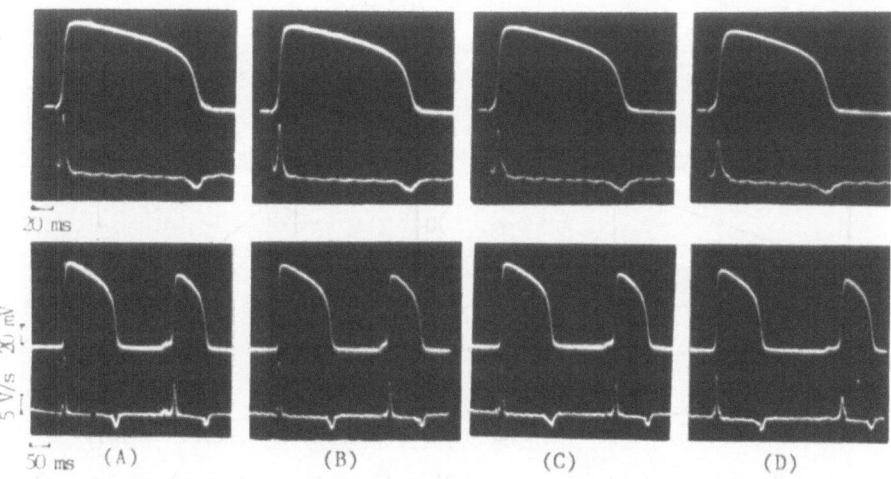

Fig. 4. Effects of sodium selenite on the slow response action potential and effective refractory period of the ventricular muscle of rabbits. Upper trace in each block: action potential; lower trace in each block: $\dot{V}_{max}$; (A) control; (B) Na_2SeO_3 0.05 mM; (C) Na_2SeO_3 0.10 mM; (D) Na_2SeO_3 0.15 mM.

Table 3. Effects of sodium selenite on the slow response action potential of ventricular muscle of rabbits (M ± SD, n = 7).

	APA (mV)	$\dot{V}_{max}$ (V/s)	APD (ms)	ERP (ms)	ERP/APD (%)
Control	77.0 ± 4.0	12.9 ± 0.8	170.7 ± 20	257 ± 38	146 ± 20
Na_2SeO_3 0.05 mM	76.0 ± 3.6* (98.7%)	11.0 ± 0.9** (85.3%)	157.0 ± 21* (91.9%)	271 ± 44** (105%)	177 ± 20* (121%)
Na_2SeO_3 0.10 mM	73.7 ± 3.7** (95.7%)	9.2 ± 1.2** (71.3%)	143.5 ± 20** (84.1%)	285 ± 54** (111%)	192 ± 36** (132%)
Na_2SeO_3 0.15 mM	70.8 ± 3.5** (91.9%)	7.4 ± 1.4** (57.4%)	127.7 ± 21** (74.8%)	320 ± 69** (124%)	247 ± 50** (169%)

*p < 0.05, *p < 0.01

no effect on the parameters of slow response action potentials of ventricular muscle of rabbits. In the presence of aspirin, the effect of sodium selenite 0.15 mM on the APD of slow response action potential only eqauled to that of sodium selenite 0.05 mM alone (Fig. 5).

Fig. 6 shows a typical blocking effects of aspirin on the electrophysiological effects of sodium selenite.

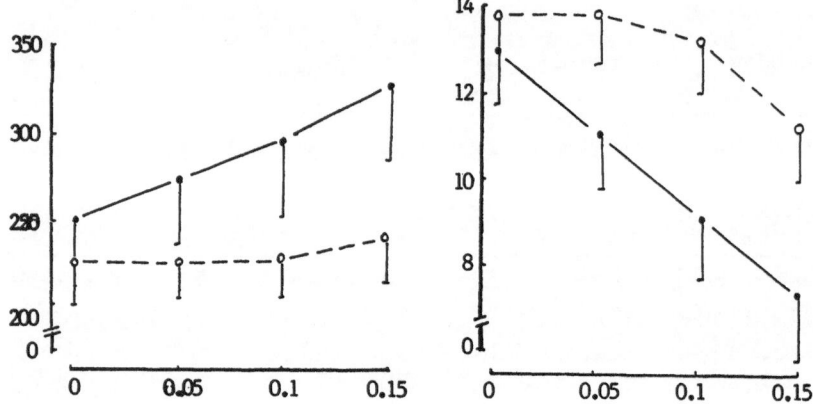

Fig. 5. Blocking effect of aspirin 24 mg/l on the electrophysiological effects of sodium selenite on the slow response action potential of rabbit ventricular muscle. Left panel: blocking effect on ERP, ordinate: ERP in ms, abscissa: concentration of Na_2SeO_3 (mM); •—• Na_2SeO_3 alone, o---o Na_2SeO_3 plus aspirin. Right panel: blocking effect on $\dot{V}_{max}$, ordinate: $\dot{V}_{max}$ (V/s), abscissa: concentration of Na_2SeO_3 (mM); •—• Na_2SeO_3 alone, o---o Na_2SeO_3 plus aspirin.

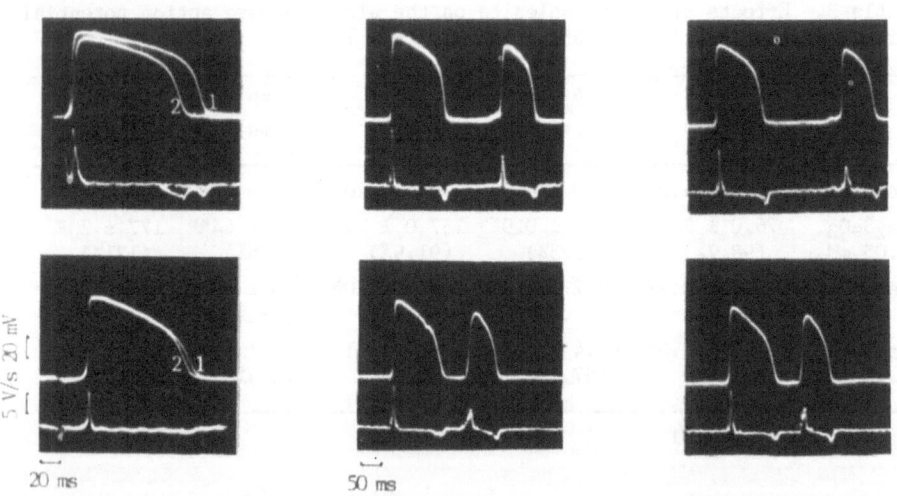

Fig. 6. Blocking effect of aspirin 24 mg/l on the electrophysiological effects of sodium selenite 0.15 mM on slow response action potential of ventricular muscle of rabbits. Upper panels: left: 1. normal APD, 2. APD in the presence of 0.15 mM Na_2SeO_3; middle: normal ERP; right: ERP in the presence of 0.15 mM Na_2SeO_3. Lower panels: left: 1. normal APD, 2. APD in the presence of 0.15 mM Na_2SeO_3 plus 24 mg/l aspirin; middle: normal ERP; right: ERP in the presence of 0.15 mM Na_2SeO_3 plus 24 mg/l aspirin.

Effects of sodium selenite and aspirin on the endogenous synthesis of prostacyclin of the perfused rabbit hearts.

Aspirin can partially block the protective and electrophysiological
effects of sodium selenite on the isolated heart and aspirin itself does
not have any effect in these respects. It is well known that aspirin is
an effective inhibitor of endogenous synthesis of prostacyclin and the
latter is the major prostanoid released from the isolated perfused rabbit
heart (6) and it may have a protecting effect on the heart against arrhythmogenesis (7).

The effects of sodium selenite and aspirin on the endogenous release
of prostacyclin from the isolated perfused heart were therefore studied.
The results are shown in Fig. 7. The stable metabolic end product of prostacyclin, 6-keto-$PGF_{1\alpha}$, was taken as a measure of prostacyclin. In the
control, the amount of 6-keto-$PGF_{1\alpha}$ released from the perfused heart was
found to be relatively constant during a twenty-minutes period. In the
presence of sodium selenite (0.05 mM), the amount of 6-keto-$PGF_{1\alpha}$ released
was increased significantly (n = 8, p < 0.05). But, in the presence of
12 mg/l aspirin, the same concentration of sodium selenite did not increase
the release of 6-keto-$PGF_{1\alpha}$, in fact, the amount of 6-keto-$PGF_{1\alpha}$ released
was decreased. These results indicate that the increase of endogenous
synthesis of prostacyclin induced by sodium selenite can be blocked by
aspirin (Fig. 7).

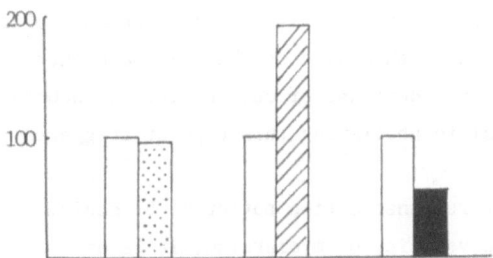

Fig. 7. Effects of sodium selenite and aspirin on the endogenous synthesis
and release of 6-keto-$PGF_{1\alpha}$ from the isolated rabbit hearts, ordinate: percentage change of 6-keto-$PGF_{1\alpha}$ concentration in the perfusate compared with
controls, abscissa: ▢ control, ▨ , ▨ , ▆ 20 min after perfusing the heart
with normal Tyrode solution, Tyrode solution containing 0.05 mM Na_2SeO_3 and
Tyrode solution containing 0.05 mM Na_2SeO_3 plus 12 mg/l aspirin respectively.

DISCUSSION

The present study shows that sodium selenite has a protective effect on the ischemic heart against ventricular arrhythmia elicited by ligation of the anterior descending coronary artery. It prolongs the effective refractory period of both fast and slow response action potentials and increases endogenous release of prostacyclin. All of the above effects can be blocked or partially blocked by adding aspirin into the perfusion fluid.

Ventricular arrhythmia induced by ischemia may be due to changes of normal and abnormal automaticity, altered conduction velocity and re-entry, or a combination of these factors. Re-entry is an important mechanism for ischemic ventricular arrhythmia. The requirements for re-entry or reexcitation are complex and mainly include: 1. existence of a closed loop conduction pathway; 2. a localized region of unidirectional block within the loop; 3. conduction time around the loop longer than the longest refractory period proximal to the region of block. The prolongation of ERP of both types of action potentials by sodium selenite is certainly effective to prevent the genesis of re-entry and to eliminate the ventricular arrhythmia.

On the other hand, the decrease of $\dot{V}_{max}$ and the shortening of the APD of the slow response action potential in the presence of sodium selenite indicate that the slow inward current (mainly Ca^{++}) could be partially blocked by this drug. As a calcium blocker, sodium selenite is useful for eliminating triggered arrhythmia. It is well known that the depolarization phase of early after-depolarization (plateau oscillation) is due to calcium inflow, so the decrease of culcium inflow by sodium selenite can eliminate this abnormal triggered activity. For delayed after-depolarization, intracellular calcium overload is the basic mechanism of this kind of abnormal pacemaker activity. So it can be supposed that the decrease of culcium inflow induced by sodium selenite would be beneficial in abolishing this type of triggered activity.

The decrease of $\dot{V}_{max}$ of the fast response action potential by sodium selenite will decrease the conduction velocity of myocardium, it is an arrhythmogenic factor for re-entry, but if the decrease of conduction velocity can induce two-way block instead of unidirectional block, it can also eliminate the re-entry. Considering the antiarrhythmic effect on the ischemic isolated heart, the effect of sodium selenite on the heart on the whole is antiarrhythmic.

Aspirin in the concentration of 24 mg/l has no effect on the electrical activity of the cardiac muscle, but it can block the electrophysiological effects of sodium selenite on the myocardium and abolish the protective effect of sodium selenite on the ischemic heart against the ventricular arrhythmia. This suggests that some intermediate reaction elicited by sodium selenite must have been blocked by aspirin. The fact that the increase of endogenous synthesis and release of prostacyclin from the isolated heart induced by sodium selenite can be reversed by adding aspirin indicates the interrelationship between the sodium selenite and endogenous prostacyclin could be an important mechanism of the antiarrhythmic effect of this drug. As we know, prostacyclin is the major prostanoid released from the isolated perfused rabbit heart and it can inhibit platelet aggregation and dilate small coronary vessels (9). It was also reported that prostacyclin has an antiarrhythmic activity in the dog. So it can be deduced that the anti-arrhythmic effect of sodium selenite in the isolated perfused rabbit heart is exerted at least partially through its ability in increasing the endo-genous synthesis and release of prostacyclin, a self-protective mechanism of ischemic cardiac muscle against arrhythmia.

SUMMARY

The results of the present study indicates that sodium selenite is an effective antiarrhythmic agent for the ischemic ventricular muscle. The main electrophysiological effects of this drug on the cardiac muscle are the prolongation of the effective refractory period and the decrease of the calcium inward current and the fast sodium current. It can increase the production of the endogenous prostacyclin. All these effects can be partially blocked by aspirin, indicating that sodium selenite–endogenous prostacyclin interrelationship is the main mechanism of sodium selenite in preventing arrhythmia.

REFERENCES

1. Chen, X. S. et al. Biological Trace Element Research 2: 91–107, 1980.
2. Westermarck, T. Acta Pharmacol. Toxicol., 41: 121–128, 1977.
3. Frost, D. V. et al. Ann. Rev. Pharmacol., 15: 259–284, 1975.
4. De Deckere, E. A. M. and Ten Hoor, P. Pflugers Arch., 370: 103–105, 1977.
5. Yilkorkals, O. et al. Prostagl. Med., 6: 427, 1981.
6. De Deckere, E. A. M., Nugteren, D. H. and Ten Hoor, P. Nature, 268: 160–163, 1977.
7. Mest, H. J. and Forste, W. Acta Biol. Med. Germ., 37: 827, 1978.
8. Kass, R. S. J. Physiol., 281: 187, 1978.
9. Coker, S. J. et al. Nature, 291: 323–324, 1981.

B. PATHOPHYSIOLOGIC ASPECTS OF ISCHEMIC INJURY

II. PATHOPHYSIOLOGIC ASPECTS OF
ISCHEMIC INJURY

6

MOLECULAR EVENTS OCCURRING DURING POST-ISCHAEMIC REPERFUSION

R. FERRARI, C. CECONI, S. CURELLO, A. CARGNONI, A. ALBERTINI, E O. VISIOLI

Cattedra di Cardiologia e Cattedra di Chimica, Universita' degli Studi di Brescia, 25100 Brescia, Italy

INTRODUCTION

The availability of techniques such as surgical reperfusion, angioplasty and thrombolysis for the restoration of blood flow to the ischaemic myocardium has revived interest in the reperfusion phenomenon (1,2,3). It is clear that reperfusion occupies a central role in tissue protection as, without it, no recovery is possible at all (4). Reperfusion, however is not necessarily beneficial and it has been reported that it can accelerate the rate of development of necrosis (4,5,6,7,8). The available data on the use of intracoronary infusion of streptokinase or urokinase for the dissolution of clot have shown recanalization rates of up 90% which are not necessarily accompained by a recovery of myocardial function. Like in animal studies, the recovery of metabolical and functional capacities of the previous ischaemic zone seems to depend on the duration of the ischaemic period (11,12,13). Thus, the biochemical events leading to the irreversibility of the ischaemic myocites and the possibility of improving recovery by acting directly during reperfusion represent a very important clinical problem.

Cause of reperfusion damage

At the present there is no simple answer to the question of what determines no recovery on reperfusion and cell death. It is not clear whether ischaemia induces cellular changes which make the events on reperfusion inevitable, or whether these events are due to reperfusion per se and are susceptible of being modified.

The problem arise from the fact that: -1) ischaemic-damage is not homogenous and many factors may combine to cause cell death; -2) severity of biochemical changes and development of necrosis are usually associated (both the processes being dependent on the duration of ischaemia) and it is impossible to establish a casual relationship; -3) the inevitability of necrosis can only be assessed by reperfusion of the ischaemic myocardium. Restoration of flow, however, might result in a numerous further negative consequences, thus directily favouring the occurrence of cell death (14,15,16,17,18).

However, it should be pointed out that the deleterious events associated with reperfusion cannot be avoided by the prolongation of an ischaemic period even in the presence of protective interventions such as pharmacological or biochemical manipulation of the ischaemic cell. These interventions, in the absence of reperfusion, do not restore normal contractile function and are able only to delay, but not to avoid, the development of injury. It is therefore difficult to believe that, with the exception of the induction of arrhythmias, reperfusion causes further injury. More likely, when not beneficial, it accelerates the rate of development of a predetermined necrosis (19).

The casual mechanism determining cell death during reperfusion is unknown. Different possible factors have been suggested as triggers of cell necrosis on reperfusion. They include: depletion of high energy phosphate (20), loss of adenine nucleotide (21) and of catecholamines (22), accumulation of calcium (17,18,23), activation of phospholipase (24) and of protease (25), detergent effect of acyl esters (26) and of lysophosphoglycerides (27), cell tearing due to contracture (28), myocardial cell swelling, and, more recently, oxygen generated free radicals (29,30,31). Often these factors are interrelated and obscure the distinction between cause and effect.

From the data shown in figures 1 and 2 it appears that there was a progression of tissue damage associated with the extension of the ischaemic period. During the early stages of ischaemia there was a rapid decline of developed pressure and a fall of CP concentration, followed by a decline of ATP content. At this stage diastolic pressure was unchanged and mitochondria had normal calcium content and function.

Extending the ischaemic period to 60 and 90 min, resulted in a progressive increase of diastolic pressure coincident with further reduction of tissue ATP. This indicates that the rate of ATP consumption exceeded the rate of ATP production. Tissue calcium was unchanged, whilst mitochondrial calcium was significantly increased, indicating that a redistribution of intracellular calcium has occurred. The finding that the ischaemic mitochondria had accumulated calcium suggests that: -1) the cytosolic calcium concentration was increased, the extramitochondrial calcium concentration being the major factor

determining calcium accumulation (18);

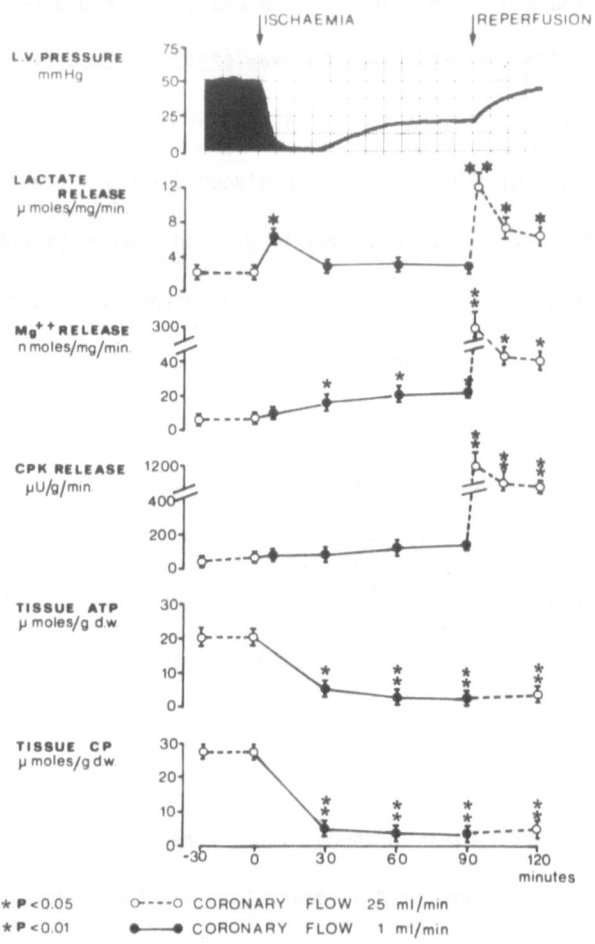

Fig. 1. Effect of ischaemia and reperfusion on mechanical and metabolic function of isolated and perfused rabbit heart. Ischaemia was induced by reducing coronary flow from 25 ml min^{-1} to 1 ml min^{-1}. Data are means $\pm$ errors of at least six experiments. Left ventricular pressures, lactate, Mg2+ and CPK release in the coronary effluent and tissue content of ATP and CP have been determined as previously described (18).

-2) the mitochondria were capable of maintaining the membrane potential which

is required to transport and to prevent the re-equilibration of calcium.

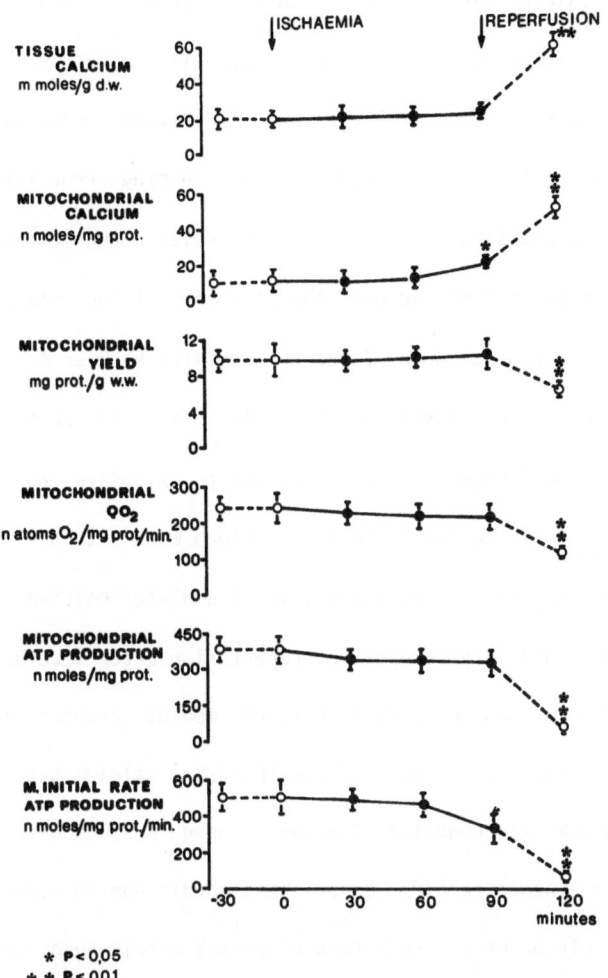

Fig. 2. Effect of ischaemia and reperfusion on mechanical and metabolic function of isolated and perfused rabbit heart. Ischaemia was induced by reducing coronary flow from 25 ml min^{-1} to 1 ml min^{-1}. Data are means $\pm$ errors of at least six experiments. Tissue and mitochondrial calcium content and mitochondrial function have been determined as previously described (42).

The alterations of intracellular calcium homeostasis are likely to be dependent on the severe ATP reduction, ATP being necessary to prevent the redistribution of calcium (16). Reperfusion of these hearts did not lead to restoration of normal function. On the contrary, it produced an increase of diastolic pressure with a very small recovery of developed pressure and no re-establishment of tissue ATP and CP concentrations. During reperfusion, there was a significant exacerbation of lactate and CPK release and massive influx of calcium. These results strongly suggest that a lesion of the cell membrane has occurred, leading to a break down of the permeability barrier to ions such as calcium and to larger molecules such as CPK. Calcium is then accumulated by the mitochondria with a consequent impairment of their oxidative phosphorilation capabilities. It has been suggested that, provided with both ADP and calcium, cardiac mitochondria will preferentially accumulate calcium prior to phosphorilating ADP (32). Therefore, on reperfusion after severe ischaemia, oxygen is restored to mitochondria whose external medium contains high level of calcium. This inevitably would stimulate mitochondrial calcium transport which, in turn, would induce mitochondrial structural damage and, as observed, a loss of the ability to synthesize ATP. Under these conditions we would expect no recovery of tissue ATP or CP and no return of normal muscle function.

These experiments provide evidence for the suggestion that a limiting factor in cell necrosis during reperfusion is related to calcium fluxes. The relative importance of this is as yet unclear and the mechanism of calcium influx remains uncertain. The observation that the influx is not reduced by administration during reperfusion of calcium antagonist agents such as verapamil (33) or nifedipine (18) supports the idea that calcium does not pass through the slow calcium channel. It seems also very unlikely that calcium uptake during reperfusion occurs by a sodium-calcium exchange mechanism (16).

The most probable explanation is that specific damage to the sarcolemma causes calcium to move down the concentration gradient. Such damage occurs within seconds after the reintroduction of the oxygenated perfusion medium and it has been suggested that it could be the consequence of oxygen toxicity (17,30,34,35).

Oxygen toxicity

For many cardiologists the concept of oxygen as a widely toxic substance seems alien. We used to consider oxygen to be of almost universal benefit in many disease situations. However there is now a convincing body of evidence suggesting that oxygen-derived free radicals may play a fundamental role in cellular damage in a wide variety of pathophysiologic processes, including injury due to radiation, inflammation and even to myocardial ischaemia and reperfusion (29,30,31,36,37).

It is well known that oxygen supplied at concentrations greater than those in normal air might damage plants, animals and aerobic bacteria (2). There is a considerable body of evidence that as much as 21% oxygen has slowly manifested damaging effects. These effects vary considerably with the type of organism used, its age and diet (38).

The inherent nature of the oxygen molecule makes it susceptible to univalent reduction reactions in the cell to form superoxide anions ($O_2^{\cdot-}$), a highly reactive free-radical (5-6). Other reactive products of oxygen metabolism can be formed from subsequent intracellular reduction of $O_2^{\cdot-}$ including oxygen peroxide (H_2O_2) and the hydroxyl radical ($\cdot OH$). Under normal conditions most of the molecular oxygen in biologic systems undergoes tetravalent reduction in the mitochondria. However, 1% or 2% leaks from this pathway to undergo univalent reduction, producing the above mentioned toxic species.

These molecules are free-radicals as they contain an odd number of electrons; as such they are quite potent oxidizing and/or reducing agents. Free radicals are also able to initiate chain reactions and are capable of various toxic activities such as the inactivation of sulphydryl enzymes, cross-linking of proteins, DNA breakdown and lipid peroxidation (35,39,40).

Different sources have been suggested to be primarely involved in the generation of oxygen free-radicals during ischaemia and reperfusion, although the primary sites of free-radicals mediated damage remain uncertain.

Within the myocardial cell the most important sites for the formation of oxygen radicals are the mitochondria. It is known that superoxide radical generation is greatest when the components of respiratory chain are in a reduced state as, for example, after ischaemia. Under these circumstances readmission of oxygen will lead to an enhance of O_2^- production by electron transport components of the ischaemic cell. In addition activated phospholipases may degrade cell membrane phospholipids, releasing arachidonic acid that can accelerate the synthesis of free-radicals intermediates by the cyclooxygenase and lipooxygenase pathways (30). From the outside of the myocardial cell is probably the enzyme xanthine oxidase the major source of oxygen free-radical formation. Ischaemia, infact, leads to the conversion of xanthine dehydrogenase into xanthine oxidase which utilizes hypoxanthine as oxidizable substrate to form uric acid and superoxide or hydrogen peroxide (35). This reaction is favoured by ischaemia which induces ATP catabolism, leading to further accumulation of hypoxanthine to serve as substrate for xanthine oxidase. Finally ischaemia triggers the activation of the complement system and generation of chemiotatic factors. As a consequence neutrophils accumulate in the vascular space of reperfused ischaemic myocardium and might cause damage through theyr ability to produce oxygen free-radicals (41).

However, in the heart there exists a series of defence mechanisms which are able to protect the cell against the cytotoxic oxygen metabolites. They include the enzymes superoxide dismutase, catalase and glutathione peroxidase plus other endogenous antioxidants such as vitamin E, ascorbic acid and cysteine (18). The basic premise for the involvement of oxygen in reperfusion damage is that ischaemia and reperfusion have altered the defence mechanisms against oxygen toxicity.

Effects of myocardial ischaemia and reperfusion on the defence mechanism against oxygen toxicity.

To investigate the possible role of oxygen in reperfusion injury, we have determined the effects of ischaemia on the activity of mitochondrial and cytosolic superoxide dismutase, the first line of defence against oxygen toxicity and of glutathione peroxidase and glutathione reductase, the second line of defence against oxygen free-radicals production (Fig. 3).

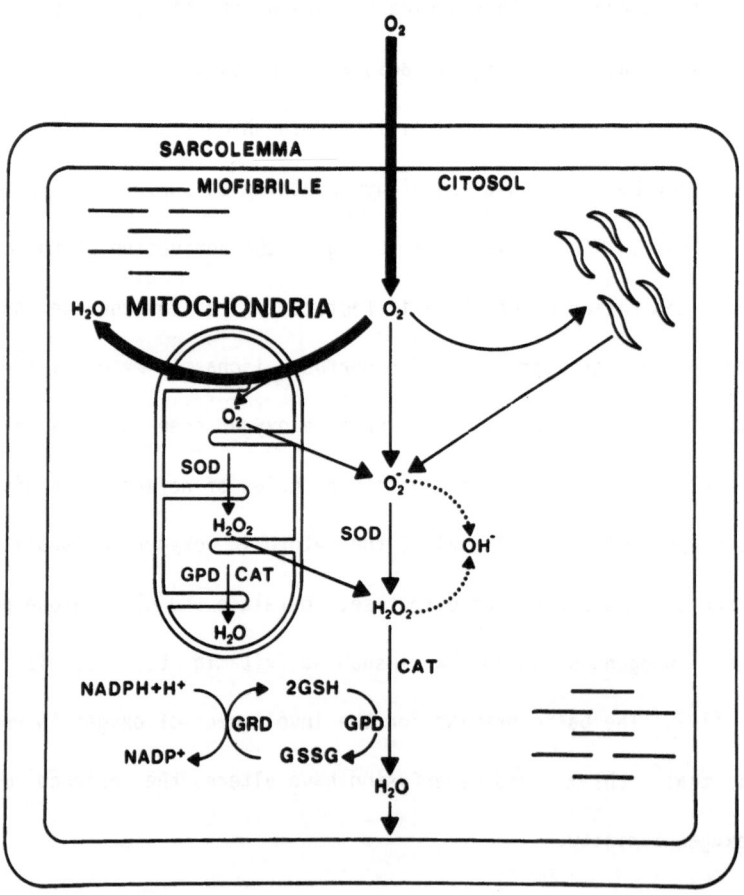

Fig. 3. Schematic representation of the myocardial defence mechanism against oxygen toxicity.

In the isolated and perfused rabbit hearts we have also measured the tissue ratio of GSH and GSSG as an index of oxidative stress. The data are shown in figure 4.

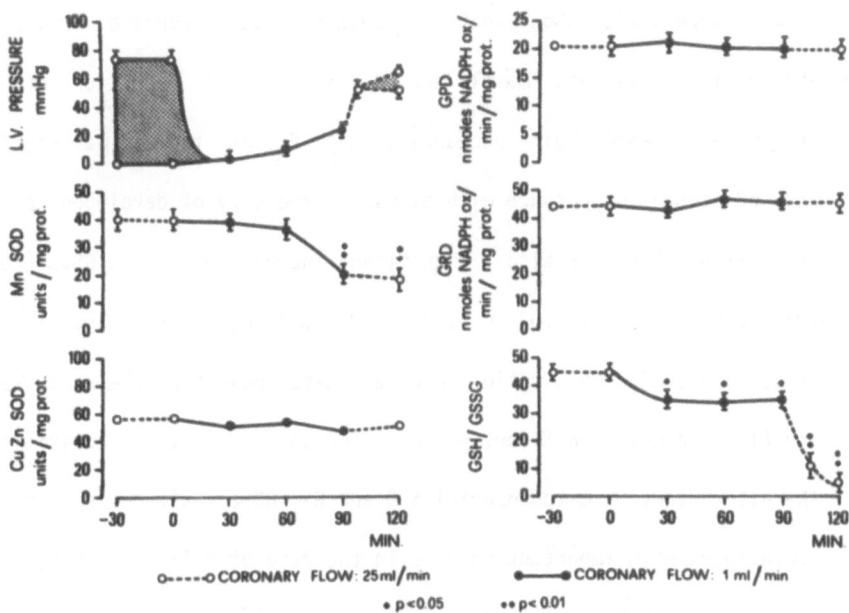

Fig. 4. Effects of ischaemia and reperfusion on superoxide dismutases, glutathione peroxidase and glutathione reductase activity and on tissue GSH/GSSG. All of the determinations were performed in the homogenate as described before (30). Results are given as means ± standard error of six experiments. P relates to the difference between values obtained after aerobic perfusion and those obtained after ischaemia and reperfusion.

Reduction of coronary flow to 1 ml/min induced a rapid decline of developed pressure, contractile activity ceasing completely 9 min after the onset of ischaemia.

Resting pressure began to rise progressively 20 min after the onset of ischaemia. 90 min of ischaemia specifically reduced the activity of mitochondrial (Mn) SOD whilst the same period of ischaemia did not affect the activity of cytosolic (Cu-Zn) SOD or of glutathione peroxidase or glutathione reductase. Figure 4 also shows that ischaemia induced a reduction in myocardial GSH/GSSG ratio. This was mainly due to a significant reduction of tissue content of GSH, GSSG being unchanged. Reperfusion induced a significant increase of diastolic pressure with almost no recovery of developed pressure. On reperfusion there was also a significant increase of tissue GSSG from the ischaemic value of 0.17 ± 0.02 to 0.55 ± 0.02 nmols/mg protein, resulting in a further decline of GSH/GSSG ratio. Figure 1 also shows that the readmission of coronary flow did not significantly modify the SOD, GRD and GPD activities.

The alterations in mitochondrial SOD and GSH/GSSG ratio during reperfusion were coincident with important changes in the rate of release of GSH and GSSG into the coronary sinus as it shown in figure 5. 120 min of ischaemia did not significantly alter the rate of GSH or GSSG release. On reperfusion, after 30 min of ischaemia, there was a small, transient increase of the rate of GSH and GSSG concentration in the coronary effluent which never exceeded the control pre-ischaemic values. Reperfusion after 60 and 90 min of ischaemia resulted in a marked and sustained release of GSH and GSSG from the heart, the rate of which was higher after 90 min of ischaemia.

These results suggest that ischaemia induces metabolic alterations capable of reducing the defence mechanisms against oxygen toxicity. The prime alteration seems to lie at the level of mitochondrial superoxide dismutase, its activity being reduced of the 50% after severe ischaemia. Under these conditions the readmission of molecular oxygen is likely to stimulate the production of $O_2^{\cdot-}$ radicals above the neutralizing capacity of mitochondrial SOD. Consequently, the second line of defence against oxygen toxicity, GPD, is likely to be highly stimulated. We found a severe alteration of the glutathione status indicating that myocardial oxidative damage has occurred and probably it has been counteracted at this level.

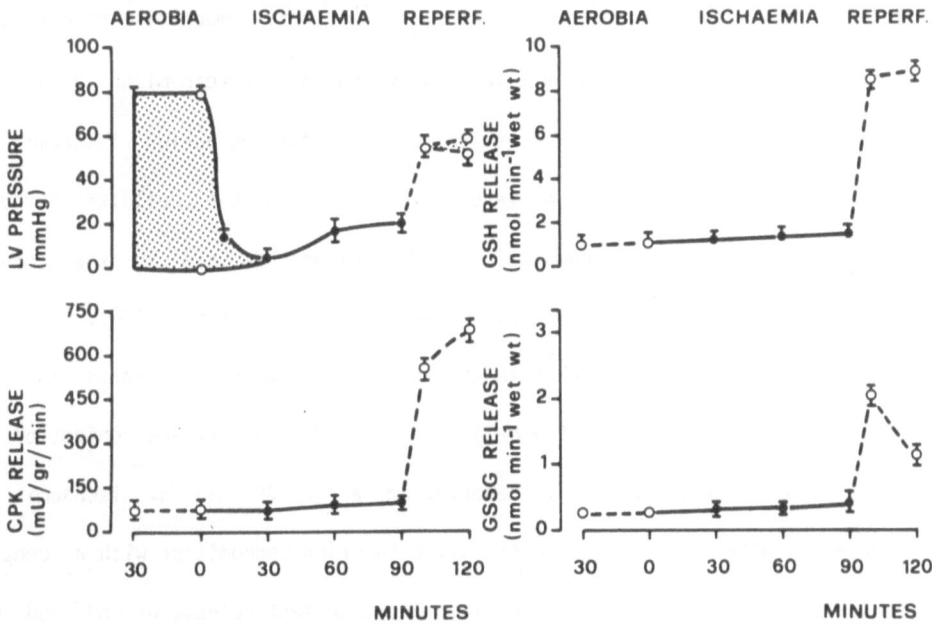

Fig. 5. Effect of ischaemia and reperfusion on systolic and diastolic pressure and on rate of GSH and GSSG release of the isolated and perfused rabbit heart. Broken lines represent aeoric perfusion and solid lines ischaemic perfusion (coronary flow 1ml/min). Ischaemia was started at time 0. The data are expressed as means ± SE of at least six separate experiments. P relates to the significance of the difference between the control and each relevant point.

There are several evidences proving that glutathione plays an important role in myocardial metabolism. Glutathione occurs predominantly intracellularly in concentrations that range from 0.5 mM to 10 mM and it is mainly in the form of GSH, being the most abundant intracellular soluble sulphydryl group. Glutathione is a key factor in the detoxification of electrophilic metabolites and reactive oxygen intermediates. Furthermore, GSH as a cosubstrate of glutathione peroxidase plays an essential protective role against oxygen free radicals and prevents peroxidation of membrane lipids, the activity of superoxide dismutase in the heart being nearly 4 times less than in liver and catalase activity being extremely low. This protective mechanism results in an increased formation of intracellular GSSG and of protein-mixed disulfides. Therefore the changes of glutathione status occurring during ischaemia and reperfusion provide important informations regarding the cellular oxidative events and a tissue accumulation and/or release of GSSG in the coronary effluent is a sensitive and accurate index of oxidative stress (30).

Our data demonstrate that in the isolated and perfused hearts ischaemia shifts the redox state of the cell towards oxidation, tissue content of GSH being significantly reduced. Reperfusion after 30 min of ischaemia was associated with a recovery of contractile function concomitant with a complete restoration of tissue GSH/GSSG ratio. The transient release of GSH and GSSG from the heart probably represents a wash out of the tripeptide rather than a reperfusion-induced exacerbation of its release from the cells. Reperfusion after 60 and 90 min of ischaemia, on the other hand, does not re-establish normal function. Under these conditions there was a further decrease of GSH/GSSG ratio (Fig. 4) with a significant increase of tissue GSSG. This finding is of importance because during reperfusion there was also a marked and sustained release of GSH and GSSG into the extracellular space, suggesting that the cellular content of GSSG was increased at least four to five fold. These data indicate that in the isolated and perfused rabbit hearts readmission of oxygen with reperfusion might result in an oxidative damage, depending on the duration of the previous ischaemic period.

All these alterations are known to cause disfunction of membrane permeability and disturbances in calcium transport. Although it is difficult to establish the time course of events occurring during post-ischaemic reperfusion, it is quite possible that the burst of oxygen free radicals generated by reperfusion will damage the cell membrane, which, in turn, will become permeable to calcium. Calcium moves into the cell because of the concentration gradient. The mitochondria would then accumulate calcium in an attempt to buffer the large influx across the sarcolemma.

This would be favoured by the ischaemic-induced reduction of the protective mechanism against oxygen toxicity.

CONCLUSION

The pathophysiology of reperfusion injury is multifactorial, involving calcium overload, altered nucleotide metabolism and impaired cell volume regulation. We have developed a different approach in the understanding of this complex biological situation and it has been extensively discussed a possible role for oxygen free radicals in reperfusion damage. Application of the basic observation discussed in this article should ultimately involve a variety of cardiovascular disorders including acute myocardial infarction, unstable angina and reperfusion during cardiopulmonary by-pass.

ACKNOWLEDGEMENTS

This study was supported by a C.N.R. Grant n. 85.00809.56. We are very grateful for the assistance of Miss Ornella del Ciello in the typing of the manuscript.

REFERENCES

1. Coley, D., Reul, G., Wukasch. D. Am. J. Cardiol. 29:575-587, 1972.
2. Furberg, D. Am. J. Cardiol. 53:626-627, 1984.
3. Mathey, D.G., Kuck, K.H., Tilsner, V., Krebber, J.J., Bleifeld, W. Circulation 67: 489-497, 1981.
4. Downey, J., Chanber, D., Roy, R., McCord, J., Hearse, D.J., Yellon, D.M. J. Mol. Cell. Cardiol. 16: 36-40, 1984.
5. Romson, J.L., Hook, B.G., Kunkel, S.L., Abrams, G.D., Schork, M.A., Lucchesi, B.R. Circulation 67:1016-1023, 1983.
6. Mannig, A.S., Hearse, D.J. J. Mol. Cell. Cardiol. 16:497-518,1984.
7. Jolly, S.R., Kane, W.J., Bailie, M.B., Abrams, G.D., Lucchesi, B.R. Circ. Res. 54:277-285, 1984.
8. Braunwald, E., Klonel, R. J. Clin. Invest. 76: 1713-1719, 1985.
9. Cooley, D., Reul, G., Wukasch, D. Am. J. Cardiol. 29:575-587, 1972
10. Baroldi, G., Milam, J., Wukasch, D., Sandiford, F., Romagnoli, A., Cooley, D. J. Mol. Cell. Cardiol. 6:395-407, 1974.
11. Ganz, W., Buchbinder, N., Marcus, H., Mondkar, A., Maddahi, J., Charuzi,

Y., O'Connor, L., Shell, W., Fishbein, M.C., Kass, R., Miyamoto, A., Swan, H.J.C. Am. Heart J. 101:4-13, 1981.

12. Mathey, D.G., Kuck, K.H., Tilsner, U., Krebber, H.J., Bleifeld, W. Circulation 67:489-497, 1981.

13. Rentrop, K.P., Blamke, H., Karsch, K.R., Kaiser, H., Leitz, K. Circulation 63: 307-317, 1981.

14. Hearse, D.J. J. Mol. Cell. Cardiol. 9: 607-616, 1977.

15. Poole-Wilson, P.A. In: Control and Manipulation of the Calcium Moviment (Ed. J.R. Parrat), Raven Press, 1985.

16. Nayler, W.G. Am. J. Phatol. 102: 262-270, 1981.

17. Ferrari, R., Ceconi, C., Curello, S., Cargnoni, A., Agnoletti, G., Boffa, G.M., Visioli, O. Eur. Heart J. 7: 3-12, 1986.

18. Ferrari, R., Albertini, A., Curello, S., Ceconi, C., Di Lisa, F., Raddino, R., Visioli, O. J. Mol. Cell. Cardiol. 18:487-498, 1986.

19. Hearse, D.J. In: Calcium antagonists and cardiovascular disease (Ed. L.H. Opie), Raven Press, New York, 1984, pp. 129-145.

20. Jenning, R.B., Hawkins, H.K., Lowe, J.E., Hill, M.C., Klottman, S., Reimer, K.A. Am. J. Pathol. 92: 187-214, 1978.

21. Reimer, K.A., Hill, M.L., Jennings, R.B. J. Mol. Cell. Cardiol. 13:229-239, 1981.

22. Gaudel, Y., Karagueuzian, H.S., De Leiris J. J. Mol. Cell. Cardiol. 11: 717-731, 1979.

23. Shen, A.C., Jennings, R.B. Am. J. Pathol. 67: 441-452, 1972.

24. Chien, K.R., Buja, L.M., Parkey, R., Bonte, F., Willerson, J.T. Clin. Res. 28:469 (abstr), 1980.

25. Ogunrd, E.A., Ferguson, A.G., Lesch, M.A. Cardiovasc. Res. 14: 254-260, 1980.

26. Vander Vausse, G.J., Prinzen, F.W., Reneman, R.S. In: Myocardial ischaemia and lipid metabolism (Eds. R. Ferrari, A.M. Katz, A. Shug and O. Visioli) Plenum Press, New York, 1980, pp. 171-184.

27. Katz, A.M., Messineo, F.C. Circ. Res. 48: 1-20, 1983.

28. Ganote, C.E., Sims, M.A. J. Mol. Cell. Cardiol. 15: 421-429.

29. Meerson, F.Z., Kagan, V.E., Kozov, Yu.P., Belkina, L.M., Arkhinpenko, Yu. V. Basic Res. Cardiol. 77: 465-485, 1982.

30. Ferrari, R., Ceconi, C., Curello, S., Guarnieri, C., Caldarera, C.M., Albertini, A., Visioli, O. J. Mol. Cell. Cardiol. 17: 937-945, 1985.

31. Werns, S.W., Shea, M.J., Lucchesi, B.R. Circulation 74: 1-5, 1986.

32. Williams, A.J., Crie, J.S., Ferrari, R. In: Advances in studies on heart metabolism (Eds. C.M. caldarera and P. Harris), Clueb, Bologna, 1982, 173-183.

33. Bourdillon, P.D.V., Poole-Wilson, P.A. Circ. res. 50: 360-368, 1982.

34. Hess, M., Manson, N. J. Mol. Cell. Cardiol. 16: 969-985, 1984.

35. McCord, J. N. Engl. J. med. 312: 159-163, 1985.

36. Hearse, D.J., Humphrey, S.M., Bullock, G.R. J. Mol. Cell. Cardiol.

18: 641-668, 1978.

37. Rao, P.S., Cohen, M.V. Mueller, H.S. J. Mol. Cell. Cardiol. 15:712-716, 1983.
38. Gershmann, R. In: Oxygen and living processes: an interdisciplinary approach (Ed. D.L. Gilbert) Springer Verlag, New York, 1981, pp. 30-60.
39. Tappel, A.L. Fed. Proc. 32: 1870-1874, 1973.
40. Freeman, B.A., Crapo, M.D. Lab. Invest. 47:412-416, 1982.
41. Engler, R.L., Schimd-Schonbeing, G.W., Paveleg, R.S. Am. J. Pathol. 111: 98-106, 1983.

7

OXIDATION OF METHIONINE IN PROTEINS OF ISOLATED RAT HEART MYOCYTES AND
TISSUE SLICES BY NEUTROPHIL-GENERATED OXYGEN FREE RADICALS

H. FLISS and G. DOCHERTY

Department of Physiology, Faculty of Health Sciences, University of
Ottawa, 451 Smyth Road, Ottawa, Ontario K1H 8M5.

INTRODUCTION

It is now well established that reperfusion of ischemic heart
tissues initiates the production of oxygen free radicals which
exacerbate the damage to the myocardium (1-3). While it is clear that a
large portion of the oxygen free radicals is formed in damaged tissue by
endogenous reactions such as the metabolism of xanthine and arachidonic
acid (4,5), it now appears likely that a major source of these free
radicals are the neutrophils which migrate into the damaged tissues
during the inflammatory response (6-8). At the site of damage, these
neutrophils can become activated and can secrete a variety of oxidants
such as superoxide anion, hydrogen peroxide, and hypochlorous acid (9).

Hypochlorous acid is one of the most highly reactive of the
neutrophil-generated oxidants (10). The production of this compound is
catalyzed by myeloperoxidase, an enzyme found in the primary granules of
neutrophils (11). Although hypochlorous acid can react with a variety
of compounds, it has a high specificity for the amino acid methionine
(12,13). Since methionine residues play a critical role in a variety of
proteins and peptides (14,15), it is possible that a significant portion
of the oxidation-related damage observed in reperfused heart is caused
by the hypochlorous acid-mediated oxidation of methionine residues in
cellular proteins. These studies were therefore undertaken with the
objectives of establishing whether methionine residues in heart proteins
are susceptible to neutrophil-mediated oxidation, and whether this
oxidation is attributable mainly to hypochlorous acid. The data
presented below suggest that the answers to both of these questions are
in the affirmative.

MATERIALS & METHODS

Methionine Determination.

An assay based on the highly specific reaction of cyanogen bromide with methionine was utilized to determine the content of oxidized methionine (methionine sulfoxide) in tissues (16). A requirement of the assay is that proteins be labelled with [^{35}S]methionine. This assay is based on the fact that cyanogen bromide reacts with methionine, but not methionine sulfoxide, to produce volatile methyl thiocyanate (17). Consequently, treatment of [^{35}S]methionine-labelled proteins with cyanogen bromide volatilizes the label from methionine residues, leaving a residue of label which corresponds directly to the initial concentration of oxidized methionine. Prior to the assay, all tissues were treated for 10 min with hot 10% trichloroacetic acid (TCA) containing 100 mM unlabelled L-methionine. The precipitated protein was washed twice with cold 10% TCA and was treated with cyanogen bromide (final concentration 6.5 mg/mL) in 70% formic acid for 1 hr at 60°C.

Myocyte Preparation.

Calcium-tolerant myocytes were isolated from rat hearts by established collagenase digestion procedures (18,19). Hearts from 300-400 g anaesthetized (80 mg sodium pentobarbital/kg body weight) male Sprague-Dawley rats were perfused for 15 min at 37°C with oxygenated MEM medium (Joklik) containing taurine (60 mM), creatine (20 mM), and HEPES (5 mM) at pH 7.3. Collagenase (Cooper Biomedical, Type CLS I) was added to a final concentration of 75 units/mL and perfusion was continued with recirculation for 35-40 min. The ventricles were cut from the softened heart, were transferred to fresh oxygenated perfusion medium containing collagenase, were minced, and were then shaken vigorously for 10 min at 37°C. The minced tissue was repeatedly drawn up into a plastic pipette to disperse the cells, and was then filtered through two layers of cheesecloth into a plastic tube. The cells were collected, and were suspended in oxygenated perfusion buffer containing 1.5% bovine serum albumin. Calcium tolerance was induced gradually by the addition, with shaking, of $CaCl_2$ in 200 µM increments at 5 min interval (viability > 85%). All buffers and media were oxygenated by bubbling with 95% O_2, 5% CO_2 gas. Cells (3.0 x 10^6) were incubated with L-[^{35}S]methionine (15 µCi) in 1 mL of Joklik medium for 2 hrs, and were washed with medium prior to exposure to oxidants.

Preparation of Heart Slices.

Hearts were removed from 300-400 g anaesthetized male
Sprague-Dawley rats and were chilled rapidly to 4°C in Krebs-Ringer
buffer (KRB). Tissue slices averaging 0.5 mm in thickness were cut from
the hearts on a Stadie-Riggs tissue slicer at 4°C (20), and were
transferred immediately to KRB at 4°C. The slices were labelled with
$[^{35}S]$methionine (15 μCi/slice) in KRB for 2 hrs at 37°C under a 95% O_2,
5% CO_2 atmosphere, and were washed twice with KRB prior to exposure to
oxidants.

Isolation of Human Neutrophils.

Heparinized (10 units/ml) venous blood was obtained from healthy
donors. Neutrophils (PMN) were isolated by centrifugation through
discontinuous gradients of Ficoll and sodium diatrizoate (21).
Contaminating erythrocytes were removed by a hypotonic wash. Cell
purity and viability were greater than 95%.

Isolation of Rat Peritoneal Neutrophils.

Rat peritoneal neutrophils were isolated according to previously
published procedures (22,23). Sprague-Dawley male 200-400 g rats were
injected intraperitoneally with 35 mL of physiological saline containing
2.0% glycogen. After 18 hrs the animals were sacrificed, the peritoneal
cavity was lavaged with 30 mL of Hank's balanced salt solution
containing heparin (5 units/mL), and the exudate was passed through
cheesecloth to remove large debris particles. The cells were pelleted
at 150 x g for 10 min, the pellet was suspended in 4 mL of Hank's, and 2
mL of suspension were layered over 3 mL of 6% Ficoll-10% sodium
diatrizoate in each of two centrifuge tubes. The cells were centrifuged
at 400 x g for 45 min at room temperature, and the pellets were
collected and subjected to a hypotonic wash to remove contaminating
erythrocytes. Cell purity and viability were greater than 95%.

Oxidants and Anti-Oxidants.

Isolated cardiac myocytes (3.0 x 10^6 in Joklik medium) and slices
(one slice per dish, in KRB), were exposed for 1 hr at 37°C to either
chemical or PMN-generated oxidants in 2.5 cm culture dishes in a total
volume of one mL. The PMN (5 x 10^6) were allowed to settle onto the
myocytes for 30 min prior to the addition of phorbol myristate acetate
(PMA, Consolidated Midland, final concentration 100 ng/mL). The
concentration of the chemical oxidants utilized, hypochlorous acid

(HClO) and hydrogen peroxide (H_2O_2), was determined spectrophotometrically at 290 nm and 230 nm respectively (24). The HClO was purchased as a commercial preparation of NaOCl (Sigma, 4-6%) and was diluted in phosphate-buffered saline (PBS), pH 7.3, prior to use. The quenching effects of anti-oxidants were established with 1 mM of dithiothreitol (DTT), glutathione (GSH), or L-methionine (MET).

Statistical Analysis.

An unpaired, one-tailed Student t-test was used. The data are presented as the mean ± SEM. Numbers in parentheses represent the number of trials.

RESULTS

The proteins in both the tissue slices and isolated myocytes contained basal levels of oxidized methionine (approximately 11% and 9%, respectively) prior to exposure to external oxidants. The possibility that this may be an artifact of the cyanogen bromide reaction cannot be ruled out at the present time. However, it is more likely that this background level of oxidized methionine, which had been observed elsewhere with other forms of methionine analysis (25-27), is caused by the continuous production of oxidants during normal cellular metabolic processes (28).

Treatment of the tissue slices and myocytes with HClO (250 μM) resulted in a dramatic increase in the concentration of oxidized methionine. The increase in the level of oxidized methionine was greater in the tissue slices (Fig. 1) than in the myocytes (Fig. 2). Preliminary data indicate that the oxidation of methionine in both slices and myocytes increases linearly with increasing HClO concentration (data not shown). The thiol reagents DTT and glutathione provided excellent protection against HClO oxidation of both slices and myocytes. Free methionine was also found to afford very good protection against hypochlorous acid (Fig. 1). The methionine residues in both the tissue slices and myocytes were considerably less sensitive to oxidation by hydrogen peroxide. Thus, while the tissue slices were approximately 10 times less sensitive to H_2O_2 than to HClO, the methionine residues in myocytes appeared to be totally impervious to 20 mM H_2O_2 (Figs. 1 and 2).

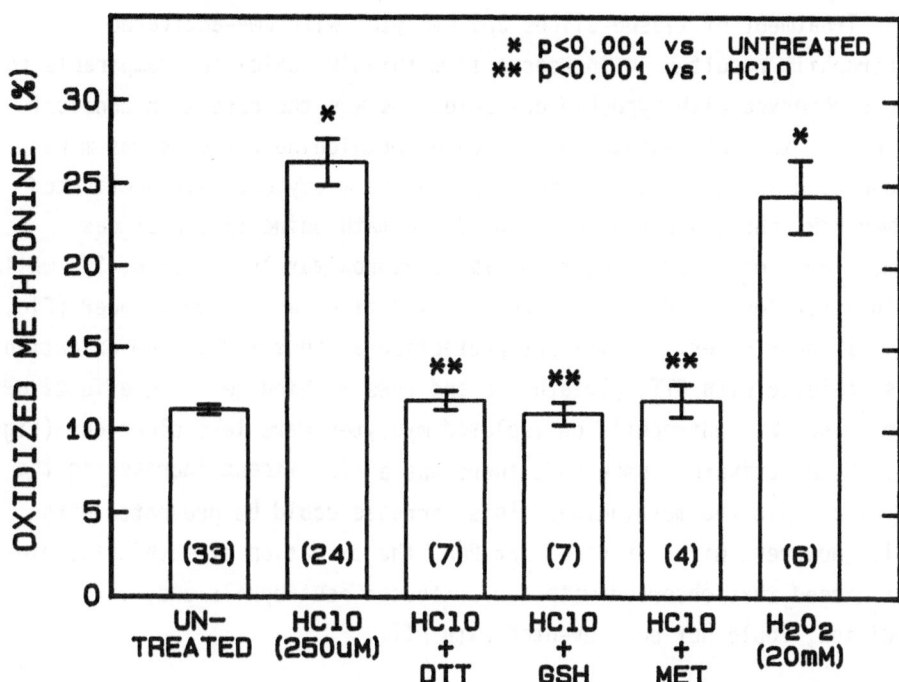

Figure 1. Chemical oxidation of slices.

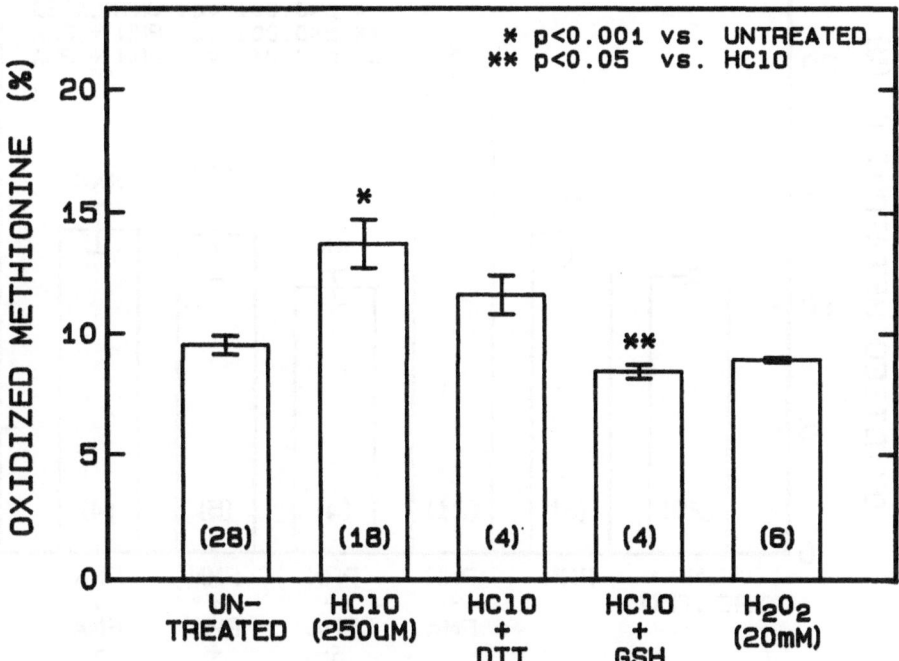

Figure 2. Chemical oxidation of myocytes.

Treatment of tissue slices and myocytes with PMA-activated neutrophils resulted in increases in methionine oxidation comparable to those observed with hypochlorous acid. As was the case with chemical oxidants, the PMN-mediated oxidation of methionine residues was more pronounced in the tissue slices than in the myocytes. With activated human PMN, the concentration of oxidized methionine in the slices almost doubled, increasing from 11% to approximately 19% (Fig. 3), while with activated rat PMN the extent of oxidation was somewhat lower (Fig. 4). In both cases, significant protection against methionine oxidation was achieved with DTT, glutathione and free methionine. The effects of human and rat neutrophils on isolated myocytes were less clear cut (Fig. 5). With activated human PMN, there was a significant increase in the level of oxidized methionine. This increase could be prevented with DTT. However, with activated rat PMN, the oxidation of methionine did not exceed that observed with non-activated neutrophils and, in addition, could not be prevented with DTT.

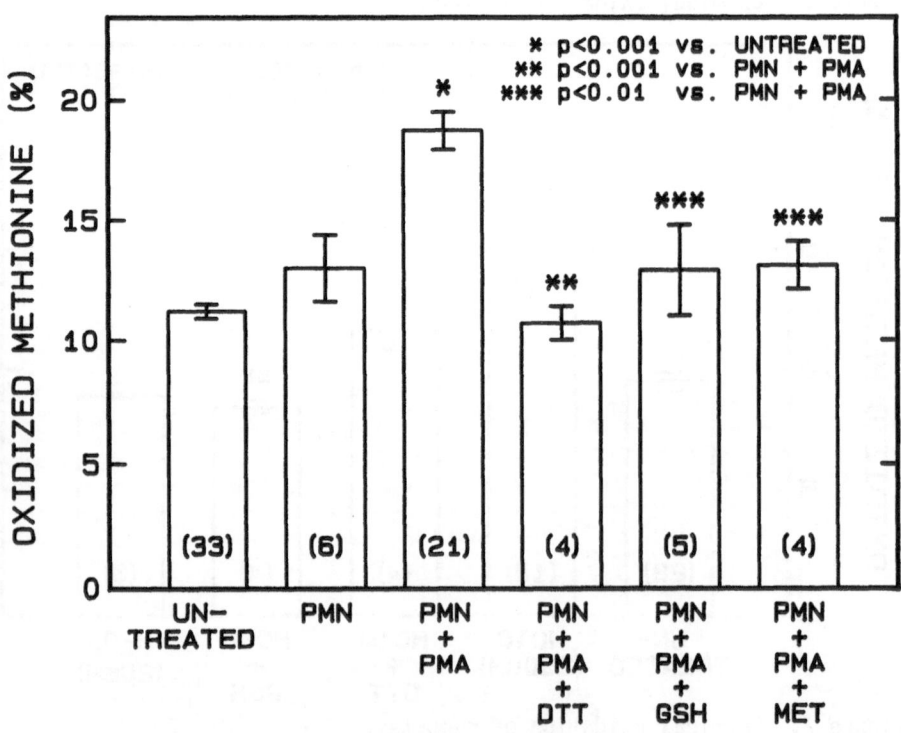

Figure 3. Oxidation of heart slices by human neutrophils.

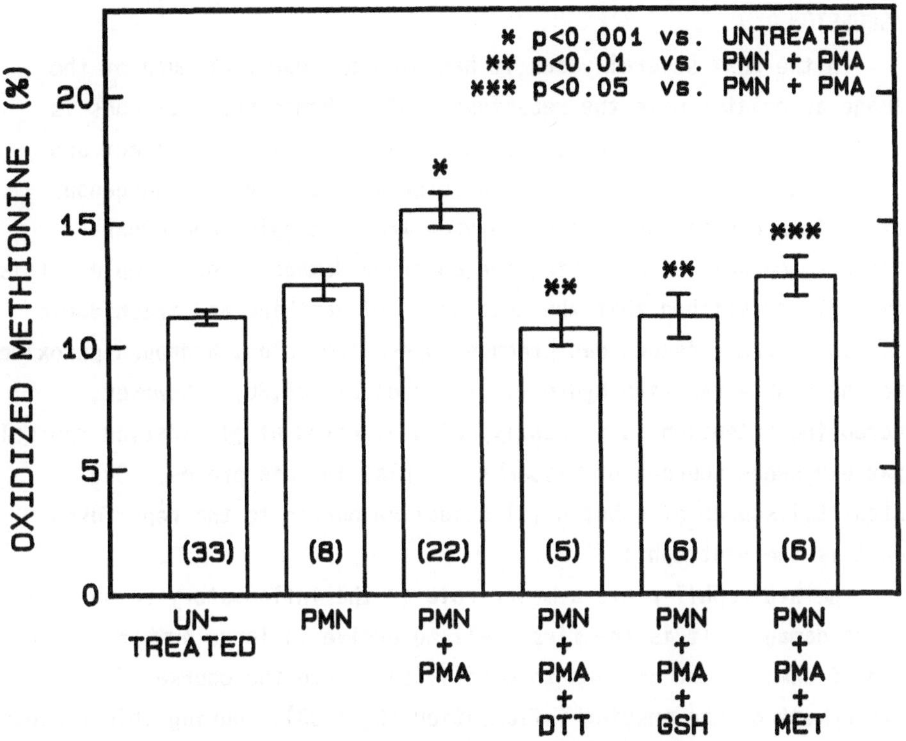

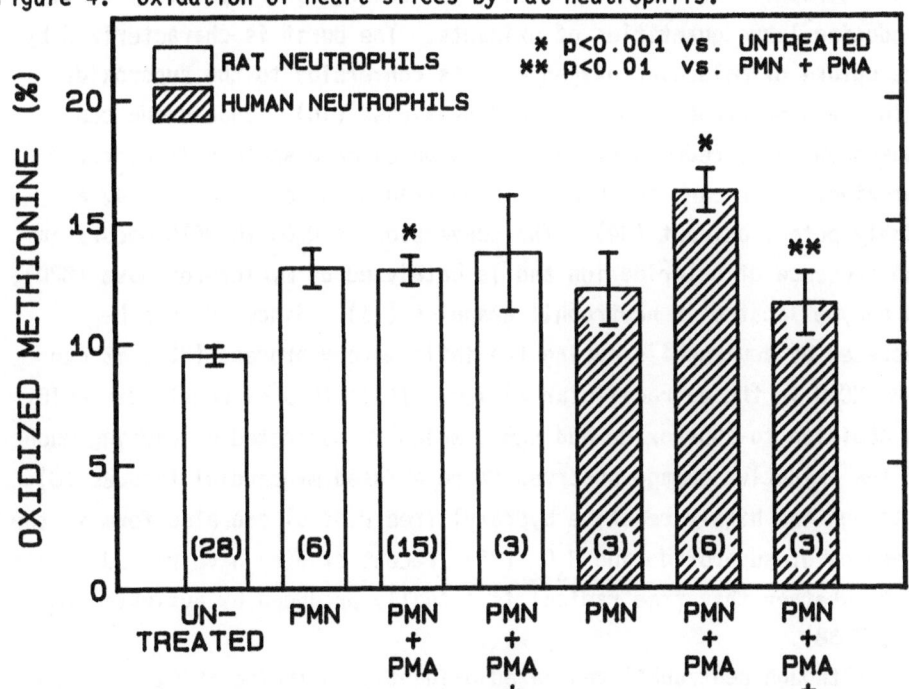

Figure 4. Oxidation of heart slices by rat neutrophils.

Figure 5. Oxidation of myocytes by human and rat neutrophils.

DISCUSSION

In the past several years it has become clear that much of the damage associated with the reperfusion of ischemic heart tissues is caused by the formation of oxidants (1-3). A variety of direct and indirect experimental approaches have shown that several endogenous metabolic processes can produce oxygen free radicals, and other oxidants, capable of effecting the observed damage. For example, it is now well established that the metabolism of xanthine and arachidonic acid in injured tissues can produce superoxide anion, hydrogen peroxide, and the highly reactive hydroxyl free radical (29,30). However, increasing attention is presently being directed at elucidating the role that exogenous sources of oxidants may play in this process. One potentital source of substantial oxidative burden to the reperfused heart is the neutrophil.

The neutrophil plays a major role in the inflammatory response to tissue damage. It is the first cell to arrive in large numbers at the site of damage, and appears to greatly influence the course of development of the ensuing inflammation (6,31-33). During this process, the neutrophil can become activated and undergo a "respiratory burst", producing large quantities of oxidants. The burst is characterized by the uptake of molecular oxygen and its conversion to the superoxide anion by a membrane-associated NADPH-oxidase (10). Superoxide can subsequently be reduced by cellular superoxide dismutase to hydrogen peroxide, which can, in turn, be converted to hypochlorous acid, a highly potent oxidant (34). The conversion of H_2O_2 to HClO occurs in the presence of chloride ion and is catalyzed by myeloperoxidase (MPO), an enzyme located in neutrophil granules (11). Since MPO can be secreted by neutrophils during the inflammatory process (35), it can form HClO in the extracellular milieu. It is this extracellular HClO, in addition to superoxide and H_2O_2, which is suspected of causing much of the oxidative damage observed in reperfused myocardial tissues (8). Although the highly reactive hydroxyl free radical can also form in the presence of superoxide and H_2O_2 (36), recent studies have raised doubts as to whether this free radical is actually produced by activated PMN (10,37,38).

Although neutrophil-generated oxidants, including HClO, have long been known to be major contributors to oxidant damage in the lungs

(39,40), they have only recently been suspected of involvement in myocardial injury (7). Recent studies indicate that the migration of neutrophils to the injured myocardium is observable in ischemic tissues prior to initiation of reperfusion (41). However, the rate of PMN influx accelerates dramatically after blood flow is re-established to the affected tissues (42). The fact that these invading neutrophils can contribute significantly to reperfusion injury in myocardium was established by indirect means. Several studies have shown that, in animals which have been rendered neutropenic by chemical or immunological means, there was a dramatic decline in the extent of observed oxidative injury (41,43).

The mechanisms of action of the PMN-secreted oxidants is not fully understood. However, it seems likely that they could cause severe damage by reacting with critical cellular components of the myocardium such as lipids and proteins. While there is strong evidence to suggest that the lipid component of cellular membranes can be oxidized (44), virtually nothing is known of the effects of these oxidants on heart proteins. The main reason for the paucity of protein- related studies was the absence, until recently, of a rapid and reliable assay for protein oxidation. Such an assay was developed recently (16). The assay facilitates the estimation of protein modification by quantitating the oxidation of methionine. Since methionine is highly susceptible to oxidants (14,15), its modification in proteins can serve as a sensitive gauge of the oxidative stress to tissues. The methionine assay was therefore used in these studies to establish the effects of chemical and PMN-derived oxidants on heart proteins.

The effects of chemical oxidation was examined with both isolated cardiac myocytes and heart tissue slices. Isolated myocytes have been shown elsewhere to react in an anomalous fashion in response to ischemic conditions. For example, unlike intact hearts, isolated myocytes do not undergo a calcium paradox or oxygen paradox during reperfusion (45). One of the objectives of these studies was, therefore, to establish whether myocyte proteins have an unusual resistance to oxidants. The data indicate that this is not the case. The proteins in both the myocytes and slices proved to be susceptible to hypochlorous acid. The concentration of HClO was chosen so as to approximate the concentration expected in the neutrophil suspensions used in these studies (46).

There appeared to be more oxidation of methionine in the slices than in the myocytes. However, a true comparison is not possible in view of the significant differences between the two model systems. The fact that the myocyte proteins were oxidized minimizes the possibility that the oxidation of methionine in the tissue slices may have occurred only in non-muscle tissue.

No attempt was made to determine the intracellular location of the oxidized proteins. Although it is possible that most of the oxidation occurred within membrane proteins, it is likely that cytoplasmic proteins were also affected. At physiological pH, hypochlorous acid consists of the non-ionized HClO and ionized hypochlorite (OCl^-) in roughly equal proportions (46,47). The non-ionized HClO can be expected to have excellent membrane penetrating properties, and should therefore be able to reach the cytoplasm.

The hypochlorous acid-induced oxidation of methionine was quenched in both myocytes and tissue slices by DTT and glutathione. The ability of thiol reagents to quench hypochlorous acid had been observed previously (12,48). Significantly, free methionine was also capable of quenching the HClO-induced oxidation of methionine in proteins. This high reactivity of methionine with HClO, which has also been observed elsewhere (12,49,50), increases the likelihood that heart proteins would be highly susceptible to oxidation by PMN-generated HClO. In contrast to the high reactivity with HClO, methionine residues in myocytes and slices were relatively non-reactive with H_2O_2. This suggests that H_2O_2, by itself, is less likely to effect significant oxidation of proteins in heart tissue than is HClO.

The fact that commercially available HClO is comparable in its action to the HClO generated by neutrophil myeloperoxidase has been established elsewhere (51). In the present studies, a similar parity in action was suggested by the fact that myocardial proteins were oxidized to a similar extent by both commercial HClO and activated PMN producing comparable amounts of HClO. The susceptibility of heart proteins to PMN-derived oxidants was investigated with both rat and human neutrophils. Studies done elsewhere have shown that rat peritoneal PMN, which migrate to the peritoneum in response to an injected irritant such as glycogen or casein, undergo a diminished respiratory burst when compared to peripheral blood PMN (52). The present investigations confirm the lowered oxidative potential of the peritoneal PMN. Both myocyte and slice proteins showed higher oxidation of methionine residues with activated human peripheral blood PMN than with peritoneal PMN. The small amount of methionine oxidation observed in both myocytes and slices with non-activated PMN is probably attributable to the low levels of activation usually observed in isolated PMN.

The PMN-induced oxidation of methionine in slices was quenched by thiol reagents and free methionine, suggesting a HClO-mediated mechanism of oxidation. In myocytes, DTT also inhibited oxidation by activated human PMN. However, the effect of rat peripheral PMN was not as clear cut in these cells since significant oxidation of methionine was found after incubation with non-activated PMN. Activation of the rat PMN with PMA did not increase the extent of oxidation. Moreover, DTT did not protect in this system. The reasons for these anomalies are not clear at the present time.

In conclusion, these data show for the first time that activated PMN can effect significant oxidation of protein in myocardial tissues. Protein modification may therefore contribute significantly to ischemia-, and reperfusion-associated damage. The reactivity of heart proteins with HClO, and their relative resistance to H_2O_2, suggests that PMN-induced oxidation of proteins is most likely attributable to the production of HClO by neutrophil myeloperoxidase at sites of myocardial injury. The high susceptibility of methionine residues to HClO suggests that oxidation of this amino acid in myocardial proteins may be of particular importance in the etiology of reperfusion injury. Methionine residues are known to play a critical role in a variety of cellular proteins (14,15). It is intriguing, for example, that a number of polypeptides involved in calcium regulation contain critical methionine residues (e.g. calmodulin (53-55), calcitonin (56), and parathyroid hormone (57)). Since a prominent component of reperfusion-associated pathology is the loss, by the myocardium, of the ability to maintain calcium homeostasis, it is possible that oxidation of methionine residues in these polypeptides by PMN-secreted HClO lies at the basis of this phenomenon.

SUMMARY

These studies investigated the effects of neutrophil-generated oxygen free radicals on myocardial proteins. Since neutrophil oxidants are suspected of playing a major role in reperfusion-associated damage in the heart, it was of interest to examine the possibility that this damage may involve protein oxidation. Utilizing a newly developed assay for methionine oxidation, these studies were able to demonstrate, for the first time, that neutrophils can cause oxidative damage in myocardial proteins. Using human or rat neutrophils which had been activated with phorbol myristate acetate, it was found that the amount of oxidized methionine in both tissue slices and isolated myocytes increased to about 20% from a basal level of approximately 10%. The oxidation of methionine could be inhibited by free methionine or thiol reagents such as dithiothreitol and glutathione. The possibility that the observed oxidation of methionine could be caused by hypochlorous acid, a highly toxic neutrophil oxidant, was tested by treating tissue slices and myocytes with hypochlorous acid at concentrations approximating those expected in the neutrophil studies. It was observed that the extent of methionine oxidation with hypochlorous acid was similar to that observed with the neutrophils. This finding, in addition to the fact that the hypochlorous acid-induced oxidation of methionine was quenched by dithiothreitol, glutathione and free methionine, suggests that the neutrophil-induced oxidation of cardiac proteins may be caused by hypochlorous acid. These findings raise the intriguing possibility that oxidation of myocardial proteins containing essential methionine residues may cause some of the reperfusion-associated damage in heart.

ACKNOWLEDGMENTS

This work was supported by a grant from the Heart and Stroke Foundation of Ontario.

REFERENCES

1. Hess, M.L. and Manson, N.H. J. Mol. Cell. Cardiol. 16: 969-985, 1984.
2. Thompson, J.A. and Hess, M.L. Prog. Cardiovascular Dis. 28: 449-462, 1986.

3. McCord, J.M., Roy, R.S. and Schaffer, S.W. Adv. Myocardiology 5: 183-189, 1985.
4. Chambers, D.E., Parks, D.A., Patterson, G., Roy, R., McCord, J.M., Yoshida, S., Parmley, L.F. and Downey, J.M. J. Mol. Cell. Cardiol. 17: 145-152, 1985.
5. Nastainczyk, W., Ullrich, V., Cadenas, E. and Sies, H. In: Oxygen Radicals in Chemistry and Biology, Walter de Gruyter & Co., Berlin, 1984, pp. 441-445.
6. Lucchesi, B.R., Romson, J.L. and Jolly, S.R. In: Therapeutic Approaches to Myocardial Infarct Size Limitation (Eds. D.J. Hearse and D.M. Yellon) Raven Press, New York, 1984, pp. 219-248.
7. Lucchesi, B.R. In: Prostaglandins and Other Eicosanoids in the Cardiovascular System (Ed. Schrör), Karger, Basel, 1985, pp. 160-171.
8. Lucchesi, B.R. and Mullane, K.M. Am. rev. Pharmacol. Toxicol. 26: 201-224, 1986.
9. Weiss, S.J. and LoBuglio, A.F. Lab. Invest. 47: 5-18, 1982.
10. Tauber, A.I. and Babior, B.M. Adv. Free Radical Biology & Medicine 1: 265-307, 1985.
11. Pember, S.O., Shapira, R. and Kinkade, J.M. Jr. Arch. Biochem. Biophys. 221: 391-403, 1983.
12. Winterbourn, C.C. Biochim. Biophys. Acta. 840: 204-210, 1985.
13. Ossanna, P.J., Test, S.T., Matheson, N.R., Regiani, S. and Weiss, S.J. J. Clin. Invest. 77: 1939-1951, 1986.
14. Brot, N. and Weissbach, H. Trend. Biochem. Sci. 7: 137-139, 1982.
15. Brot, N. and Weissbach, H. Arch. Biochem. Biophys. 223: 271-281, 1983.
16. Fliss, H., Weissbach, H. and Brot, N. Proc. Natl. Acad. Sci. USA 80: 7160-7164, 1983.
17. Gross, E. Methods Enzymol. 11: 238-255, 1967.
18. Hohl, C.M., Altschuld, R.A. and Brierley, G.P. Arch. Biochem. Biophys. 221: 197-205, 1983.
19. Farmer, B.B., Mancina, M., Williams, E.S. and Watanabe, A.M. Life Sci. 33: 1-18, 1983.
20. Grochowski, E.C., Ganote, C.E., Hill, M.L. and Jennings, R.B. J. Mol. Cell. Cardiol. 8: 173-187, 1976.
21. Boyum, A. Scand. J. Clin. Lab. Invest. 21(Suppl. 97): 77-89, 1968.
22. Calamai, E.G. and Spitznagel, J.K. Lab. Invest. 46: 597-604, 1982.
23. Hodinka, R.L. and Modrzakowski, M.C. Infect. Immunity 40: 139-146, 1983.
24. Brestel, E.P. Biochem. Biophys. Res. Commun. 126: 482-488, 1985.
25. Parish, C.R. and Stanley, P. Immunochemistry 9: 853-872, 1972.
26. Kikuchi, Y., Yamiya, N., Nozawa, T. and Hatano, M. Eur. J. Biochem. 125: 575-577, 1982.
27. Sanchez, J., Nikolan, B.J. and Stumpf, P.K. Plant Physiol. 73: 619-623, 1983.
28. Halliwell, B. and Gutteridge, J.M.C. Free radicals in biology and medicine. Clarendon Press, Oxford, 1985.
29. Jones, D.P. In: Oxidative Stress (Ed. H. Sies) Academic Press, New York, 1985, pp. 151-195.
30. Flohé, L., Beckmann, R., Giertz, H. and Loschen, G. In: Oxidative Stress (Ed. H. Sies) Academic Press, New York, 1985, pp. 403-435.

31. Weiss, S.J., Lampert, M.B. and Test, S.T. Science 222: 625-628, 1983.
32. El-Hag, A., Lipsky, P.E., Bennett, M. and Clark, R.A. J. Immunol. 136: 3420-3426, 1986.
33. Mullane, K.M., Kraemer, R. and Smith, B. J. Pharmacol. Methods 14: 157-167, 1985.
34. Clark, R.A. In: Adv. Inflammation Res., Vol 5, (Ed. G. Weissmann) Raven Press, New York, 1983, pp. 107-146.
35. Klebanoff, S.J. and Clark, R.A. The neutrophil:function and clinical disorders, Elsevier-North Holland, Amsterdam, 1978.
36. Hess, M.L., Rowe, G.T., Caplan, M., Romson, J.L. and Lucchesi, B. In: Adv. myocardiology, vol 5 (Eds. P. Harris and P.A. Poole-Wilson) Plenum, New York, 1985, pp. 159-175.
37. Green, T.R., Fellman, J.H. and Eicher, A.L. FEBS Lett. 192: 33-36, 1985.
38. Britigan, B.E., Rosen, G.M., Chai, Y. and Cohen, M.S. J. Biol. Chem. 261: 4426-4431, 1986.
39. Hammond, B., Kontos, H.A. and Hess, M.L. Can. J. Physiol. Pharmacol. 63: 173-187, 1985.
40. Johnson, K.J., Fantone, J.C. III, Kaplan, J. and Ward, P.A. J. Clin. Invest. 67: 983-993, 1981.
41. Mullane, K.M., Read, N., Salmon, J.A. and Moncada, S. J. Pharmacol. Exp. Ther. 228: 510-522, 1984.
42. Engler, R.L., Dahlgren, M.D., Peterson, M.A., Dobbs, A. and Schmid-Schönbein, G.W. Am. J. Physiol. 251: H93-H100, 1986.
43. Romson, J.L., Hook, B.G., Kunkel, S.L., Abrams, G.D., Schork, M.A. and Lucchesi, B.R. Circulation 67: 1016-1023, 1983.
44. Sepe, S.M. and Clark, R.A. J. Immunol. 134: 1888-1895, 1985.
45. Piper, H.M., Spahr, R., Hutter, J.F. and Spieckermann, P.G. Basic Res. Cardiol. 80(Suppl. 2): 159-163, 1985.
46. Severns, C., Collins-Lech, C. and Sohnle, P.G. J. Lab. Clin. Med. 107: 29-35, 1986.
47. Ushijima, Y. and Nakano, M. Biochem. Biophys. Res. Commun. 93: 1232-1237, 1980.
48. Cuperns, R.A., Muijsers, A.O. and Wever, R. Arthritis Rheumatism 28: 1228-1233, 1985.
49. Matheson, N.R. and Travis, J. Biochemistry 24: 1941-1945, 1985.
50. Tsan, M.-F. and Chen, J.W. J. Clin. Invest. 65: 1041-1050, 1980.
51. Clark, R.A. J. Immunol. 136: 4617-4622, 1986.
52. Zimmerli, W., Lew, P.D., Cohen, H.J. and Waldvogel, F.A. Infect. Immunity 46: 625-630, 1984.
53. Walsh, M. and Stevens, T.C. Biochemistry 16: 2742-2749, 1977.
54. Walsh, M. and Stevens, T.C. Biochemistry 16: 3924-3930, 1977.
55. Babu, Y.S., Sack, J.S., Greenhough, T.J., Bugg, C.E., Means, A.R. and Cook, W.J. Nature 315: 37-40, 1985.
56. Tobler, P.H., Tschopp, F.A., Dambacher, M.A., Born, W. and Fischer, J.A. J. Clin. Endocrinol. Metab. 57: 749-754, 1983.
57. Frelinger, A.L. and Zull, J.E. J. Biol. Chem. 259: 5507-5513, 1984.

8

PHOSPHOLIPID METABOLISM IN HEART MEMBRANES

K.J.KAKO AND M.KATO
Department of Physiology, University of Ottawa, Ottawa, Ontario, K1H 8M5.

INTRODUCTION

Tremendous advances have been made over the past decade in our understanding of the structure and function of cell membrane systems. The membrane systems of the heart muscle, such as sarcolemma, sarcoplasmic reticulum and mitochondria, regulate contractile function as well as heart metabolism. Dhalla, Ziegelhoffer and Harrow published a review in 1977 (1), wherein they stated that "the exact mechanisms of changes in Ca^{2+} movements between various membrane systems and myofilaments seem to reside in the orientation of different phospholipid and protein molecules within a given membrane system. Further studies on the basic architecture of membrane systems under different experimental conditions is thus considered to be valuable in understanding the exact participation of sarcolemmal, sarcotubular system and mitochondria in regulating myocardial function."

In this review, results of recent research dealing with relationships between membrane lipids and membrane functions will be discussed. It should be pointed out here that lucid theoretical analyses of the role played by lipids and their metabolites in ischemic membranes were presented by Katz and Messineo in 1981 (2) and by Corr, Gross and Sobel in 1984 (3).

MEMBRANE STRUCTURE

Among various proposals, the most well accepted structure of the membrane is Singer and Nicholson's fluid mosaic model. In this model, a bilayer of lipids is aligned so as to contain their hydrophobic tails in the middle of the bilayer, while their hydrophilic heads face the two surfaces of a membrane. Membrane proteins are embedded in the bilayer lipids, their hydrophobic part positioned at the hydrophobic mid-section of the membrane (4,5). For example, the alpha subunit of (Na^+K^+)ATPase, Ca^{2+} activated ATPase and erythrocyte glycoprotein all show a conformation, in which a long polypeptide chain of the molecule traverses back and forth through the membrane bilayer (4,6,7). The most precisely known structure is the bacteriorhodopsin molecule with 7 rod structures traversing the membrane, proposed by Henderson and others (8). The proximity and hence close contacts of the protein with surrounding lipids are important factors in their interaction. Certain amounts of surrounding lipids may form a special microenvironment for a membrane protein (lipid domaine).

When membrane bilayer is sliced horizontally through the hydrophobic midlayer by the freeze fracture technique, a large number of intramembranous particles become visible. Deguchi, Jorgensen and Maunsbach carried out an electron microscopic examination of (Na^+K^+)ATPase purified from the kidney medulla (9). They calculated the number and area of the ATPase molecules, which corresponded reasonably well with the number and area of intramembranous particles observed by electron microscopy. However, a greater number of intramembranous particles is found in the natural membrane, and thus, it does not appear to be entirely accounted for by the postulated quantity of protein molecules.

Attempts to correlate membrane functions with the detailed compositions of membrane lipids have been hampered by the complexity of molecular structures of phospholipid. Cardiac sarcolemma is composed of many different phospholipids; 75 % of the total phospholipids were composed of choline and ethanolamine phospholipids, nearly 50 % of which consist of vinyl ether lipids (10). Phosphatidylinositol, which comprises only 6 % of the total, plays a crucial function as a signal transducer. Other minor components, lyso phospholipids, may be causally related to the dysrhythmia that is associated with myocardial infarction (3).

Moreover, widely different fatty acid and positional distributions in individual phospholipids have been disclosed. For example, the stereospecific fatty acid distribution found in the phosphatidylcholine molecule is quite different from that found in the phosphatidylethanolamine molecule, and different fatty acid tails exhibit different stereo-chemical configurations (5,10). Choline plasmalogens contain predominantly the vinyl ether of palmitic aldehyde, while ethanolamine plasmalogens are composed predominantly of the vinyl ethers

of stearic and oleic aldehydes, as well as of arachidonic acid at the
sn-2 position. However, the precise functional significance of the large
number of phospholipids differing in their molecular structures is not
known. In addition to the complexity of phospholipid molecular structure,
the distribution of phospholipid in the membrane is topologically
non-homogeneous, adding further difficulties in examining the correlation
between membrane function and lipid composition (11,12). Finally, the
membrane lipids are in a dynamic equilibrium, i.e., their composition
continuously changes with respect to space and time. The movement of
lipids within the membrane is particularly accelerated by interventions
which induce alterations in the membrane lipid composition (11,12).

Interactions between membrane lipids and membrane enzymes have
been investigated, among others, by van Deenen's laboratory in the 1970s
(12). The principal approaches taken were i) to modify the lipid
composition by various phospholipases or phospholipid exchange proteins,
and ii) to supplement delipidated membrane enzymes with various purified
lipids. These approaches have been adopted recently in investigations of
cardiac sarcolemmal membranes.

We will focus our attention on the effect of lipid changes on the
functions of (Na^+K^+)ATPase, $(Ca^{2+}Mg^{2+})$ATPase, Ca^{2+}
transport and Na^+/Ca^{2+} antiporter.

EFFECTS OF CARNITINE & COA ESTERS

Neely and his associates found that the levels of carnitine and
CoA esters of fatty acids were increased in ischemic perfused rat heart
(3). Therefore, effects of these intermediates on the membrane enzymes
were investigated by several laboratories.

Pitts and Okhuysen's results indicated linear inhibition of
(Na^+K^+)ATPase of the purified bovine heart membrane by increasing
concentrations of palmitylcarnitine (13). The results were obtained by
using a partially purified enzyme preparation. By contrast, a study using
vesicular sarcolemmal preparations revealed that palmitylcarnitine,
acting as a surface-active agent, unmasked the latent
(Na^+K^+)ATPase activity, and hence the potentiation of activities
were observed when its concentration was low, and when the membrane
preparation was tightly sealed. Higher concentrations of

palmitylcarnitine were inhibitory (14). Ouabain binding as well as adenylate cyclase activities were inhibited likewise by increasing concentrations of palmitylcarnitine (14,15).

An unmasking effect was evident in the experiment, in which the action of arachidonyl–CoA, not a carnitine ester, was examined by Owens, Kennett and Weglicki (16). Thus, low concentrations of arachidonyl–CoA stimulated and its high concentrations inhibited the activity of the sarcolemmal fraction prepared from the canine myocytes.

The effect of carnitine and CoA esters may not be specific to one enzyme, because their action was found to be similar when other membrane functions were tested. Thus, when Ca^{2+} stimulated ATPase, Ca^{2+} binding and Ca^{2+} uptake of cardiac sarcoplasmic reticulum were assayed in the presence of increasing concentrations of palmitylcarnitine, these activities were proportionally inhibited (16,17).

From the available evidence, therefore, it is safe to conclude that carnitine and CoA esters of fatty acids impair various functions of the membrane. However, the question of whether or not the concentration of palmitylcarnitine, particularly its local concentration adjacent to the membrane, is raised in ischemic cells to a level that is inhibitory to the enzyme activity, has not been completely resolved (13,22).

EFFECTS OF ACIDIC LIPIDS

Purified $(Na^+ K^+)$ATPase requires acidic phospholipid for optimal function (6). Carafoli and his associates succeeded in purifying Ca^{2+} ATPase, first, from red blood cells and then, from heart muscle (18). When the purified, solubilized ATPase was reconstituted with an acidic phospholipid, i.e., phosphatidylserine or phosphatidylinositol, the enzyme showed a high affinity towards Ca^{2+}, whereas it showed a low affinity when the enzyme was reconstituted with phosphatidylcholine liposomes. Both Vmax and Km were affected by the species of the phospholipid. The enzyme with a low affinity state was shifted to a higher affinity state by calmodulin (18). It appears that the accessibility of the active site of the ATPase to Ca^{2+} is increased by a conformational change of the molecule induced by acidic phospholipids or calmodulin.

Philipson and his associates have investigated in detail the interrelationship between changes in lipid composition and the Na^+/Ca^{2+} exchange function of sarcolemmal membrane. Clostridium phospholipase C hydrolyzed preferentially phosphatidylcholine, phosphatidylethanolamine and sphingomyelin of the sarcolemmal membrane, but phosphatidylserine and phosphatidylinositol were less affected. Therefore, following treatment with phospholipase C, the sarcolemmal membrane contained a relatively greater proportion of phosphatidylserine and phosphatidylinositol, two acidic phospholipids, although the total quantity of phospholipid was decreased. Philipson's group found that such a treatment enhanced the rate of Na^+ dependent Ca^{2+} uptake by the cardiac sarcolemmal membrane. On the other hand, (Na^+K^+)ATPase activity was not potentiated by the lipase treatment (19).

Phospholipase D converts membrane glycero phospholipids to phosphatidic acid. An increase in proportion of the acidic to other phospholipids by the enzyme treatment again augmented exclusively the Na^+/Ca^{2+} exchange activity of heart sarcolemma (20). The enhanced Ca^{2+} flux as a result of an increase in acidic phospholipid was accompanied by the augmentation of contractility in a cardiac muscle preparation (21).

Similarly, addition of fatty acids, expecially unsaturated fatty acids, or anionic amphiphilic compounds, such as dodecyl sulfate, increased the rate of Na^+ dependent Ca^{2+} uptake by cardiac sarcolemmal vesicles. Likewise, passive Ca^{2+} permeability of the membrane was increased by the presence of unsaturated fatty acids (21,22). These results suggest that the negative charge facilitates binding of Ca^{2+} to the Na^+/Ca^{2+} exchanger, and that the exchanger is extremely susceptible to membrane perturbations. Philipson and Ward conclude that fatty acids which accumulate during myocardial ischemia are sufficient in quantities to alter sarcolemmal Ca^{2+} transport (21).

EFFECTS OF METHYLATION

Phosphatidylcholine is mostly synthesized via the CDP choline pathway in the cell. However, it can be formed by methylation of phosphatidylethanolamine. Axelrod, Hirata and others' work showed that such methylation of phosphatidylethanolamine was associated with a variety of intensified cellular activities (23). The methylating enzymes are localized asymmetrically in the membrane, thus, facilitate the translocation of phospholipids from the cytoplasmic side to the outer surface of the membrane. It is postulated that the methylation of phospholipid serves as the role of signal transduction for many cell surface receptors, for example, for neurotransmitters, immunoglobulin, etc.(23).

Therefore, the effects of phospholipid methylation on activities of the Ca^{2+} regulating membrane enzymes were studied recently. Chauhan and Kalra used kidney cortex membrane and found that ATP—dependent Ca^{2+} uptake was increased by methylation, induced by the incubation with S—adenosyl methione (24).

The work carried out by Dhalla and his associates showed that both Ca^{2+} ATPase activities and phospholipid methylation of the cardiac sarcoplasmic reticular fraction were increased by adenosyl methionine and inhibited by methyl acetimidate, an inhibitor of methylation (25). Similarly, both Ca^{2+} ATPase and ATP—dependent Ca^{2+} accumulation of sarcolemmal membrane was stimulated by the administration of 10 - 150 μM of adenosyl methionine (26).

Results obtained by Boyle et al. indicate that the suppression of methylation by feeding a choline deficient diet plus injections of methylation inhibitors, cycloleucine and periodate—oxidized adenosine, resulted in a lowering of the ratio of phosphatidylcholine to phosphatidylethanolamine of the mouse liver microsomes, concurrently with the reduction of microsomal Ca^{2+} ATPase activities and Ca^{2+} uptake (27). Other microsomal enzymes, NADH—cytochrome c reductase, cytochrome P 450 reductase, etc. were not affected.

These results suggest that N—methylation of membrane phospholipids may play an important role in the modulation of Ca^{2+} transport mechanisms and hence the contractility of the heart.

CHANGES IN MYOCARDIAL ISCHEMIA

The results thus far discussed indicate that the modification of membrane phospholipid compositions alters the essential membrane functions, represented as activities of (Na^+K^+)ATPase and

Ca^{2+} ATPase, as well as rates of Ca^{2+} transport and Na^+/Ca^{2+} exchange. It is reasonable to expect, therefore, that such modifications of membrane components, and hence functions, take place in the ischemic myocardium.

Chien, Farber and colleagues, presented evidence which demonstrated that the degradation of phospholipids occurred in the ischemic liver and heart, together with impairment of some membrane functions. The phospholipid content of the sarcoplasmic reticulum was decreased several hours following left ventricular ischemia in rats, simultaneously with the decrease in Ca^{2+} uptake by the sarcoplasmic reticulum. Chlorpromazine protected against the loss of phospholipids, the inhibition of Ca^{2+} uptake and the increased Ca^{2+} permeability of the sarcoplasmic reticulum. The results suggest that the accelerated catabolism of membrane phospholipid by phospholipases is the critical factor in the development of ischemic irreversible membrane malfunction (28).

The Ca^{2+} transport by the heart membranes was measured by Daly et al. by using rat heart Langendorff perfusion. It was found that 60 minutes ischemia reduced the rate of Ca^{2+} uptake by the Na^+/Ca^{2+} exchange of the sarcolemmal fraction. However, passive permeability properties of the sarcolemma as measured by Ca^{2+} efflux from preloaded vesicles was not altered by hypoxia, ischemia or reperfusion (29). Bersohn et al. demonstrated also a depression of sarcolemmal Na^+/Ca^{2+} exchange activities in the rabbit heart rendered ischemic from 5 minutes to 2 hours. Activities of (Na^+K^+)ATPase and adenylate cyclase of the sarcolemmal membrane were also depressed during ischemia (30). A recent report from Bing's laboratory indicates that ATP-dependent sarcolemmal Ca^{2+} uptake and endogenous phosphorylation were both significantly decreased by repeated coronary occlusion, which lasted for a total period of 18 minutes, followed by reperfusion in the isolated dog heart experiment (31).

We carried out experiments in which a branch of the left anterior descending coronary artery was occluded for 1.5 hours followed by 3 hours reperfusion in anesthetized open-chested dogs. Sarcolemmal fractions were purified by the method of Reeves and Sutko. The activities of (Na^+K^+)ATPase of sarcolemmal fractions isolated from the ischemic

Fig.1. Effect of
Ischemia/Reperfusion on
Activities of (Na⁺K⁺)ATPase
and p-Nitrophenyl Phosphatase
(pNPPase), and Phospholipid
Contents of Dog Heart
Sarcolemmal Preparation.
        Sarcolemmal
fractions were prepared by
the method of Reeves and
Sutko from endocardial (End)
and epicardial (Epi) layers
of the left ventricle
following a 1.5 h ischemia
and 3 h reperfusion period.
Nisoldipine was given
intravenously at a dose of
5 µg/kg twice. The ATPase
activity is expressed as
µmole Pi/mg protein.h,
p-NPPase as nmole
nitrophenol/mg.h, and
phospholipid as nmole/mg
(n = 4).

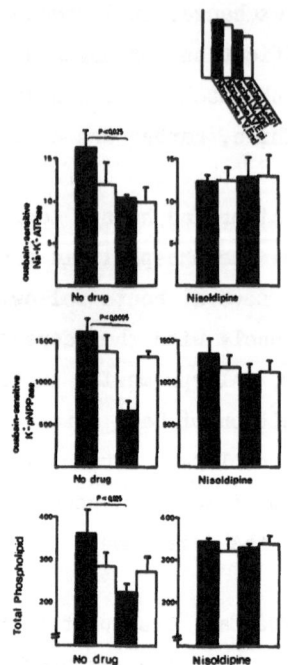

subendocardial muscle layers were significantly decreased in comparison
to those from non-ischemic areas (Fig.1). Treatment of dogs with
Nisoldipine prevented the enzyme depression. There was no significant
difference between enzyme activities of ischemic and non-ischemic
subepicardial muscle layers (32).

        Activities of K⁺ stimulated p-nitrophenyl phosphatase and
phospholipid contents of sarcolemmal fractions isolated from ischemic
subendocardial layers were significantly decreased, as compared to those
of non-ischemic subendocardial layers. Nisoldipine (5 µg/kg twice by an
intravenous injection) corrected the enzyme dysfunction and alteration in
membrane composition (Fig.1)(32).

        Our results further indicated that phospholipid compositions of
the sarcolemmal fraction and the mitochondrial fraction were modified by
ischemia in the dog myocardium (Fig.2). Once again significant decreases
in phosphatidylcholine and phosphatidylethanolamine of the ischemic heart
muscle were observed (33).

Fig.2. Effect of Ischemia on the Phospholipid Composition of Sarcolemmal and Mitochondrial Fractions of Dog Hearts.

Subcellular fractions were prepared from dog ventricles following 3 h coronary occlusion. Phospholipids were extracted and analyzed by thin-layer chromatography. Abbreviations are PC (phosphatidylcholine), PE (phosphatidylethanolamine), S (sphingomyelin), C (cardiolipin), PS (phosphatidylserine), PI (phosphatidylinositol) and empty columns (miscellaneous lipids). The number of assays was 4 each.

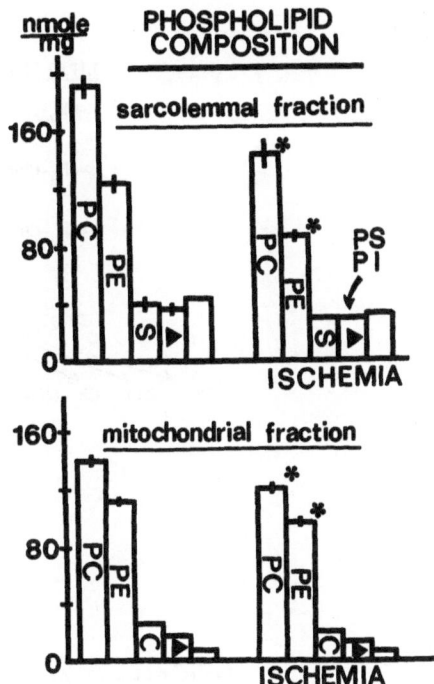

FREE RADICAL EFFECTS

In order to help in elucidating the mechanism responsible for these changes in membrane structures and functions, we felt it necessary to examine the recently proposed hypothesis that the generation of oxygen free radicals induces lipid peroxidation and hence membrane dysfunction during the development of ischemia-reperfusion tissue injury (34,35).

Postulated steps of the lipid peroxidation reaction are illustrated in Fig.3. Long chain polyunsaturated fatty acids are oxidized, particularly by the action of oxygen free radicals, and degraded, via a chain reaction, ultimately to short chain fragments. When such oxidative catabolism takes place in the membrane lipid bilayer, its consequences are grave, as free radical damage results in fatty acid oxidation, aldehyde formation, amino acid oxidation, cross-linking of proteins and lipids, protein strand scission, etc., resulting in impairments of the permeability, substrate and ion transports, and receptor function of membranes (34,35,36).

Fig.3.

**Lipid
Peroxi-
dation
Reaction**

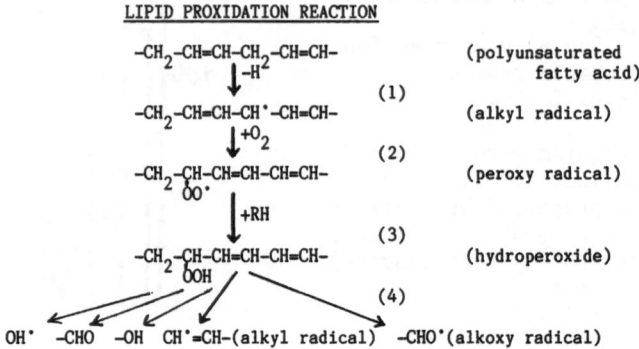

LIPID PROXIDATION REACTION

$-CH_2-CH=CH-CH_2-CH=CH-$ (polyunsaturated fatty acid)

    ↓ $-H$ (1)

$-CH_2-CH=CH-CH^\cdot-CH=CH-$ (alkyl radical)

    ↓ $+O_2$ (2)

$-CH_2-\underset{OO^\cdot}{CH}-CH=CH-CH=CH-$ (peroxy radical)

    ↓ $+RH$ (3)

$-CH_2-\underset{OOH}{CH}-CH=CH-CH=CH-$ (hydroperoxide)

     (4)

$OH^\cdot$ $-CHO$ $-OH$ $CH^\cdot=CH-$(alkyl radical) $-CHO^\cdot$(alkoxy radical)

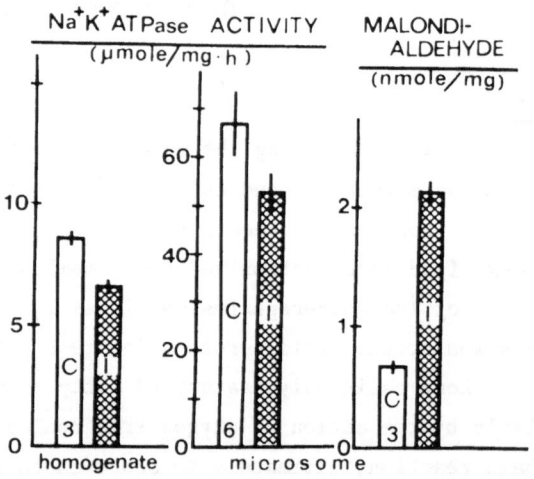

**Fig.4. Effect of Ischemia/Reperfusion on the $(Na^+K^+)ATPase$
Activity and Malondialdehyde (MDA) Content in the Dog Kidney.**
     Homogenates and microsomal fractions were prepared from the outer
medulla of dog kidney rendered ischemic (2 h) followed by reperfusion (15
min). The MDA content of the microsomal fraction was determined by a
thiobarbituric acid method. Abbreviations are, C (contralateral kidney)
and İ (ischemic-reperfused kidney). Numbers of experiments are indicated
in the columns.

In our recent experiment, in which we adopted a dog kidney ischemia (2 hours)-reperfusion (15 minutes) model, we obtained results indicating depression of $(Na^+ K^+)$ATPase of both homogenates and microsomal fraction prepared from the outer medulla, as well as the enhanced production of malondialdehyde (Fig.4)(37).

We examined in addition the effect of lipid antioxidants in our in vitro experiments, which were carried out by using membrane-bound $(Na^+ K^+)$ATPase preparations of the kidney medulla. In these experiments, we adopted a mixture of 0.5 mM (or 50 mM) H_2O_2, 0.1 mM $FeCl_3$ and 1 mM ADP as a free radical generating system (37).

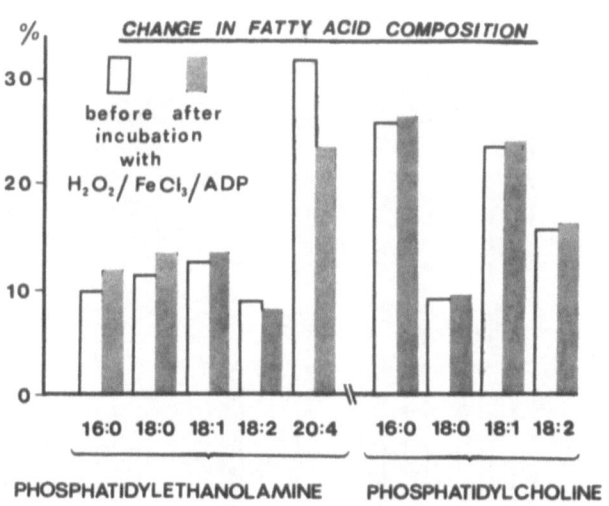

Fig.5. Change in Fatty Acid Composition of Membrane Phospholipids Induced by Hydroxyl Radicals.
      Purified porcine kidney membrane preparations were incubated for 15 min in the presence of 50 mM H_2O_2, 0.1 mM $FeCl_3$, 1.0 mM ADP and Tris buffer, pH 7.5. Phospholipids were extracted, separated and analyzed by gas chromatography. Fatty acids are designated by the chain lengths and the number of double bonds. The compositions are shown in % of total fatty acids (n = 2). It is evident that arachidonic acid in the ethanolamine phospholipid was decreased by lipid peroxidation.

Incubation of the membrane preparation in the presence of the free radical generating system reduced the content of polyunsaturated fatty acids of ethanolamine glycero phospholipids, most likely 1-alkenyl-2-acyl species. The fatty acid composition of choline phosphoglyceride remained unchanged (Fig.5). The incubation suppressed the activity of $(Na^+ K^+)$ATPase and concurrently augmented lipid peroxidation, as indicated as malondialdehyde accumulation (Fig.6)(37). When an antioxidant, butylated hydroxytoluene or propyl gallate, was present in the incubation mixture containing the free radical generating system, lipid peroxidation was prevented and the impaired $(Na^+ K^+)$ATPase activity was partially restored (Fig.6). These results suggest that the inhibition of lipid peroxidation may prevent the deterioration of

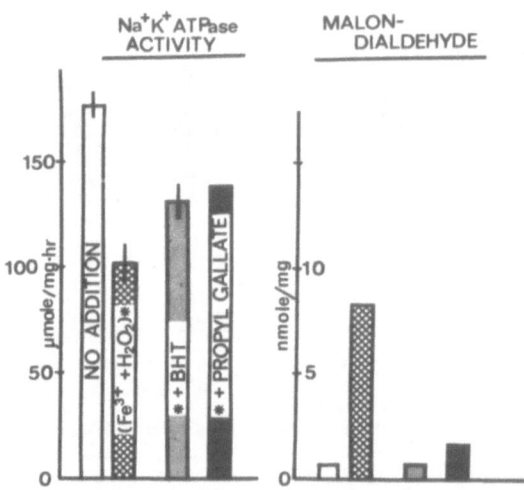

Fig.6. The Effect of Lipid Antioxidants on Kidney Membrane $(Na^+ K^+)$ATPase Activities and Malondialdehyde Formation.
        Membrane-bound ATPase was prepared by the method of Jorgensen, and was incubated in the presence of 0.5 mM H_2O_2, 0.1 mM $FeCl_3$ and 1.0 mM ADP (*), plus 2 mM butylated hydroxytoluene (BHT) or 2 mM propyl gallate. Numbers of experiments were 9 (control), 5 (*), 3 (BHT) and 2 (propyl gallate).

membrane functions caused by the generation of reactive intermediates by the univalent reduction of oxygen.

In conclusion, this review of recent work reveals that alterations in the membrane phospholipids and lipid intermediates can either potentiate or inhibit membrane functions, such as ATPases and Ca^{2+} transport. Although membrane phospholipids are ultimately reduced and their metabolites accumulate in myocardial cell ischemia, the precise causal relationship between these metabolic derangements and the ischemic membrane dysfunction is as yet to be elucidated. Similarly, the role played by lipid peroxidation in the pathogenesis of membrane damage in ischemia-reperfusion injury must be further investigated.

ACKNOWLEDGEMENTS

The work was supported by grants from the Medical Research Council (Personnel support to KJK), Uehara Foundation (Personnel support to MK), Heart & Stroke Foundation of Ontario, and J.P.Bickell Foundation. The assistance of C.Kako, K.Takahashi and S.C.Vasdev is gratefully acknowledged. Nisoldipine, BAY K 5552, was kindly supplied by Dr.A.Scriabine of Miles Lab.Inc.,New Haven,CT.

REFERENCES

1. Dhalla,NS, Ziegelhoffer,A, Harrow,JAC. Can.J.Physiol.Pharmac. 55,1211-1233 (1977)
2. Katz,AM, Messineo,FC. Circ.Res. 48,1-16 (1981)
3. Corr,PB, Gross,RW, Sobel,BE. Circ.Res. 55,135-154 (1984)
4. Benga,G, Holmes,RP. Prog.Biophys.Mol.Biol. 43,195-257 (1984)
5. Gomperts,B. The Plasma Membrane, Academic Press, 1-219 (1977)
6. Jorgensen,PL. Biochim.Biophys.Acta 694,27-68 (1982)
7. Finean,JB. Membranes and Their Cellular Function, Blackwell, 1-227 (1984)
8. Robertson,RN. The Lively Membranes, Cambridge Univ.Press, 1-206 (1983)
9. Deguchi,N, Jorgensen,PL, Maunsbach,AB. J.Cell Biol. 75,619-634 (1977)
10.Gross,RW. Biochemistry 23,158-165 (1984)
11.Kako,KJ. Med.Res.Rev.(in press, 1986)

12.van Deenen,LLM. FEBS Letters 123,3-15 (1981)

13.Pitts,BJR, Okhuysen,CH. Am.J.Physiol 247,H840-846 (1984)

14.Abe,M, Yamazaki,N, Suzuki,Y, Kobayashi,A, Ohta,H. J.Mol.Cell.Cardiol. 16,239-245 (1984)

15.Adams,RJ, Cohen,DW, Gupte,S, Johnson,JD, Wallick,ET, Wang,T, Schwartz,A. J.Biol.Chem. 254,12404-12410 (1979)

16.Owens,K, Kennett,FF, Weglicki,WB. Am.J.Physiol. 242,H456-461 (1982)

17.Pitts,BJR, Tate,CA, van Winkle,WB, Wood,JM, Entman,ML. Life Sci. 23,391-402 (1978)

18.Carafoli,E, Zurini,M. Biochim.Biophys.Acta 683,279-301 (1982)

19.Philipson,KD, Frank,JS, Nishimoto,AY. J.Biol.Chem. 258,5905-5910 (1983)

20.Philipson,KD. Ann.Rev.Physiol. 47,561-571 (1985)

21.Philipson,KD, Ward,R. J.Biol.Chem. 260,9666-9671 (1985)

22.Ashavaid,TF, Covin,RA, Messineo,FC, MacAlister,T, Katz,AM. J.Mol.Cell.Cardiol. 17,851-861 (1985)

23.Hirata,F, Axelrod,J. Science 209,1082-1090 (1980)

24.Chauhan,VPS, Kalra,VK. Biochim.Biophys.Acta 727,185-195 (1983)

25.Ganguly,PK, Panagia,V, Okumura,K, Dhalla,NS. Biochem.Biophys.Res.Comm. 130,472-478 (1985)

26.Panagia,V, Okumura,K, Makino,N, Dhalla,NS. Biochim.Biophys.Acta 856,383-387 (1986)

27.Boyle,DM, Suarez,CP, Dean,WL. Cell Calcium 5,475-485 (1984)

28.Chien,KR, Pfau,RG, Farber,JL. Am.J.Pathol. 97,505-530 (1979)

29.Daly,MJ, Elz,JS, Nayler,WG. Am.J.Physiol. 247,H237-243 (1984)

30.Bersohn,MM, Philipson,KD, Fukushima,JY. Am.J.Physiol. 242,C288-295 (1982)

31.Chemnitius,JM, Sasaki,Y, Burger,W, Bing,RJ. J.Mol.Cell.Cardiol. 17,1139-1150 (1985)

32.Takahashi,H, Kako,KJ. Biochem.Med. 31,271-286 (1984)

33 Vasdev,SC, Biro,GP, Narbaitz,R, Kako,KJ. Can.J.Biochem. 58,1112-1119 (1980)

34.Freeman,BA, Crapo,JD. Lab.Invest. 47,412-426 (1982)

35.Kako,KJ. Jikei Med.J. 32,609-639 (1985)

36.Kako,KJ. Can.J.Cardiol. 2,184-194 (1986)

37.Kako,KJ. unpublished observation, also, Abstr. X.World Congr.Cardiol. (1986)

9

MODELS OF INJURY OF CARDIOVASCULAR MEMBRANES BY AMPHIPHILES AND FREE RADICALS

W. B. WEGLICKI, I. T. MAK, B. F. DICKENS and J. H. KRAMER

Department of Medicine, George Washington University School of Medicine, Washington DC 20037

INTRODUCTION

Current evidence from ultrastructural, biochemical and electrophysiological studies suggest that membrane damage is an early event in ischemic myocardial injury (1-3). Previous investigations (4-8) suggest that sarcolemmal, microsomal and lysosomal structural and functional integrity may be compromised by any one or combinations of mechanisms that may be active during ischemia. During ischemia, cellular membranes may be subjected to perturbations by accumulated lipid metabolites, elevated levels of free radicals and activated lipolytic enzymes. We have investigated the molecular nature of several injurious processes in vitro in an effort to determine the potential sequence of events leading to ischemic membrane damage. Incubation of highly purified hepatic lysosomes at acid pH results in loss of lysosomal latency and leakage of lysosomal lipases. When the sarcolemmal (SL) membranes from canine myocytes were incubated with the soluble lysosomal enzymes, the membrane phospholipids were differentially hydrolyzed. In the presence of a $\cdot O_2^-$ driven (derived from dihydroxy-fumarate) iron catalyzed-free radical generating system, the SL membrane fluidity was altered. The peroxidation of the SL membrane was accompanied by a selective loss of phospholipids and the membrane-bound Na,K-ATPase was also inactivated. Furthermore, free radical-mediated SL membrane injuries were potentiated by acidosis and by micromolar concentration of lipid amphiphiles (palmitoyl-CoA, palmitoyl-carnitine and lyso-PC). In addition, incubation of the lysosomes with the free radical system resulted in a significant production of lyso-PC and lyso-PE suggesting that free radical-triggered lipolysis might occur in the lysosome. Thus, these in vitro studies provide model systems for assessment of subcellular membrane injury during ischemia under highly controlled conditions.

METHODS

   Adult canine myocytes were isolated from ventricular tissue by collagenase digestion and the native (no detergent treatment) myocytic sarcolemmal fractions were obtained after differential and sucrose density centrifugation (9). The sarcolemmal fractions were enriched 50-fold in p-nitrophenyl phosphatase activity (10) and Na,K-ATPase activity was 67.0 ± 6.1 umol/mg protein/hr as determined at $37^{\circ}C$ and pH 7.2 by a spectrophotometric-coupled enzyme method (11). Protein concentration was determined according to the method of Lowry et al (12).

   Rat hepatic lysosomes were isolated by the free flow electrophoresis procedure described previously (13). Lysosomes were enriched 40-60 fold in N-acetyl-β-glucosaminidase activity. The lipases used for hydrolyzing sarcolemmal lipids were obtained from the soluble portion (lysosol) of the lysosomal system (14).

   "Membrane fluidity" was monitored by fluorescence polarization of the probe 1,6-diphenyl, 1-3-5-hexatriene (DPH). The probe was added to the sarcolemmal membranes in a minimum volume of tetrahydrofuran at a ratio of 1/500 probe to phospholipid molecules. The fluorescence polarization was measured using a custom built fluorometer as previously described (15). Membrane phospholipids were extracted and analyzed (16). The amphiphilic agents employed in this investigation were L-palmitoyl carnitine, L-palmitoyl CoA, lysophosphatidylcholine, palmitic and oleic acids (P-L. Biochemicals, Milwaukee, Wisconsin); all were dissolved (under N_2 gas) in membrane incubation buffer composed of 120 mM KCL, 50 mM sucrose and 10 mM potassium phosphate, pH 7.2. In some studies, aliquots of sarcolemma (75-100 ug/ml, final) were preincubated with each lipid amphiphile at specified concentrations for 10 min at $37^{\circ}C$. The peroxidation reactions were initiated by the introduction of an exogenous free radical generating system composed of dihydroxyfumarate (DHF) and Fe^{3+}-ADP. The final concentrations of these components as well as additional incubation conditions, are described in the appropriate tables and figure legends. The rates of lipid peroxidation were assayed as malondialdehyde (MDA) formation using the thiobarbituric acid procedure (13). Statistical analyses were performed by unpaired Student's t-test.

RESULTS AND DISCUSSION

   At the first ISHR meeting in Winnipeg, we presented (17) the first evidence of significant accumulation of arachidonic acid in ischemic cardiac tissue (Control - 3.5%; ischemia - 18.5%). Since arachidonate (20:4) was primarily associated with myocardial phospholipids (Table 1) we suggested

Table 1. Percent Fatty Acid Composition of Phospholipids and Triglycerides in Canine Myocardium

Fatty Acid	Phospholipid	Trigylceride
16:0	8.4	15.3
16:0DMA	3.6	--
16.1	--	2.3
18:0	21.2	2.1
18:0DMA	2.1	--
18.1	18.8	47.9
18.2	18.1	14.2
18:3	--	0.4
20:4	27.7	0.4

that the ischemia-associated increase in arachidonate represented release from membrane pools. However, it still remains unclear from which cell types of the myocardium or from which class of lipids the arachidonate arises. The potential importance of phospholipases A in the loss of membrane lipids during ischemia prompted us to begin a systematic study of the subcellular location and characterization of phospholipases in myocardial tissue. A partial summary of some of the characterizations of myocardial phospholipases is presented in Table 2. In general, the acid-

Table 2. Phospholipases A of Canine Myocardium

Fraction	PLA	pH Optimum	Ca^{++}	EDTA
Mitochondrial	A_2	9.5	++++	0
Lysosomal	$A_2 > A_1$	4.5	+++	++
Sarcolemmal	A_2	7.0	+++	0
Microsomal	A_2	7.0	++	0

active phospholipases are localized in the lysosomes and are active even in the absence of added calcium. The other myocardial phospholipases are in the microsomes, plasmalemma and mitochondria, and are generally active at neutral to alkaline pH; they require calcium in the millimolar range for maximal activation.

The high specific activity of lysosomal phospholipases suggested that

they might participate in the degradation of phospholipids and using immuno-
histochemical techniques (18) it was suggested that the loss of lysosomal
membrane integrity might be an early event in myocardial ischemia. The
early decrease in myocardial pH associated with ischemia may render
subcellular membranes susceptible to lipolysis by lysosomal lipases released
during the loss of lysosomal integrity. We postulated that during the
acidosis accompanying ischemia, while cytosolic calcium is in the micromolar
range, lysosomal phospholipases are activated, resulting in the loss of
lysosomal latency; the released lysosomal phospholipases may then
participate in the production of arachidonic and other free fatty acids from
subcellular membrane phospholipids (14). We began to test this hypothesis
by studies of isolated lysosomes from cardiac and hepatic sources. For this
purpose it would have been ideal to have highly purified and intact cardiac
lysosomes. We utilized the technique of free flow electrophoresis for the
separation of subcellular organelles, and this procedure allowed us to
obtain better than 50-fold enriched 'native' hepatic lysosomes which were
relatively free of contamination by mitochondria and microsomes (13,19);
unfortunately, the same procedure could only enrich cardiac lysosomes up to
15-fold above the homogenate. Using the highly purified hepatic lysosomes,
the effects of acidosis on lysosomal lipolysis and latency were studied.
Incubation of the lysosomes at pH 5.0, in the absences of added calcium at
37°C for 30 minutes resulted in dramatic increases in lysophosphatidylcholine, lysophosphatidylethanolamine and free fatty acids; concomitantly,
the latency of the lysosome was lost. Thus, lysosomal membrane phospholipid
degradation could easily account for the observed loss of latency in
myocardial ischemia. Since the release of lipases from lysosomes adjacent
to the sarcolemma may occur, the lipids of the sarcolemma could be potential
targets of lysosomal phospholipases. By first isolating the lysosomes, it
was possible to begin to sort out the contributions of the soluble portion
of the lysosome, the lysosol; it was found that the lysosol contained a very
active phospholipase A_2 which we used for further studies of phospholipase A
attack of cardiac membranes. Isolated sarcolemmal preparations from canine
hearts were used as a "myocardial substrate" for the hydrolysis by lysosomal
phospholipases A. When the sarcolemmal membranes were incubated with the
lysosol, hydrolysis of phosphatidylcholine and phosphatidylethanolamine was
noted (Table 3), with significant ($P<0.05$) production of their respective
lysophospholipids; significant increase in arachidonic acid was observed.

A pH of 5.0 was chosen for this study, although the reported pH of the intracellular cytosol during ischemia would be higher (20); however the pH in the region of the negatively charged sarcolemmal membrane should be lower than that of the cytosol.

Table 3. Alterations in Phospholipid Concentrations Following Incubations of Sarcolemma with Lysosol (nM lipid phosphorous/mg SL protein)

Phospholipid	Sarcolemma + Lysosol	
	0°	37°
Phosphatidylcholine	491	482
Phosphatidylethanolamine	290	282
Phosphatidylserine	79.6	66.3
Phosphatidylinositol	57.3	59.2
Sphingomyelin	221	170
Cardiolipin	9.0	11.0
Lysophosphatidylcholine	6.8	21.6**
Lysophosphatidylethanolamine	7.8	22.8**

In recent years, numerous studies have strongly suggested the participation of oxygen free radicals (i.e. $\cdot O_2^-$, H_2O_2 and $\cdot OH$) in the pathogenesis of myocardial ischemic injury (21,22). Therefore we designed experiments to determine which lipids of the sarcolemma were most susceptible to exogenously added free radicals. Significant losses of sarcolemmal phosphatidylcholine (40%) and phosphatidylethanolamine (65%) occur within 30 minutes of exposure to this exogenous free radical generating system. Membrane physical properties, as measured by changes in the fluorescence polarization of DPH, were dramatically altered by exposure to the exogenous free radical generating systems (Fig. 1). The observed increase in membrane polarization correlates with a decrease in "membrane fluidity". Since there is a known correlation between membrane structure and membrane-bound enzyme function, we investigated the effects of free radicals on membrane-bound enzymes. Significant losses of Na,K-ATPase activity could be observed (Table 4) concurrent with the free radical-induced losses of sarcolemmal membrane phospholipids, production of MDA and changes in membrane fluidity.

Lower pH favors the formation of the protonated form of $\cdot O_2^-$ (23), the perhydroxyl radical [HO_2^-], which is a stronger oxidant than $\cdot O_2^-$ and

Table 4. Time Course of Free Radical-Mediated Injury of Myocytic Sarcolemma

Exposure time (min)	Na,K-ATPase activity (% inhibition)	MDA formed (nmol/mg prot)
0.2	5.6 + 4.0	1.6 + 0.2
5	55.5 + 3.6	55.0 + 5.0
20	70.0 + 5.2	81.3 + 8.6
45	80.5 + 3.1	127.0 + 8.0
90	90.5 + 2.7	138.5 + 7.2

Values are means ± SD of 4-7 preparations. Prior to assay, sarcolemmal membranes (100 ug/ml) were incubated (pH 7.2) overtime in the pressence of the free radical generating system consisting of 3.3 mM DHF plus 0.1 mM $FeCl_3$ chelated by 1 mM ADP.

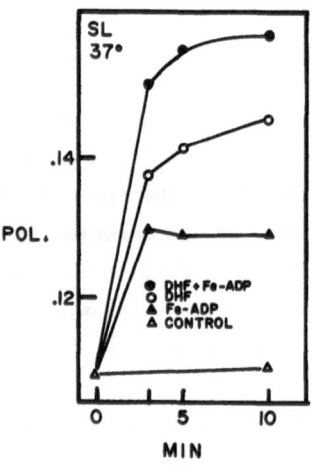

Fig. 1. Time course of the influence of exogenous free radical generating systems on sarcolemmal membrane fluidity. Membranes were labeled with DPH and membrane fluidity determined with and without various radical generating systems.

partitions better into lipid and the hydrophobic domains of proteins. Furthermore, a recent study indicated that low pH accelerated the conversion of $\cdot O_2^-$ to the highly reactive $\cdot OH$ in the presence of Fe^{3+} (24). Our data show that lower pH potentiaties free radical-induced loss in membrane-bound enzymatic function of the canine sarcolemma; as shown in Figure 2, at pH 7.2, incubation of isolated canine sarcolemma with a free radical generating system (DHF + Fe^{3+}-ADP) for 45 min resulted in 50% loss of Na,K-ATPase activity. However, incubation at pH 6.0-6.4 under the same condition resulted in 75% loss in activity of the enzyme, and lowering pH to 6.0-6.4

alone did not change the ATPase activity; these data indicate that acidosis potentiates the free radical-induced loss of membrane enzyme function in vitro.

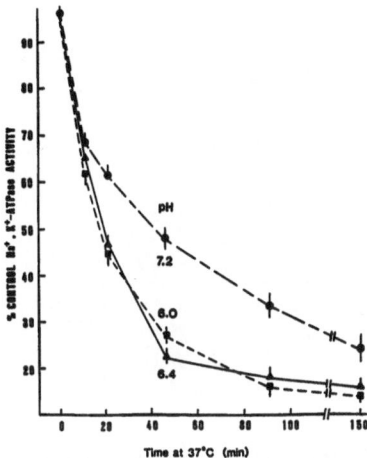

Fig. 2. Time course of the influence of pH on free radical-mediated inhibition of sarcolemmal Na,K ATPase. Prior to assay, sarcolemma membranes (100 ug/ml) were incubated at the pH indicated in the presence of the free radical generating system (0.83 mM DHF plus 0.025 mM $FeCl_3$ chelated by 0.25 mM ADP). Values are means of 5-8 experiments and are expressed as % change $\pm$ SE from control activity (100%) at the appropriate pH and incubation time.

It has been known that lysophosphatidylglycerides and long chain acyl carnitines accumulate in ischemic tissue and both have been reported to be arrhythmogenic (25). We have observed that lysophosphatidylcholine accelerates peroxidation in sarcolemmal membranes induced by a $\cdot O_2^-$ driven Fe^{3+} catalyzed free radical systems in concentration from 10 to 100 uM in a time-dependent manner (7). Similarly, palmitoyl carnitine and other lipid amphiphiles were found to promote sarcolemmal lipid peroxidation achieving maximal stimulation at 50 uM (Fig 3). It is interesting that free fatty acids (16:0 and 18:1) had no effect on this lipid peroxidation (data not shown). Preliminary studies suggest that palmitoyl carnitine and lysophosphatidylcholine are able to promote sarcolemmal lipid peroxidation even when exposed to low and and otherwise non-injurious levels of the exogenous free radical generating system (data not shown). Since the levels of the lipid amphiphiles used are within the levels found in ischemic tissues our findings may represent a novel mechanism of injury, but the relevance of this model to the situation in situ still needs to be determined.

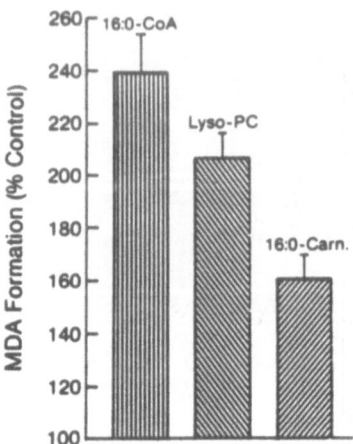

Fig. 3. Effects of various lipid amphiphiles on sarcolemmal lipid peroxidation. Sarcolemmal samples were preincubated at 37°C with the indicated amphiphiles (each at 50 uM) for 10 minutes before the additions of Fe^{3+}-ATP and DHF at the concentrations described in figure legend 2. After 20 minutes of incubation, samples were assayed for MDA formation and expressed as % relative to the controls in the absence of amphiphiles. Values are means ± SE of 3-8 preparations.

We continue to utilize our "free flow electrophoresis lysosomes" as models of biological membrane injury. When free radicals are produced in vitro, rapid loss of lysosomal latency and production of malondialdehyde (MDA) can be observed. It is of interest that phosphatidylcholine and phosphatidylethanolamine remain the most susceptible lipids to free radical injury (Table 5). We tested the hypothesis that free radicals may enhance the process of lipolysis in lysosomes. At pH 6.0, after incubation for 30 minutes under conditions where no lipolysis would occur in normal lysosomes, a significant production of lysophosphatidylcholine and lysophosphatidylethanolamine could be seen with a decrease in phosphatidylcholine and phosphatidylethanolamine (Table 5). The expected products of deacylation (free fatty acids) were not found in the lipid soluble phase and it was postulated that free radical peroxidation products (of the unsaturated acyl chains in the sn-2 position of phospholipids) enhanced deacylation and release of the remaining peroxidized acyl moiety into the water soluble extract. Thus, although the expected stoichiometry was not demonstrated, we postulate that free radical-triggered lipolysis occurred.

Table 5. Free Radical-Induced Changes in the Major Phospholipids of Hepatic Lysosomes.

	Mole Percent of Control Lipid Phosphorous		
Phospholipid	Control	10 min	20 min
Phosphatidylcholine	55.2	46.0**	43.4**
Phosphatidylethanolamine	21.4	11.6**	9.3**
Lysophosphatidylcholine	1.6	5.3*	6.1**
Lysophosphatidylethanolamine	0.4	1.3	2.6*

* = P < 0.05, ** = P < 0.01

Thus, we have attempted to determine the cellular and molecular sources of the breakdown of myocardial phospholipids during myocardial ischemia. Studies at the cellular and subcellular levels confirm the potential for phospholipase attack of lysosomal membranes, previously peroxidized membranes and the enhancement by amphiphiles of this peroxidative reaction. Although the complex sequence of events leading to cardiovascular membrane damage during myocardial ischemia in vivo remains uncertain, the models of injury considered in this study may by themselves, or in concert with other events, elicit potentially deleterious consequences to the ischemic, reperfused myocardium.

REFERENCES
1. Jennings, R.B., Ganote, C.E., Reimer, K.A. Am. J. Pathol. 81:179-194, 1975.
2. Corr, P.B., Lee, B.I., Sobel, B.E. Acta Med. Scand. 651:59-69, 1981.
3. Ashraf, M., Halverson, C.A. Am. J. Pathol. 88:583-594, 1977.
4. Weglicki, W.B., Kramer, J.H., Franson, R.C., Pang, D.C., Owens, K. In Pathobiology of Cardiovascular Injury: Advances in Myocardiology, Vol. 7 (Eds. L. Stone and W.B. Weglicki), Martinus Nijhoff Publishing Co., Hihgham, MA, 1985, pp. 258-272.
5. Kramer, J.H., Mak, I.T., Weglicki, W.B. (1984) Circ. Res. 55:120-124, 1984.
6. Kramer, J.H., Weglicki, W.B. Am. J. Physiol. 248:H75-H81, 1985.
7. Mak, I.T., Kramer, J.H., Weglicki, W.B. J. Biol. Chem. 261:1153-1157, 1986.
8. Weglicki, W.B., Dickens, B.F., Mak, I.T., Kramer, J.H. Life Chem. Reports 3:189-198, 1985.
9. Weglicki, W.B., Owens, K, Kennett, F.F., Kessner, A., Harris, L., Wise, R.M., Vahouny, G.V. J. Biol. Chem. 255:3605-3609, 1980.
10. Skou, J.C. Biochim. Biophys. Acta 339:258-273, 1974.

11. Owens, K., Kennett, F.F., Weglicki, W.B. Am. J. Physiol. 242:H456-H461, 1982.
12. Lowry, O.H., Rosebrough, N.J., Farr, A.L., Randall, R.J. J. Biol. Chem. 193:265-275, 1951.
13. Mak, I.T., Misra, H.P., Weglicki, W.B. J. Biol. Chem. 258:13733-13737, 1983.
14. Beckman, J.H., Owens, K., Knauer, T.E., Weglicki, W.B. Am. J. Physiol. 242:H652-H656, 1982.
15. Spanier, A.M, Dickens, B.F. and Weglicki, W.B. Am. J. Physiol. 249: H20-H28, 1985.
16. Weglicki, W.B., Dickens, B.F., and Mak, I.T. BBRC 126:229-235, 1984.
17. Weglicki, W.B., Owens, K., Urschel, C.W., and Sonnenblick, E.H.: In: Recent Advances in Studies of Cardiac Structure and Metabolism, 3:781, 1974.
18. Decker, R.S., Poole, A.R., Crie, J.S., Dingle, J.T., and Wilderenthal, K. Am. J. Pathol. 98:445-456, 1980.
19. Beckman, J.K., Owens, K., and Weglicki, W.B. Lipids 16:796-799, 1981.
20. Cobbe, S.M. and Poole-Wilson, P.A. J. Mol. Cell. Cardiol. 12:745-760, 1980.
21. Guarnieri, C., Flamingni, F., and Coldarera, C.M. J. Mol. Cell. Cardiol. 12:797-808, 1980.
22. Meerson, F.Z., Kagan, V.E., Kozlov, Y.P., Belkina, L.M., Arkhipenko, Y.V. Basic Res. Cardiol. 77:465-485, 1982.
23. Fee, J.A., In: Metal Ion-Activation of Dioxygen (Ed. T. G. Spiro), John Wiley and Son Inc., New York, 1980, pp 173-237.
24. Backer, M.S. and Gebicki, J.M. Arch. Biochem. Biophys. 234:258-264, 1984.
25. Corr, P.B., Gross, R.W., and Sobel, B.E. Circ. Res. 55:135-154, 1984.

10

INABILITY OF SUPEROXIDE DISMUTASE AND CATALASE TO INHIBIT CALCIUM INFLUX ON
REOXYGENATION OF RABBIT MYOCARDIUM

P.A.POOLE-WILSON, M.A.TONES[*]

Department of Cardiac Medicine, Cardiothoracic Institute and National Heart
Hospital, 2 Beaumont Street, London W1N 2DX, UK.
[*]Present address, Department of Biochemistry, University Hospital Medical
School, Clifton Boulevard, Nottingham NG7 2UH, UK.

INTRODUCTION

On reoxygenation (1) or reperfusion (2) of heart muscle after a period
of hypoxia or ischaemia, sufficient to cause a change in resting tension,
there is a sudden release of cytosolic enzymes, a loss of ionic homeostasis,
an increased influx of calcium (1,3,4,5) and a failure of recovery of
mechanical function. These events have been interpreted as indicating
further damage to heart muscle associated with reoxygenation or reperfusion.
The damage can be partly circumvented by perfusing the myocardium with a
solution containing low calcium for several minutes; mechanical and
biochemical recovery is enhanced (6,7,8).

The mechanism of damage on reoxygenation or reperfusion is uncertain.
It has been suggested that sudden swelling due to a raised intracellular
osmotic pressure (9) or forces on cells caused by contraction of adjacent
cells (10) disrupt the cell membrane. Alternately calcium may move into the
myocardium in exchange for sodium (11) or due to damage of the cell membrane
by oxygen radicals (1,12). Scavengers of radicals have been shown to reduce
myocardial infarct size and prevent myocardial damage (13) although in other
reports (14) no benefit was seen. Most previous studies have been performed
on in vivo models of myocardial ischaemia in which the mode or site of action
of radical scavengers is difficult, if not impossible, to determine. It
cannot be excluded that the effects of scavengers are primarily on the
vascular system, and consequent haemodynamic changes and alterations of
coronary flow affect infarct size and markers of ischaemia.

The present experiments were undertaken to investigate whether the
radical scavengers, superoxide dismutase and catalase, could alter the

calcium influx which has been shown to occur on reoxygenation or reperfusion
in an isolated preparation of rabbit heart muscle perfused at constant flow
(1,4,5).

MATERIALS AND METHODS

The experimental preparation was the arterially perfused
interventricular septum of the rabbit heart. The experimental techniques
have been described previously (1,4,5). Male New Zealand white rabbits (2-4
kg) were heparinised and anaesthetised with sodium pentobarbitone. The heart
was removed. The septal artery was cannulated and the triangular
interventricular septum was held by two pairs of forceps and tension recorded
from the apex (Statham, UC2). Septa were perfused at a mean rate of 1.6
$ml.min^{-1}.g^{-1}$ wet tissue. Temperature was maintained at $35^{o}C$ and the septa
were electrically stimulated at 90 $beats.min^{-1}$.

The perfusate contained in mM: Na^+ 143, K^+ 5.0, Ca^{2+} 1.8, Mg^{2+} 1.0, Cl^-
117, $H_2PO_4^-$ 0.4, HCO_3^- 28.0, D-glucose 11.1. The solution was gassed with
95% oxygen and 5% CO_2 and had a pH of 7.35. For hypoxic and substrate free
perfusion the solution was equilibrated with 95% and 5% CO_2 and D-mannitol
was used instead of D-glucose.

$^{47}Ca^{2+}$ and ^{51}Cr-EDTA were added to the perfusate and the uptake of these
two isotopes recorded simultaneously so as to follow the uptake of calcium
and changes in the extracellular space respectively. Counts were recorded
each minute by placing a sodium iodide crystal (8 x 5 cm, type 1258/3E,
Harshaw, Holland) attached to a counter (J and P Engineering, Reading)
immediately in front of the muscle. Windows were chosen on the counter so
that the two isotopes could be separated. A correction was made for the
crossover of $^{47}Ca^{2+}$ counts into the window for ^{51}Cr-EDTA.

Superoxide dismutase and catalase (150 $units.ml^{-1}$) were added ten
minutes before reoxygenation and continued for 10 or 20 minutes into the
period of reoxygenation after 30 or 45 minutes of hypoxia respectively. The
enzyme solutions were filtered immediately before use.

Malondialdyhyde was assayed using the method of Kornburst and Mavis (15)
by the thiobarbituric acid reaction which generates a chromogen with an
absorbance at 535 nm. Oxidised and reduced glutathione were measured by the
method of Tietze (16). Angiotensin converting enzyme was measured with an
assay based on the conversion of hippuryl-glycyl-glycine to hippuric acid.

RESULTS

The activity of the enzyme preparations was confirmed by demonstrating
that the reduction of ferricytochrome C by a mixture of xanthine and xanthine

oxidase (17) could be prevented by superoxide dismutase at a concentration of
1.5 U.ml^{-1} and partially reduced by catalase at a concentration of 15 U.ml^{-1}.

The release of malondialdehyde into the coronary effluent from the septa
was sought. There was no detectable release under either control or hypoxic
conditions or on reoxygenation. In contrast, exposure of four septa to
cumene hydroperoxide (100 µM) caused an increased release of malondialdehyde
reaching a peak rate of 0.9 mmol.min^{-1}.g^{-1} wet tissue after 15 minutes (Fig.
1).

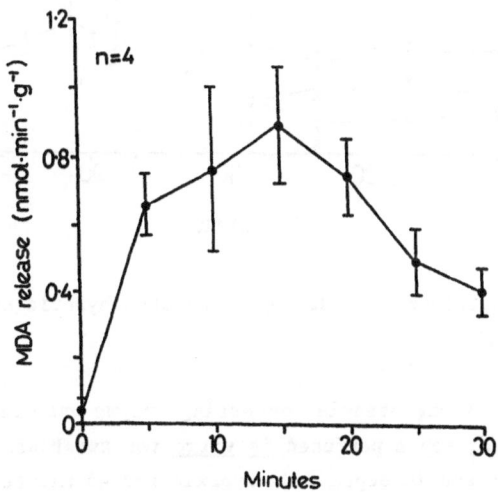

Fig. 1.   Effect of perfusion with 100 µm cumene hydroperoxide on
release of malondialdehyde into the coronary effluent (n=4).

The release of glutathione in this preparation during and after 45
minutes of hypoxia is shown in Fig. 2. Under control conditions the release
of total glutathione was approximately 0.4 µg.min^{-1}.g^{-1} wet tissue. 35% of
glutathione was in the reduced form (GSH). The rather high proportion of
oxidised glutathione (GSSG) may be due to the fact that the preparations are
perfused with a solution having a very high PO$_2$, and as a consequence are
subject to a certain degree of oxidative stress under control conditions.
Hypoxia caused a large increase in the rate of release of both GSSG
(oxidised form) and GSH which was significant after 30 minutes (P<0.05).
The increased release of GSH was greater than that of GSSG. Reoxygenation
caused a further increase in the rate of release of glutathione and this was
accounted for by an increased release of GSH rather than GSSG.

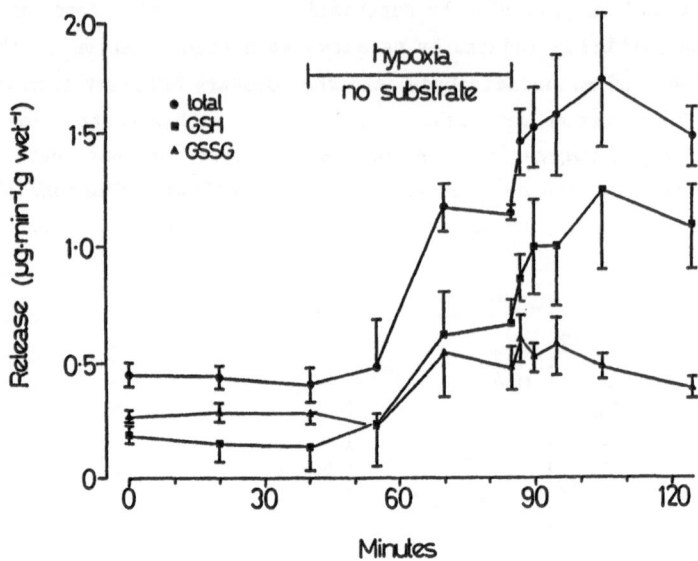

Fig. 2. Glutathione loss during 45 minutes hypoxia and reoxygenation
(n=4).

The activity of angiotensin converting enzyme was measured in fresh
septa free of blood, septa perfused _in vitro_ for two hours or more under
control conditions and in septa made hypoxic for 45 minutes and reoxygenated
for 40 minutes. The activities were in U.mg protein^{-1} 131 ± 11 (n = 4), 134
± 7 (n=5), 130 ± 2 (n = 3), respectively.

Fig. 3 and Fig. 4 show the effect of the combination of superoxide
dismutase and catalase on the uptake of $^{47}Ca^{2+}$ after 45 minutes of hypoxia.
The uptake of calcium in comparison to control experiments in the absence of
the two enzymes was no different after 30 minutes (n = 5) or after 45 minutes
of hypoxia (n = 4) (Fig. 5).

DISCUSSION
These experiments show that superoxide dismutase and catalase do not
inhibit the influx of calcium which occurs on reoxygenation after a
substantial period of hypoxic substrate free perfusion in this preparation.
Several characteristics of the preparation are relevant to this observation.

The activity of angiotension converting enzyme was similar in fresh
tissue to that subjected to hypoxia and reoxygenation suggesting that the

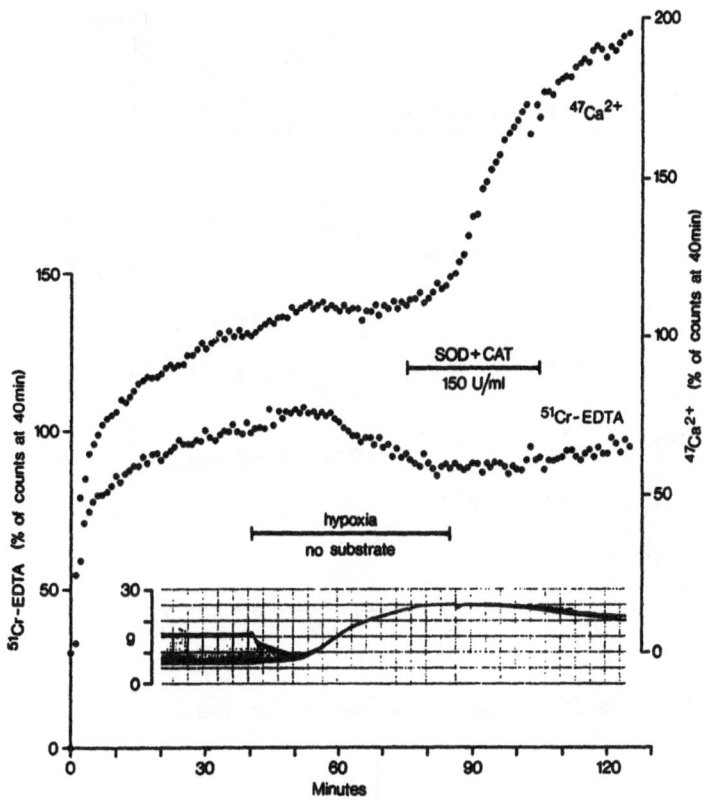

Fig. 3. Single example of effect of superoxide dismutase and
catalase on the uptake of ^{51}Cr-EDTA and ^{47}Ca^{2+} during 45
minutes of substrate free hypoxia and reoxygenation.

endothelium in the vasculature was still intact. This is an important
observation, as the endothelium is thought to be the location of xanthine
oxidase, possibly an important source of superoxide radicals under hypoxic or
reoxygenated conditions. The release of GSH and GSSG under control conditions
was similar to that reported in the isolated rat heart (18,19). The
mechanism responsible for increased release of both GSH and GSSG during
hypoxia is unknown but observations similar to ours have been reported
previously (18). The absence of a further increase of GSSG release on
reoxygenation despite an increased GSH release indicates that reoxygenation
does not cause an increase in glutathione peroxidase metabolism of lipid
peroxides. Membrane bound fatty acid peroxides can only be metabolised by
glutathione peroxidase after being released from the phospholipid by

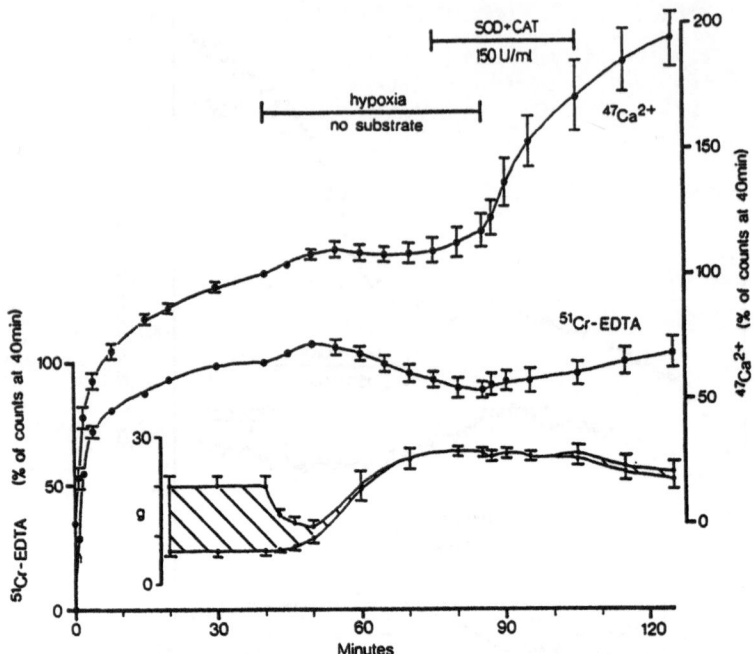

Fig. 4. Mean results of four experiments like Fig.3.

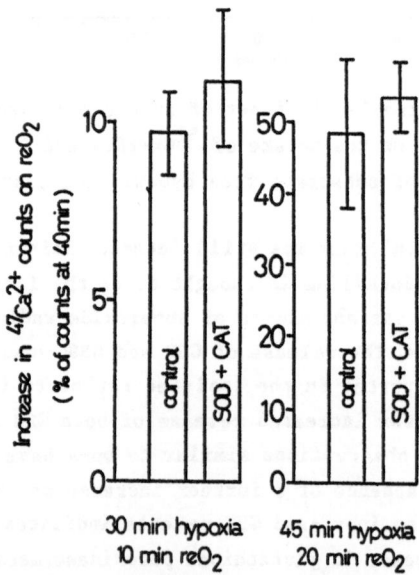

Fig. 5. Effect of superoxide dismutase and catalase on reoxygenation
induced uptake of $^{47}Ca^{2+}$.

phospholipase A_2 (20). This raises the possibility that peroxidation of membrane lipids could cause increased flux through glutathione peroxidase only if phospholipase A_2 was active also.

We were unable to detect appreciable release of malondialdehyde from preparations under control, hypoxic, or reoxygenated conditions, the detection limit of the assay being of the order of 0.1 nmol/ml. In contrast, the presence of cumene hydroperoxide caused a large release of malondialdehyde from the tissue (Fig. 1.). There are two possibilities. First, lipid peroxidation does not occur on reoxygenation and therefore has no role to play in the calcium uptake which occurs at that time. Second, lipid peroxidation does occur but the amount of malondialdyhyde released is below the detection limit of the assay used.

Gauduel and Duvelleroy (21) reported that superoxide dismutase and catalase reduced enzyme release and malondialdyhyde release from the isolated rat heart reoxygenated after 60 minutes of hypoxia at 37°C. Some of this effect may have been due to alterations of coronary flow which doubled in enzyme treated hearts. The authors assumed that the increased coronary flow was the result of protection of the heart but it could not be ruled out that the protection of the heart was a consequence of increased coronary flow brought about as a direct effect of superoxide dismutase. The release of malondialdyhyde reported was 1.5 $nmol.min^{-1}.g^{-1}$.wet tissue which is 50% greater than the maximum release found in the present preparation when treated with cumene hydroperoxide (see Fig. 1). Therefore, a similar release would have been easily detectable in our experiments. We cannot exclude the possibility that the difference in results may be accounted for by species, differences of temperature, the absence of substrate in our experiments and the fact that Gauduel and Duvelleroy (21) used the potassium arrested heart undertaking no mechanical work.

In the preparation used in this study the calcium uptake on reoxygenation is due to an increased influx (1,4,5). The cell membrane appears not to be disrupted since the extracellular marker ^{51}Cr-EDTA does not gain access to the intracellular fluid (1,4,5), the uptake can be inhibited by small cations such as nickel (1), an increased release of potassium does not occur on reoxygenation (unpublished), and the release of enzymes from the myocardium on reoxygenation is small (approximately 2% of the total tissue content) (1,5). Additionally, alteration of the calcium content of the perfusate at the time of reperfusion can improve mechanical recovery indicating that the myocardial cells are not irreversibly damaged in the sense that the sarcolemma had been totally destroyed (7). The increased calcium uptake might be due to sodium calcium exchange (11) although in this preparation we have not been able to obtain evidence to support that concept (22). We have previously reported that hydroperoxides causes a calcium influx without disruption of the cell membrane identical to that observed during hypoxia (23). Importantly, this influx is also blocked by nickel ions. These observations strongly suggest that radical formation is an important potential mechanism for the uptake of calcium on reoxygenation. Radical formation during and after ischemia has been directly demonstrated (24).

The present experiments showed that the addition of two radical scavengers to the perfusate did not prevent the uptake of calcium and might therefore be construed as evidence against the uptake of calcium being due to radical damage. Radicals in the context of ischaemia and hypoxia may be formed from white cells, from the activity of xanthine oxidase on xanthine in endothelial cells, from mitochondria or directly in the cell membrane. Since we have shown that the endothelium is intact in this preparation it is possible that the two enzymes did not reach the sarcolemma or did not reach the intracellular space and prevent radicals perhaps formed in mitochondria or in the cell membrane itself causing damage.

Previous reports suggest that these scavengers can reduce myocardial infarct size in the intact dog (13). In such an experimental model it may be that radicals formed by white cells are of particular importance in contrast to the present experiments where white cells were absent from the perfusate. Radicals may also be formed in endothelial cells of the dog by the action of xanthine oxidase (12). Recent studies undertaken since the present experiments were performed have shown that xanthine oxidase is present in the endothelium of dog and rat but absent in rabbit. This observation might explain the positive results obtained with radical scavengers in dog (13) and rat (20), and the lack of any effect in rabbit (the present study).

The present experiments show that the calcium influx and the lack of mechanical recovery on reoxygenation can occur even in the presence of superoxide dismutase and catalase and suggest that if the formation of radicals is important in causing damage to the rabbit myocardium it cannot always be prevented by the addition of extracellular scavengers. It seems likely that the protective effects of enzymatic scavengers against cellular damage may depend on the relative contributions of leucocytes and endothelial cell generated radicals versus those produced within the myocyte itself.

REFERENCES

1 Poole-Wilson, P.A. In: Control and manipulation of calcium movement. (Ed. J.R. Parratt) Raven Press, New York, 1985, pp. 325-340.

2 Hearse, D.J. J. Mol. Cell. Cardiol. 9:605-616, 1977.

3 Shen, A.C., Jennings, R.B. Am. J. Pathol. 67:441-452, 1972.

4 Poole-Wilson, P.A., Harding, D.P., Bourdillon, P.D.V., Tones, M.A. J. Mol. Cell. Cardiol. 16:175-187, 1984.

5 Bourdillon, P.D.V., Poole-Wilson, P.A. Cardiov. Res. 15:121-130, 1981.

6 Chappell, S.P., Lewis, M.J., Henderson, A.H. Cardiov. Res. 19:299-303, 1985.

7 Shine, K.I., Douglas, A.M. J. Mol. Cell. Cardiol. 15:252-260, 1983.

8 Kuroda, H., Ishiguro, S., Mori, T. J. Mol. Cell. Cardiol. 18:625-633, 1986.

9 Steenbergen, C., Hill, M.L., Jennings, R.B. Circ. Res. 57:864-875, 1985.

10 Ganote, C.E., Kaltenbach, J.P. J. Mol. Cell. Cardiol. 11:389-406, 1979.

11 Lazdunski, M., Frelin, C., Vigne, P. J. Mol. Cell. Cardiol. 17:1029-1042, 1985.

12 McCord, J.M., Roy, R.S. Can. J. Physiol. Pharmacol. 60:1346-1352, 1982.

13 Jolly, S.R., Kane, W.J., Bailie, M.B., Abrams, G.D., Lucchesi, B.R. Circ. Res. 54:227-285, 1984.

14 Gallagher, K.P., Buda, A.J., Pace, D., Gerren, R.A., Shlafer, M. Circulation. 73:1065-1076, 1986.

15 Kornburst, D.J., Mavis, R.D. Lipids. 15:315-322, 1980.

16 Tietze, F. Anal. Biochem. 27:502-522, 1969.

17 McCord, J.M., Fridovich, I. J. Biol. Chem. 244:6049-6055, 1969.

18 Guarnieri, C., Flamigni, F., Calderera, C.M. J. Mol. Cell. Cardiol. 12:797-808, 1980.

19 Tamura, M., Oshino, N., Chance, B. J. Biochem. 92:1009-1013, 1982.

20 Grossman, A., Wendel, A. Eur. J. Biochem. 135:549-552, 1983.

21 Gaudel, Y., Duvelleroy, M.A. J. Mol. Cell. Cardiol. 16:459-470, 1984.

22 Tones, M.A., Poole-Wilson, P.A. J. Mol. Cell. Cardiol. 18(suppl1):216,1986.

23 Tones, M.A., Poole-Wilson, P.A. Cardiov. Res. 19:228-236, 1985.

24 Rao, P.S., Cohen, M.V., Mueller, H.S. J. Mol. Cell. Cardiol. 15:713-716, 1983.

11

CATECHOLAMINE RELEASE IN MYOCARDIAL ISCHEMIA AND ITS CLINICAL IMPLICATIONS

W. KÜBLER, R. DIETZ, W. MÄURER and A. SCHÖMIG

Abteilung Innere Medizin III (Kardiologie) University of Heidelberg/ Germany

The occurrence of myocardial necrosis (1) and of ventricular tachyarrhythmias (2) has been related to high local concentrations of noradrenaline during ischemia. The positive results of secondary prevention beta-blocker trials after myocardial infarction and of recent studies of beta-blocker treatment in acute moycardial infarction (ISIS I study) may support this concept. Cardiac catecholamine release was, therefore, investigated in patients with ischemic heart disease and in animal experiments.

I. EXPERIMENTAL STUDIES

Local metabolic factors of cardiac catecholamine release during ischemia were investigated in the isolated perfused rat heart. Without sympathetic stimulation, no increase in net noradrenaline release can be detected in periods of ischemia ranging up to 10 min (3,5). After prolongation of the ischemic period beyond 10 min increasing amounts of noradrenaline are released (4,5). After 60 min of ischemia the cardiac catecholamine stores are depleted by more than 60 %. The amount of noradrenaline in the venous effluent during reperfusion decreases exponentially with time indicating a wash out process (6). Similar results could be obtained for adrenaline and deaminated metabolites such as DOPEG.

Catecholamine net release was further investigated after different periods of ischemia with and without desipramine, an inhibitor of neuronal reuptake, the main

inactivation process for neuronally released
catecholamines. Under areobic control conditions and at the
beginning of ischemia net catecholamine release is either
not influenced or increased in the presence of desipramine.
After more than 10 min of ischemia, however, desipramine
reduces cardiac catecholamine release, whereas after 60 min
desipramine has no effect on cardiac noradrenaline release.
Similar results were obtained with cocaine another
inhibitor of neuronal uptake(5).

In order to test the effect of sympathetic stimulation
on cardiac catecholamine release the left stellate ganglion
was electrically stimulated (7) during an aerobic control
period and during 1 min of ischemia. Under these conditions
cardiac catecholamine net release is greatly reduced in the
ischemic experiments due to delayed wash out and hence
increased reuptake. Inhibition of neuronal uptake by
desipramine, therefore, greatly increases catecholamine net
discharge, mainly at the beginning of ischemia due to
cessation of blood flow. By extension of the ischemic
period to 10 min, however, this effect of desipramine, i.
e. increased catecholamine net release, is markedly
attenuated. During an ischemic period of 20 min desipramine
even greatly reduces net catecholamine release; this can be
observed both in experiments with and without sympathetic
stimulation.

Under aerobic conditions the neuronal uptake blocker
desipramine greatly increases noradrenaline release, the
same holds true for yohimbine, a presynaptic alpha 2
blocker. The local anaesthetic lidocaine, however, greatly
reduces stimulation induced catecholamine release under
aerobic conditions; this indicates that exocytosis is the
mechanism of neurotransmitter release. After 20 min of
ischemia other mechanisms are operating: neither yohimbine
nor lidocaine affect catecholamine release, whereas the
neuronal uptake blocker desipramine now greatly reduces
noradrenaline release.

Fig. 1: Evaluation of cardiac catecholamine uptake in patients by simultaneous determination of coronary blood flow and of the arterio- coronaryvenous noradrenaline difference. The example on the left panel shows a patient in whom symdrome X was excluded by determination of coronary reserve; on the right panel a patient with severely impaired LV- function is revealed.

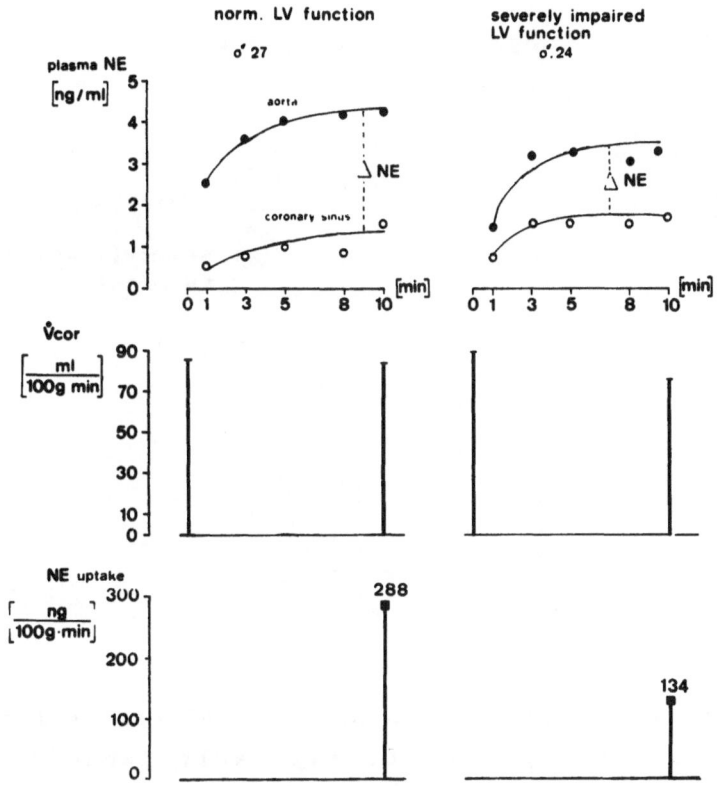

The data presented are summarized in Table 1 (for further details see (5)):

During phase I of myocardial ischemia lasting for approximately 10 min in the rat heart, the release mechanism of noradrenaline is not altered compared to aerobic control conditions. Noradrenaline release can be increased by sympathetic stimulation. During phase I neuronal uptake is still active and its inhibition by neuronal uptake blockers, therefore, augments noradrenaline release during this phase. Also the normal modulation of exocytosis, e. g. by alpha 2 receptors is maintained as

Fig. 2: Mean values and standard deviation for cardiac
noradrenaline uptake in patients with normal LV- function
(patients in whom syndrome X was excluded by determination
of coronary reserve) (n = 11) and in patients with severely
depressed LV- function (n = 11). Cardiac catecholamine
uptake was evaluated by simultaneous determination of
coronary blood flow and arterio- coronaryvenous
noradrenaline differences.

myocardial NE uptake

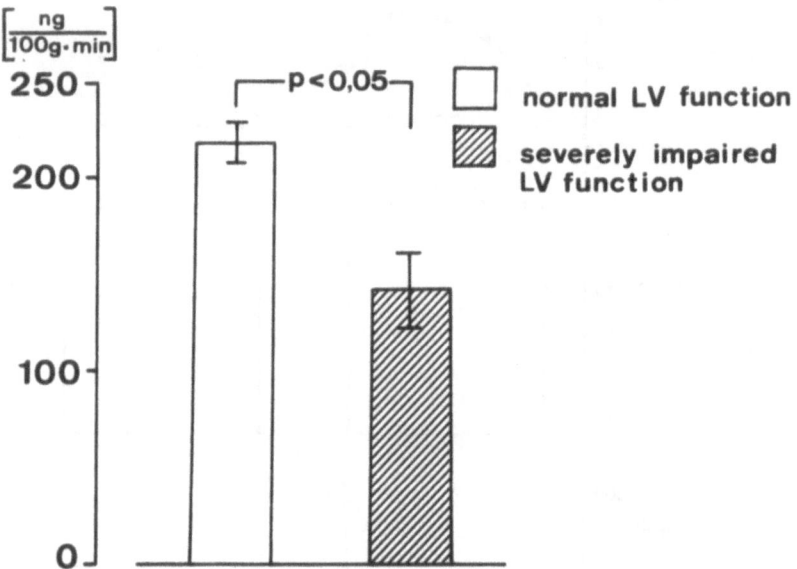

indicated by the effect of alpha 2 blockers. All these
findings indicate, that during early ischemia the
predominant mechanism of noradrenaline release is
exocytosis like under aerobic conditions. There is,
however, a quantitative difference: the response of
catecholamine release to sympathetic stimulation is
attenuated already after 3 - 4 min of ischemia.

During phase II lasting for about 15 - 40 min of
ischemia in the rat heart noradrenaline release is
augmented, and not affected by sympathetic stimulation. In
contrast to phase I, blockade of neuronal uptake leads to a
marked decrease in noradrenaline release. These findings
indicate carrier mediated efflux as main mechanism of
noradrenaline release during phase II.

Fig. 3: Catecholamine net release in normals (patients in whom syndrome X was exluded) and in patients with coronary heart disease during atrial pacing stress test (upper panel) and during isometric exercise by handgrip (lower panel). On the ordinate maximal coronary flow is given.

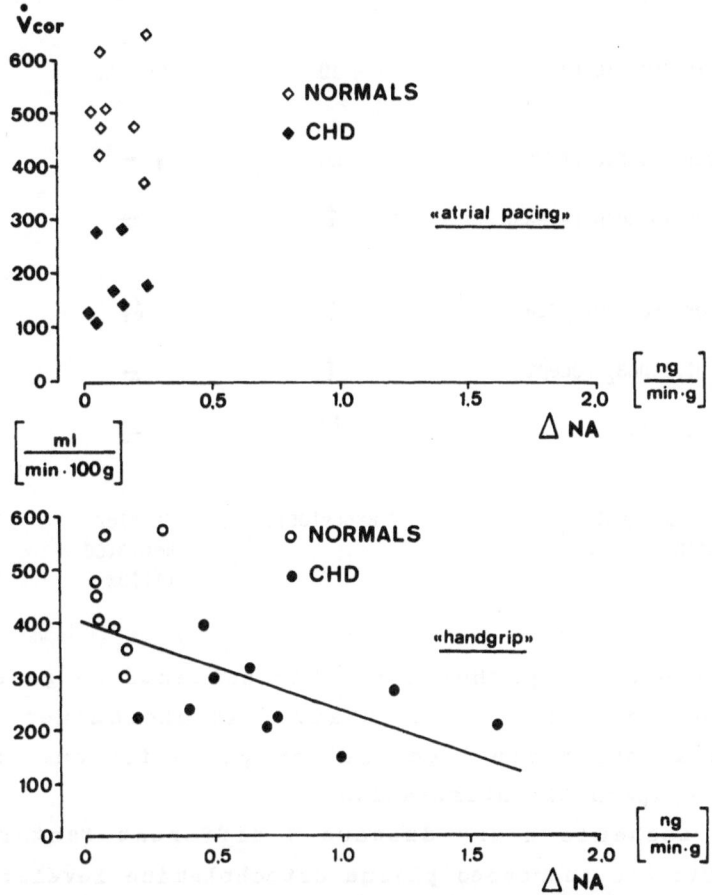

During the IIIrd and last phase beyond 40 min of ischemia in the rat heart, noradrenaline release is greatly augmented but not affected by neuronal uptake blockers. Leakage due to membrane damage can be assumed as the predominant release process.

II. CLINICAL STUDIES

In patients with ischemic heart disease the situation is even more complex. Neither local catecholamine concentrations at the cardiac receptor site nor cardiac sympathetic nerve stimulation can be measured. The

Table 1: Phases of cardiac catecholamine release during different periods of ischemia

	Phase 1	Phase 2	Phase 3
time of ischemia (min)	- 10	15 - 40	40 -
spontaneous release of NA	=	↑ - ↑↑	↑↑↑
stimulation induced release	↑	=	
blockade of neuronal uptake	↑	↓↓	=
blockade of alpha$_2$ receptors	↑	=	
local anesthetics	↓↓	=	
predominant mechanism of noradrenaline release	exocytosis	carrier mediated efflux	leakage

evaluation of sympathetic tone in patients is generally based on the evaluation of plasma catecholamines. Their concentrations reflect general sympathetic tone but not cardiac sympathetic stimulation.

In ischemic heart disease 4 different factors may contribute to increased plasma catecholamine levels:
1) Emotional factors
2) Hemodynamic factors
3) Metabolic factors
4) Therapeutic factors

1) EMOTIONAL FACTORS: Anxiety, fear, and pain may induce sympathetic overactivity. These factors are difficult to be quantitated in individual patients and may never reach a steady state under clinical conditions as they are influenced by therapeutics, such as e. g. morphine and/or antianginal drugs.

Table 2:   Summary of the data in form of a working hypothesis.

Catecholamine Release		Anginal Attack		Infarcting Myocardium		
		transient (PTCA)	severe	reversible (intervention)	irreversible damage	ischemic cardiomyop.
Experiment. Mechanisms (local)	Exocytosis	+	+			
	Carrier med.		+	+		
	Leakage				+	
Clinical Factors (Plasma levels)	Emotional	?	+	+	+	
	Hemodyn.		(+)	(+)	+	+
	Metabolic	?	+	+	+	
	Therapeutic			+		

2) HEMODYNAMIC FACTORS: Due to previous myocardial necrosis in many patients with ischemic heart disease left ventricular (LV) function is markedly impaired. This leads likewise to increased plasma catecholamine levels.

Different animal models of heart failure reveal increased catecholamine overflow due to marked reduction in neuronal reuptake in the heart (9,10). Also in patients cardiac catecholamine net uptake or net release can be quantitated by simultaneous determination of coronary blood flow - using the argon method - and of arterio-coronaryvenous differences of noradrenaline. In patients with severely impaired LV function noradrenaline uptake is markedly reduced as can be seen from the example given in Fig 1. In Fig. 2 the data obtained in controls and in patients with severely impaired LV function are summarized, a significant reduction in cardiac noradrenaline uptake is seen in the patients' group.

In patients with impaired LV- function increased

plasma catecholamine levels are most likely more related to peripheral underperfusion than to depressed LV- function itself. Plasma noradrenaline levels show no strong inverse relationship to LV ejection fraction but a rather good correlation to reduced cardiac index. The same holds true for adrenaline.

3) METABOLIC FACTORS: For the diagnosis of ischemic heart disease stress tests are often applied. These, too, modulate cardiac catecholamine release. As can be seen from the results presented in Fig. 3 atrial pacing stress test up to a heart rate of 120 beats/min does not significantly influence cardiac catecholamine release in patients with coronary heart disease compared to the controls. Isometric stress by handgrip, however, augments cardiac noradrenaline overflow in the patients' group. There is a negative correlation between maximal coronary blood flow and noradrenaline release: the more reduced the maximal coronary blood flow, the higher the noradrenaline release. These studies, however, do not allow firm conclusions concerning the trigger mechanisms, e. g. ischemia and/or reflexes.

Reversible acute myocardial ischemia is induced in patients during percutaneous transluminal coronary angioplasty (PTCA) when a coronary stenosis is dilated by insufflation of a balloon catheter. Preliminary data of our group indicate that during this rather short occlusion period of 20 - 40 sec no net release of noradrenaline can be observed. This finding is in agreement with the results obtained in animal experiments (see paragraph I).

4) THERAPEUTIC FACTORS: It is well known that antianginal drugs modulate directly, or more often indirectly sympathetic tone. Apart from these pharmacological effects other factors are operating too.

The most promising approach to infarct limitation is

from a theoretical and probably also from a practical point
of view early reperfusion to reestablish blood supply and
oxygen availability. After succesful reperfusion the plasma
catecholamine levels show distinct changes: Whereas those
patients without succesful reperfusion reveal markedly
elelvated plasma noradrenaline levels for the first 20 hrs
after onset of symptoms, patients with succesful
reperfusion show a pronounced decrease in the previously
elevated noradrenaline levels after myocardial blood supply
has been reestablished. The same holds true for adrenaline.
The data reveal that after succesful reperfusion sympathoneuronal and sympathoadrenal activities are markedly
attenuated. This can hardly exclusively be explained by
improvement of cardiac performance and of peripheral
circulation. Other mechanisms, mainly reflexes originating
from the ischemic area have to be assumed to be operating
too. In essence the marked attenuation of the increased
sympathoneuronal and sympathoadrenal activities reveal that
succesful reperfusion may have additional beneficial
effects apart from wash out of ischemic metabolites and of
restauration of oxygen availability.

IN CONCLUSION:
    In Table 2 the data are summarized in form of a
working hypothesis.
    During short periods of transient ischemia, e. g.
during PTCA, lasting only for 20 - 40 sec exocytosis as the
main mechanism of cardiac catecholamine release is
maintained.
    During a severe anginal attack lasting for more than
10 min apart from exocytosis carrier mediated efflux can be
assumed to be operating locally in the ischemic area. The
rise in plasma catecholamines is mainly related to
emotional and metabolic factors and most likely to
hemodynamic factors too.
    Infarcting myocardium is generally caused by coronary

thrombosis; this can be derived from the results of thrombolytic therapy in acute myocardial infarction. During reversible damage, e. g. due to very early reperfusion, carrier mediated efflux has to be assumed as the predominant mechanism of local catecholamine release. Plasma catecholamine levels are not only influenced by emotional, hemodynamic and metabolic factors, but also by the therapeutic intervention itself probably mediated by reflexes.

In myocardial infarction with irreversible damage leakage is the ultimate mechanism of local catecholamine release. Plasma catecholamine levels are influenced by emotional, hemodynamic and metabolic factors.

Lastly, in ischemic cardiomyopathy, i. e. in severely impaired cardiac function due to extended previous myocardial infarctions increased plasma catecholamine levels are mainly caused by hemodynamic factors related to reduced neuronal uptake and to peripheral underperfusion.

These studies were supported by a grant from the Deutsche Forschungsgemeinschaft within the SFB 320, Herzfunktion und ihre Regulation, University of Heidelberg.

REFERENCES:

1. Sakai, K. and Spieckermann, P. G. Effects of reserpine and propranolol on anoxia induced enzyme release from the isolated perfused guinea pig heart. Naunyn Schmiedebergs Arch. Pharmacol. 291: 123- 130, 1975.

2. Corr, P. B. and Gillis, R. A. Autonomic neural influences on the dysrhythmias resulting from myocardial infarction. Circ. Res. 43: 1- 9, 1978.

3. Dietz, R., Schömig, A., Strasser, R. and Kübler, W. Catecholamines in myocardial hypoxia and ischemia. In: Catecholamines and the Heart (Eds. Delius, W., Gerlach, E., Grobecker, H. and Kübler, W.), Springer Verlag, Berlin, Heidelberg, New York, 1981, pp. 201- 208.

4. Schömig, A., Dietz, R., Strasser, R., Dart, A. M. and Kübler W. Noradrenaline release and inactivation in myocardial ischemia. In: Advances in Studies on Heart Metabolism (Eds. Calderera, C. M. and Harris, P.), CLUEB, Bologna, 1982, pp. 239 - 244.

5. Schömig, A., Dart, A. M., Dietz, R., Mayer, E. and Kübler W. Release of endogenous catecholamines in the ischemic myocardium of the rat. Locally mediated release. Circ. Res. 55: 689 - 701, 1984.

6. Schömig, A., Dart, A. M., Dietz, R., Kübler, W. and Mayer, E. Paradoxical role of neuronal uptake for the locally mediated release of endogenous noradrenaline in the ischemic myocardium. J. Cardiovasc. Pharmacol. 7: 40 - 44, 1985.

7. Dart, A. M., Schömig, A., Dietz, R., Mayer, E. and Kübler, W. Release of endogenous catecholamines in the ischemic myocardium of the rat. Effect of sympathetic nerve stimulation. Circ. Res. 55: 702 - 706, 1984.

8. Mäurer, W., Tschada, R., Manthey, J., Ablasser, A. and Kübler, W. Catecholamines in patients with heart failure. In: Catecholamines and the Heart (Eds. Delius, W., Gerlach, E., Grobecker, H. and Kübler W.), Springer Verlag, Berlin, Heidelberg, New York, 1981, pp. 417 - 428.

9. Dietz, R., Schömig, A., Strasser, R., Mäurer, W., Manthey, J. and Kübler W. Humoral adaptation mechanisms in heart failure. In: Congestive Cardiomyopathy (Eds. Goodwin, J. F., Hjalmarson, A. and Olsen E. G. J.), Mölndal, Sweden, 1981, pp. 128 - 137.

10. Kübler, W., Dietz, R., Mäurer, W. and Schömig, A. Metabolic aspects of compensatory mechanisms in cardiac failure. In: Cardiac Glycosides 1785- 1985 (Eds. Erdmann, E., Greeff, K. and Skou, J. C.), Steinkopff Verlag, Darmstadt, Springer Verlag, New York, 1986, pp. 417- 428.

11. Schömig, A., Ness, G., Mayer, E., Katus, H. and Dietz, R. Sympathetic activity in patients with acute myocardial infarction before and after intracoronary thrombolytic therapy. Eur. Heart J. 5: 39 A 144, 1984.

12

CORONARY BLOOD FLOW IN MYOCARDIAL STRESS WITH CATECHOLAMINE ADMINISTRATION
IN THE DOG

R.M. BERNE, J.M. GIDDAY, H.E. HILL, R. RUBIO

Department of Physiology, University of Virginia School of Medicine,
Charlottesville, Virginia 22908 U.S.A.

INTRODUCTION

When the oxygen supply to the myocardium is inadequate for its needs,
adenosine formation and release as well as coronary blood flow increase(1).
This holds true whether oxygen supply is reduced or oxygen demand is
increased. Furthermore, adenosine release and coronary blood flow
correlate well over a wide range of cardiac metabolic activity (2).
With use of an adenosine uptake blocker (dipyridamole) adenosine release
and coronary blood flow still show good correlation but both variables
become independent of myocardial oxygen consumption (3).

One of the chief problems with these studies has been the inability
to determine the periarteriolar concentration of adenosine. Crude
estimates of the interstitial fluid concentrations have been made by
sampling tissue, venous effluents, cardiac lymph and pericardial infusates
(fluid injected into the pericardial sac and left in contact with the heart
for fixed periods of time during control and experimental conditions).
However, all of these methods have serious drawbacks.

RESULTS AND DISCUSSION

Recently, we have devised a method which appears to provide a
reasonable measure of myocardial interstitial fluid adenosine levels in
the dog heart (4). A round plastic chamber (either 1 cm^2 or 2 cm^2) is
placed on the epicardial surface of the left ventricle of the open chest
dog and held in position with four radial sutures. A fluid-tight seal is
made with a thin layer of silicone grease and 100 µl or 200 µl of Krebs-
Henseleit solution are placed in the 1 cm^2 or 2 cm^2 chambers, respectively.
The average depth of the fluid in the chamber is 1 mm and it is continuously
stirred by the movements of the beating heart. Removal and analysis of
the chamber fluid for adenosine after different contact times with the

epicardial surface of the heart revealed a rapid increase in the adenosine
concentration in the first 4 to 6 minutes. Thereafter, the adenosine
levels remained constant as long as measured (over 1 hour). In most
experiments adenosine was measured by HPLC alone, but when adenosine levels
were very low we combined HPLC with enzymatic conversion of adenosine to
uric acid and quantified the uric acid by electrochemical detection (5).

Cardiac stress was imposed by intravenous infusion of catecholamines.
In pentobarbital-anesthetized open chest dogs, the parietal pericardium
was opened and served as a cradle for the heart. In the first series of
experiments in which dobutamine (10 µg/kg/min) was infused, the control
chamber adenosine concentrations averaged 83 pmoles/ml and increased
significantly with dobutamine administration (Table 1). The change in
dP/dt served as an index of myocardial oxygen consumption and showed a
greater than threefold increase with dobutamine. Chamber adenosine levels
and dP/dt returned to control levels after cessation of the dobutamine
infusion (4).

A second series of experiments was carried out with the same procedure
except that norepinephrine (0.1 µg/kg/min) was given intravenously and
left anterior descendens coronary blood flow was measured (6). Myocardial
adenosine release and coronary blood flow were augmented to approximately
the same degree by norepinephrine and returned to control levels when the
infusion was discontinued (Table 2).

The results of these experiments are consonant with a role for
adenosine in the regulation of coronary blood flow in cardiac stress
produced by catecholamine administration. To what extent chamber adenosine
concentrations reflect myocardial interstitial fluid concentrations is
unknown. However, the facts that 1) adenosine levels reach a plateau in
4-6 minutes irrespective of the metabolic activity of the heart and 2)
the visceral pericardium does not constitute a diffusion barrier (as judged
from the observation that the rate of disappearance of ^{3}H-sucrose is the
same in the presence or absence of the visceral pericardium) support the
concept that chamber adenosine concentrations come into equilibrium with
the myocardial interstitial fluid, at least in the region of the
epicardium.

Table 1. Effect of Dobutamine on dP/dt and Adenosine Release from the Epicardial Surface of the Left Ventricle of the Dog Heart.

Dog #	RATE OF VENTRICULAR PRESSURE DEVELOPMENT (dP/dt) mm Hg/sec			CHAMBER ADENOSINE AT EQUILIBRIUM pmoles/ml		
	Control	Dobutamine	Recovery	Control	Dobutamine	Recovery
1	-	-	-	96	181	72
2	1939	7215	1587	106	185	63
3	1429	8063	1683	82	136	73
4	5016	12024	3016	66	247	93
5	1968	7682	1711	68	185	71
6	1936	10793	1904	79	124	75
Mean±S.E.	2458	9155	1980	82.8±6.4	176.3±17.8	74.5±4.0

Table 2. Effect of Norepinephrine on Coronary Blood Flow and Adenosine Release from the Epicardial Surface of the Left Ventricle of the Dog Heart.

Dog #	CORONARY BLOOD FLOW ml/min/100 g			CHAMBER ADENOSINE AT EQUILIBRIUM pmoles/ml		
	Control	Norepi-nephrine	Recovery	Control	Norepi-nephrine	Recovery
1	57	103	50	36	109	27
2	16	31	14	48	129	51
3	48	102	44	84	172	138
4	32	64	31	35	163	73
5	24	105	21	88	329	120
6	16	44	16	39	117	34
7	23	74	21	53	121	43
Mean±S.E.	31±6	75±11	28±5	55±8	163±29	69±16

SUMMARY

Intravenous administration of catecholamines produce increases in dP/dt, coronary blood flow and adenosine release from the epicardial surface of the left ventricle of the dog.

REFERENCES

1. Berne, R.M. Circ. Res. 47:807-813, 1980.
2. Knabb, R.M., Ely, S.W., Bacchus, A.N., Rubio, R. and Berne, R.M. Circ. Res. 53:33-41, 1983.
3. Knabb, R., Gidday, J.M., Ely, S.W., Rubio, R. and Berne, R.M. Am. J. Physiol. 247:H804-H810, 1984.
4. Gidday, J.M., Van Cleeff, S., Rubio, R. and Berne, R.M. The Physiologist 28:340, 1985.
5. Berne, R.M., Curnish, R.R., Gidday, J.M. and Rubio, R. J. Liquid Chromatography 9:113-119, 1986.
6. Hill, H.E., Gidday, J.M., Rubio, R. and Berne, R.M. Federation Proc. 45: 533, 1986.

13

MORPHOMETRIC ANALYSIS OF REGIONAL MYOCARDIAL PERFUSION IN RATS AS MEASURED
BY NON-RADIOACTIVE MICROSPHERES

M. KORPAN AND K. RAKUSAN

Department of Physiology, University of Ottawa, Ottawa, Canada K1H 8M5

INTRODUCTION

The radioactive microsphere technique is the most accurate method
currently available for measuring regional myocardial perfusion in
experimental animals. It is based on the principle that microspheres
distribute in proportion to regional myocardial blood flow if the basic
criteria of the technique are satisfied (1). However, this assumption is
not substantiated since microsphere distribution is determined indirectly
from measurements of tissue radioactivity. Furthermore, the use of
relatively large tissue samples for accurate measurements decreases
spatial resolution and, therefore, prevents studies of regional myocardial
perfusion in smaller animals.

These limitations may be overcome with the use of carbonized non-
radioactive polysterene microspheres. Unlabelled spheres have previously
been used in rats to measure single glomerular blood flow (2), and blood
flow distribution within skeletal muscle (3) and ventricular myocardium
(4). Methods using non-radioactive microspheres have also been developed
which permit the quantification of total organ blood flow (5, 6).
Unlabelled spheres have the advantage of being visually detected in
histological preparations, making such measurements possible. Additional
problems associated with a radioactive label (e.g. radiation hazards,
radioactivity leaching into the suspending medium, energy overlap between
different labels, accurate determination of the total number of microspheres injected, and reference sample withdrawal) are also eliminated.

In this report we describe a morphometric technique using non-
radioactive microspheres to determine regional myocardial blood flow
distribution with a high degree of spatial resolution in anesthetized
rats. Particular consideration was made to the effect of injection site
and the number of microspheres injected on microsphere aggregation.

METHODS

Two experimental series were carried out. In the first series, non-radioactive microspheres were injected either into the left ventricle (n=10) or the left atrium (n=10). In both groups, a large percentage of microsphere aggregates was found, and shown to distort estimates of myocardial blood flow distribution. This may have resulted from injection of a very large number of spheres. Thus, the occurence of aggregation following left atrial injection of a standard number of spheres (approximately the median of the values reported for studies on rats) was the basis for the second experimental series (n=6).

Animal Preparation.

Sprague-Dawley rats weighing 230-494 g were anesthetized with sodium pentobarbital (45 mg/kg, i.p.). Anesthesia was maintained throughout the experimental procedure with supplementary doses as required.

For left ventricular injection, a smooth-tipped polyethylene cannula (PE-10), stabilized by a metal stylet, was inserted into the right carotid artery, and advanced into the left ventricular cavity. The metal stylet was then removed, and the cannula flushed with 0.2 ml of heparinized saline (12.5 mg%).

For left atrial injection, Wicker and Tarazi's (7) method of left atrial catheterization in anesthetized rats was used, with moderate modifications. The rats were catheterized via a tracheostomy and ventilated with room air. Following palpation, the left atrium was exposed by small lateral thoracotomy and gently supported with forceps. A bevel-tipped, balloon-tipped polyethylene cannula (PE-10), stabilized by a metal stylet, was inserted into the left atrium by puncture. The metal stylet was removed, and the cannula flushed with 0.2 ml of heparinized saline (12.5 mg%). The chest wall was then closed, taking care not to disturb the protruding cannula, as quick turns of the cannula can result in obstruction of its tip, or in complete displacement. The lungs were then expanded by positive pressure, and the animal disconnected from the respirator.

Following cannulation, a minute volume of blood was withdrawn into the cannula to ascertain a properly positioned and unobstructed tip, and immediately replaced (this verification process was repeated prior to, and intermittently during, microsphere injection). Proper placement of the cannula was further verified at necropsy.

Preparation and Injection of Microspheres.

Non-radioactive, carbonized, plastic microspheres (9.3 ± 0.4 μm in diameter) were obtained from New England Nuclear (Boston, MA) suspended in 0.9% saline and 0.01% Tween 80. In the first experimental series, approximately 5×10^6 microspheres suspended in 1.0 ml of saline were injected over 1 min, and the cannula was flushed with 1.0 ml of saline over the following minute. Immediately prior to injection, the microsphere suspension was vortexed for 5 min, and then ultrasonicated for 45-60 min to disperse microsphere aggregates. In the second series, microspheres were mixed, injected, and flushed according to the protocol developed by Flaim et al. (8). Approximately 1.5×10^5 microspheres suspended in 0.5 ml of saline were injected over 15 sec, and flushed in with 1.0 ml of saline over the next 15 sec. Immediately prior to injection, the microsphere suspension was vortexed for 5 sec, and then ultrasonicated for 30 sec. In both series, care was taken to execute the injections in a smooth and consistent manner.

Five min following injection, the hearts were arrested by an intra-arterial injection of saturated KCl and excised. The apex and base were removed. The remaining tissue was then rapidly frozen in liquid N_2, and placed in a cryostat (IEC Minotome Microtome-Cryostat) for equilibration at -18° to -20°C for 30-60 min.

Morphometric Analysis.

The sampling technique for the first experimental series is shown in Fig. 1. Four transverse sections of 16 μm thickness were obtained non-sequentially from the midventricular level (Fig. 1i), fixed (5% acetic acid, 95% absolute alcohol) for 1 min, and stained with periodic acid-Schiff. Each section was then projected from a distance of 3.3 m onto a vertical surface. Three regions of the left ventricular free wall (anterior, lateral, and posterior) were sampled per section (Fig. 1ii). A plastic measuring device was placed along each sampling site to count concurrently the number of muscle fibers across the wall and the number of microspheres within a 10 cm wide range, which corresponds to approximately 850 μm of myocardial tissue. Two data sets were compiled for each sampling site. For one data set all the microspheres counted, whether they occurred singly or as aggregates, were recorded, with the assumption that aggregation was due to random distribution of single spheres within the capillaries. For the second data set each aggregate was counted as

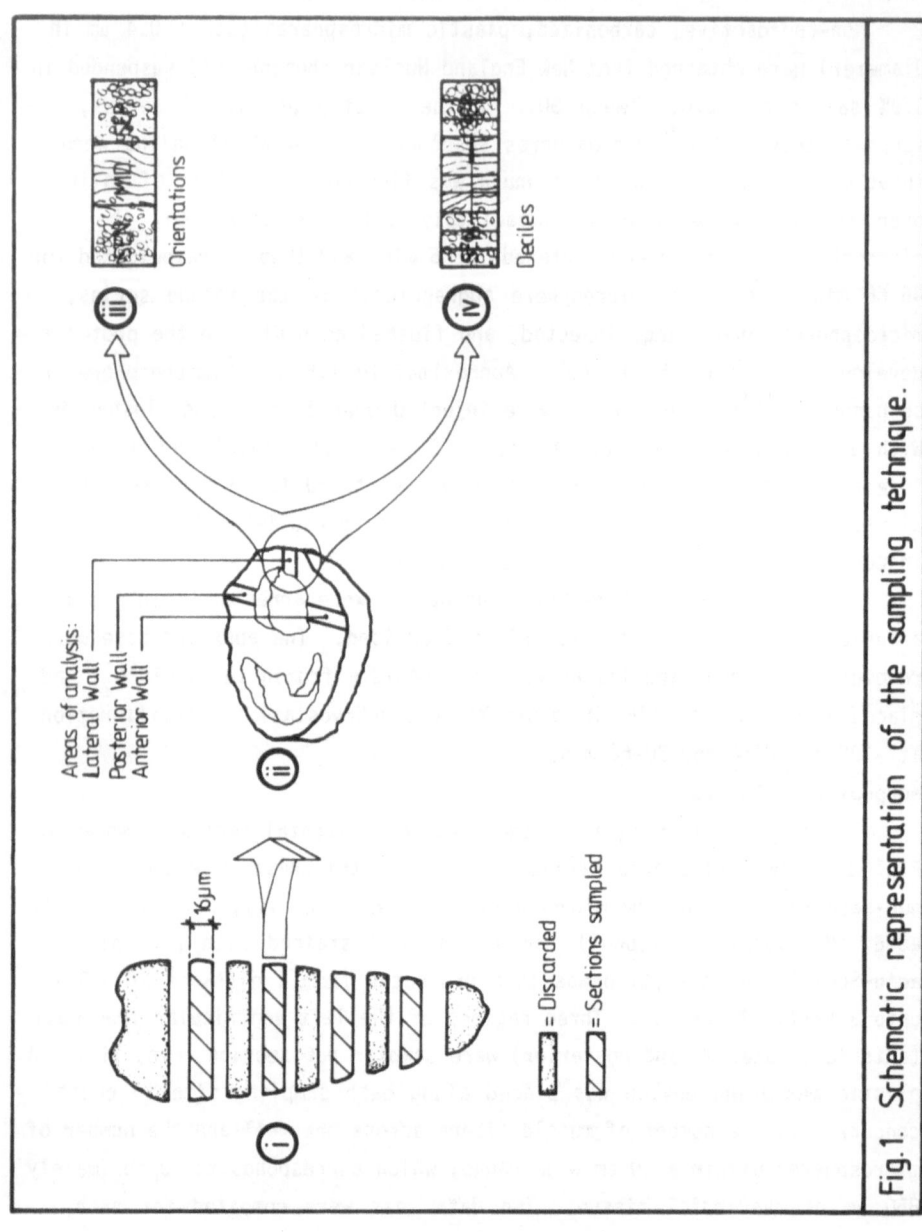

Fig.1. Schematic representation of the sampling technique.

1 microsphere, with the assumption that it entered the capillary as an aggregate due to inadequate mixing either prior to, or following injection.

Transmural myocardial blood flow distribution was expressed by the number of microspheres in subendocardial (SEN), midwall (MID), and subepicardial (SEP) layers divided according to muscle fiber orientation (Fig. 1iii), and by the number of microspheres in deciles of the wall thickness according to the total number of layers (Fig. 1iv). Afterwards, two corresponding SEN/SEP ratios were calculated for each sampling site. First, a SEN/SEP ratio was determined from the distribution of microspheres in SEN and SEP layers divided according to orientation. A second type of SEN/SEP ratio was determined from the distribution of microspheres in 2 equal zones of the left ventricular wall thickness divided according to the total number of layers, with the inner half representing the SEN and the outer half representing the SEP.

For the second experimental series, the ventricular myocardium was cut transversely into 20 μm thick sections. Every fourth section was fixed and stained as previously described. Each of 45 serial sections per heart was then projected onto a vertical surface, and the number of microspheres located singly and as aggregates in SEN, MID, and SEP layers of the left ventricle (free wall + septum) was counted. Due to the time factor involved, the number of muscle fiber layers across the left ventricular wall was not determined and, therefore, microsphere distribution in deciles of the wall thickness was not evaluated.

Data were analyzed using split-plot factorial analysis of variance (9). Variances were compared by the Levine test. The criterion for statistical significance was $p < 0.05$. Measured parameters were then averaged for animals in each group. All data were calculated from these averaged values and expressed as Mean ± SEM.

RESULTS
Effect of injection site on microsphere distribution in the left ventricular wall.

The adequacy of mixing of microspheres injected into the left ventricle or the left atrium may be determined from the data presented in Fig. 2. The average number of microspheres per decile of the left ventricular wall thickness was higher following left ventricular injection

compared with left atrial injection, although the total number of microspheres injected was similar for both injection sites. Body weights
between the 2 groups of animals were also similar (302 ± 55 g (Mean ± SD),
left ventricular injection; 342 ± 86 g (Mean ± SD), left atrial
injection). It is, therefore, assumed that heart weights were comparable.

The difference in the number of microspheres was more pronounced when
all the microspheres per aggregate were counted. This may be attributed
to the significantly greater degree of microsphere aggregation with left
ventricular injection (33%) than with left atrial injection (24%).
However, both injection sites were associated with a significant degree of
aggregation.

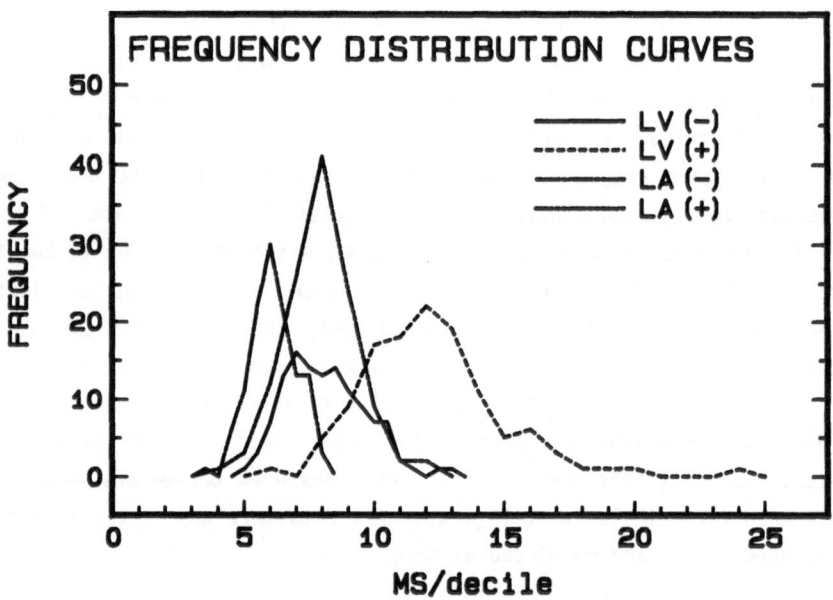

Fig. 2. Variation in the distribution of the number of microspheres per
decile of the left ventricular wall thickness in animals receiving left
ventricular or left atrial microsphere injection.
LV = left ventricular injection; LA = left atrial injection; (-) = each
aggregate was counted as 1 microsphere; (+) = all microspheres per
aggregate were counted; MS = microspheres.

Variability in the data was also significantly greater with left ventricular injection than with left atrial injection. For either site of injection, variability was highest when all microspheres per aggregate were counted. The coefficients of variation (i.e., the SD expressed as the percentage of the mean) for left ventricular and left atrial injection, respectively, were 18.5% and 14.8% when microsphere aggregates were counted as single spheres, and 22.3% and 16.3% when all microspheres per aggregate were counted.

The effect of injection site on microsphere distribution in deciles of the left ventricular wall thickness is presented in Fig. 3 (upper panel). When all microspheres were counted, minor transmural inequalities of microsphere distribution were observed following left atrial injection, but these were not statistically significant (SEN/SEP = 1.09 ± 0.04). With left ventricular injection, the pattern of microsphere distribution approximated a sine wave; microspheres were predominant in the subendocardium, with a slight decrease in the number of spheres in the deepest subendocardial layer, and were present in the least amount in the subepicardium, with a slight increase in the outermost subepicardial layer. However, significant differences were not indicated, probably due to the large variability in measurements in the deepest subendocardial layers. On the other hand, the SEN/SEP ratio calculated from these data (1.29 ± 0.06) was significantly higher than for left atrial injection, indicating relative subendocardial overperfusion.

When microsphere aggregates were counted as single spheres, transmural microsphere distribution was uniform following both left ventricular (SEN/SEP = 1.17 ± 0.05) and left atrial (SEN/SEP = 1.06 ± 0.07) injection. Thus, the proportion of microspheres present as aggregates was highest in the subendocardial layers and decreased gradually towards the subepicardium, as shown in Fig. 3 (lower panel). The decrease was more pronounced following left ventricular injection (r = -0.93; slope of regression line = -1.03) than with left atrial injection (r = -0.72; slope of regression line = -0.71).

Similar results were obtained when transmural microsphere distribution was measured in subendocardial, midwall, and subepicardial layers of the left ventricular wall divided according to muscle fiber orientation. SEN/SEP ratios for left ventricular and left atrial injection, respectively, were 1.49 ± 0.15 and 1.06 ± 0.08 when all microspheres per aggregate were counted, and 1.19 ± 0.09 and 0.98 ± 0.05 when microsphere aggregates were counted as single spheres.

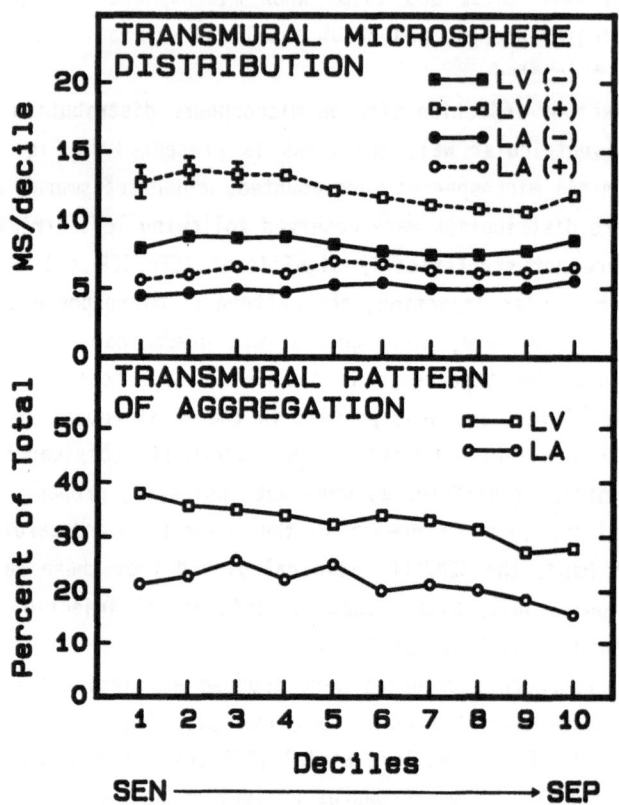

Fig. 3. Upper panel: The effect of injection site on microsphere distribution in deciles of the left ventricular wall thickness. Mean ± SEM. Lower panel: Percentage of the total number of microspheres per decile present as aggregates. Data were calculated from mean values shown in the upper panel. LV = left ventricular injection; LA = left atrial injection; (-) = each aggregate was counted as 1 microsphere; (+) = all microspheres per aggregate were counted; MS = microspheres; SEN = subendocardium; SEP = subepicardium.

Effect of injection of a standard number of microspheres on microsphere aggregation

Of the total number of microspheres counted, 93.1% were found as individual spheres, and 6.9% (maximum 9.1%) were present as aggregates. Most aggregates consisted of two spheres (83.8%), but aggregates of up to a maximum of 6 spheres were also observed.

There were no statistically significant differences between the distribution of microspheres located singly or as aggregates among the 45 transverse sections. However, the transmural distribution of single spheres was slightly, but significantly, different from that of microsphere aggregates. Of the total number of microspheres present in each muscle fiber orientation, aggregation was highest in the subendocardium (7.2%) as compared to the midwall (6.8%) and subepicardium (6.7%). Regardless, the relative error imposed is small, since the subendocardial/subepicardial ratio is not altered when aggregates are included in the calculation (SEN/SEP = 1.34).

DISCUSSION

A method to determine the regional distribution of non-radioactive microspheres in rat myocardium has been proposed by Vetterlein (10). This method involves counting and mapping of unlabelled spheres in various planes of 1 mm thick tissue sections made transparent with sodium hydroxide. Although a high spatial resolution can be achieved, the pattern of microsphere distribution cannot be related to the myocardial morphology. This may be limiting, especially when measuring regional myocardial perfusion under conditions in which the myocardial morphology is altered (e.g. hypertrophy, infarction). Furthermore, the tissue thickness necessitates constant focussing and refocussing of microspheres in the various planes. Data collection may, therefore, be subject to error. Vetterlein (10) did not report quantitative data on regional microsphere distribution, and we are not aware of any subsequent use of this technique. Therefore, the present morphometric method was developed to accurately measure regional myocardial perfusion in rats by ensuring that the structural integrity of the myocardium was maintained, and that other potential sources for error were eliminated.

To minimize the variability related to random microsphere distribution, it was necessary to inject a very large number of spheres.

Accurate determination of myocardial blood flow distribution also requires that microspheres be completely mixed with the blood before entering the coronary circulation. An injection site most distal to the first arterial branching theoretically should result in the most adequate mixing. Wicker and Tarazi (7, 11) have shown that microspheres injected into the left ventricle are inadequately mixed, based on their finding that coronary blood flow determinations in rats are significantly less variable with left atrial injection compared with left ventricular injection. However, this finding has not been universally accepted (e.g. 8). Since the above observations were based on measurements of tissue radioactivity, we reassessed the effect of injection site on microsphere distribution.

The present results confirm that microspheres injected into the left atrium are more uniformly distributed in the aortic root, resulting in more accurate determination of regional myocardial blood flow distribution. Inadequate mixing with left ventricular injection is indicated by 1) the greater delivery of microspheres to the coronary circulation, 2) the greater variability in the number of microspheres per unit of tissue, and 3) the greater degree of microsphere aggregation, with preferential location of aggregates in the subendocardium.

Preferential streaming of a large number of microspheres due to inadequate mixing may in part explain why mean values of coronary blood flow are generally higher with left ventricular injection compared with left atrial injection (11, 12), especially at fast injection rates (13). The greater interaction between microspheres at higher concentrations (14) would also increase the percentage of the microspheres injected entering the coronary circulation as aggregates. Microspheres aggregates, in turn, would preferentially lodge in the subendocardial layers due to axial streaming, resulting in overestimation of subendocardial flow. Aggregation due to random distribution of single spheres within the coronary vasculature also increases with increasing numbers of microspheres entering the coronary circulation (15). This would, at least in part, account for the significantly higher degree of aggregation across the left ventricular wall following left ventricular injection. Single spheres lodged in very close proximity at the ostia of branching vessels may also appear as aggregates in cross-section (16). Although it is not possible to distinguish the cause of microsphere aggregation following left ventricular injection with the present technique, it is probable that all of these factors are involved, and result in overestimation of coronary blood flow.

It has been suggested that the catheter position, rather than the injection site, is the critical factor influencing the degree of mixing of microspheres in anesthetized rats (12). However, the relatively large diameter catheter used for left ventricular injection in the above study may have modified the pattern of blood flow in the aortic root to some degree, resulting in more variable streaming of microspheres. Smaller catheters, as used in the present study, appear to have a negligible effect on microsphere streaming; variability in coronary blood flow measurements following left atrial injection is unaltered when a second catheter is placed in the left ventricle via the right carotid artery (17).

Although mixing of microspheres following left ventricular injection was shown to be inadequate for accurate measurements of regional myocardial perfusion, the significant degree of aggregation observed following left atrial injection of a large number of spheres was also more pronounced in the subendocardial layers. It may be inferred that left atrial injection also results in incomplete mixing of microspheres in the aortic root. Alternatively, the uneven distribution of microsphere aggregates could result from myocardial blood flow alterations which may occur secondary to injection of a large number of spheres in rats (13, 18, 19). Therefore, we examined the transmural distribution of aggregates following an injection protocol generally used for myocardial blood flow determinations in rats with the radioactive microsphere technique. Although the percentage of microspheres present as aggregates was significantly lower with this injection, suggesting that the occurrence of aggregation with left atrial injection is largely due to the interaction of single spheres within the coronary vessels, the uneven pattern of aggregation still persisted. These results indicate that left atrial injection of up to 5×10^6 microspheres causes no significant changes in regional myocardial flows. This view is supported by a study (20) in which transmural myocardial blood flow distribution measured with radioactive microspheres remained unaltered following serial left atrial injections totalling 48×10^6 spheres in dogs. Thus, microspheres are not completely mixed when injected into the left atrium. However, this is significantly less pronounced compared with left ventricular injection.

In conclusion, estimates of myocardial blood flow distribution which are based on measurements of tissue radioactivity may be distorted by various degrees due to the uneven distribution of microsphere aggregates. The degree of error, which indicates the adequacy of mixing of micro- spheres with blood, was shown to depend on the site of microsphere injection. In addition, the occurrence of aggregates within the coronary vasculature and, thus, the probability of overestimating total myocardial blood flow values, also increases with increasing numbers of microspheres entering the coronary circulation. This was shown to be a function of both the injection site and the total number of microspheres injected. If a sufficient degree of aggregation occurs in the larger coronary vessels, total myocardial blood flow may actually be decreased. Thus, the results of the present study indicate that left ventricular injection of micro- spheres is unsuitable for determining myocardial blood flow and its transmural distribution. For more accurate measurements, left atrial injection is recommended. Furthermore, the number of microspheres injected should be minimized, while assuring delivery of an adequate number of microspheres to each tissue sample. However, this necessitates an increased number of experiments to compensate for the larger degree of variability associated with injecting less microspheres.

SUMMARY

We have developed a morphometric technique for measuring regional myocardial blood flow distribution with a high spatial resolution in rats. The technique involves injection of non-radioactive microspheres and subsequent sectioning of the tissue to be studied, allowing for direct visualization of microspheres and muscle fibers. Because microsphere aggregation has been shown to be a significant problem, and may alter both estimates of total myocardial blood flow and its transmural distribution, we evaluated the effect of injection site (left ventricle vs. left atrium) and the number of microspheres injected (5×10^6 vs. 1.5×10^5) on micro- sphere aggregation in the left ventricle of anesthetized rats. Aggregation varied around 28% following left ventricular or left atrial injection of the larger microsphere dose, and was more pronounced in the subendocardium, especially following left ventricular injection. With left atrial injection of the smaller microsphere dose, the degree of aggregation was significantly lower (7%), but the uneven distribution of aggregates persisted. These results suggest that the degree of aggregation and the transmural distribution of aggregates must be considered when interpreting data which are based on measurements of tissue radioactivity.

ACKNOWLEDGEMENTS

This work was supported by the Ontario Heart and Stroke Foundation.

REFERENCES

1. Heymann, M.A., Payne, B.D., Hoffman, J.I.E. and Rudolph, A.M. Prog. Cardiovasc. Dis. 20: 55-79, 1977.
2. Poujeol, P., Chabardès, D., Bonvalet, J.P. and de Rouffignac, C. Pflügers Arch. 357: 291-301, 1975.
3. Wisnes, A. and Kirkebo, A. Acta Physiol. Scand. 96: 256-266, 1976.
4. Vetterlein, F. and Schmidt, G. Basic Res. Cardiol. 75: 526-536, 1980.
5. Vetterlein, F., Halfter, R. and Schmidt, G. Arzneim.-Forsch. 29: 747-751, 1979.
6. Shell, W., Kligerman, M., Chang, B.-L., See, J., Meerbaum, S. and Corday, E. Circ. 72 (Supp. III): 191, 1985.
7. Wicker, P. and Tarazi, R.C. Am. J. Physiol. 242: H94-H97, 1982.
8. Flaim, S.F., Nellis, S.H., Toggart, E.J., Drexler, H., Kanda, K. and Newman, E.D. J. Pharmacol. Methods 11: 1-39, 1984.
9. Kirk, R.E. Experimental design: procedures for the behavioural sciences. 2nd ed. Brooks/Cole Pub. Co., Monterey, Calif., 1982.
10. Vetterlein, F. Basic Res. Cardiol. 70: 401-405, 1975.
11. Wicker, P. and Tarazi, R.C. Cardiovasc. Res. 16: 580-586, 1982.
12. Kobrin, I., Kardon, M.B., Oigman, W., Pegram, B.L. and Frohlich, E.D. Am. J. Physiol. 247: H35-H39, 1984.
13. Tuma, R.F., Vasthare, U.S., Irion, G.L. and Wiedeman, M.P. Am. J. Physiol. 250: H137-H143, 1986.
14. Phibbs, R.H. and Dong, L. Can. J. Physiol. Pharmacol. 48: 415-421, 1970.
15. Harell, G.S., Dickhoner, W.A. and Breiman, R.S. Microvasc. Res. 13: 203-210, 1977.
16. Eng, C., Cho, S., Factor, S.M., Sonnenblick, E.H. and Kirk, E.S. Circ. Res. 54: 74-82, 1984.
17. Wicker, P. Personal communication.
18. Stanek, K.A., Smith, T.L., Murphy, W.R. and Coleman, T.G. Am. J. Physiol. 245: H920-H923, 1983.
19. Tsuchiya, M., Walsh, G.M. and Frohlich, E.D. Am. J. Physiol. 233: H617-H621, 1977.
20. Baer, R.W., Payne, B.D., Verrier, E.D., Vlahakes, G.J., Molodowitch, D., Uhlig, P.N. and Hoffman, J.I.E. Am. J. Physiol. 246: H418-H434, 1984.

14

PROSTAGLANDINS AND DEFECTS IN VASCULAR FUNCTION

Dennis B. McNamara, John A. Bellan, Philip R. Mayeux, Morris D. Kerstein*,
Albert L. Hyman*, Philip J. Kadowitz and Daniel S. Rush*

Departments of Pharmacology and Surgery*, Tulane University School of
Medicine, New Orleans, Louisiana

INTRODUCTION

Atherosclerotic arterial lesions have been reported to exhibit
altered arachidonic acid metabolism (1-4). These alterations have
consistently involved decreases in arterial prostacyclin (prostaglandin
I_2 or PGI_2) synthesis; arterial thromboxane A_2 (TXA_2) formation (3)
and increased PGE_2 formation (2) have also been associated with atherosclerotic lesions. Conversely, it has been recently reported that total
urinary excretion of 2,3-dinor-6-keto-$PGF_{1\alpha}$, one of the metabolites of
PGI_2 produced in vivo, is higher in patients with severe atherosclerosis
than normal subjects (5). It was suggested that there was an increase
in PGI_2 formation due to stimulation of PGI_2 synthetase as there may be
increased platelet-endothelial interactions in patients with severe
atherosclerosis. The present study reports that there are graduated
decreases in human arterial PGI_2 synthetase activity within atherosclerotic plaque but that these decreases are focal, as the arterial
regions immediately adjacent to the plaque exhibit normal PGI_2 synthetase
activity.

MATERIALS AND METHODS

Atheromatous carotid plaques were removed from patients with
cerebrovascular insufficiency by standard carotid endarterectomy.
Carotid specimens were then dissected into the following fractions:
1) grossly nonatheromatous intimal surface adjacent (proximal and distal)
to the carotid plaque, 2) subintimal carotid plaque, 3) atherosclerotic
arterial surface overlying carotid plaque at the point of arterial
stenosis, and 4) any gross areas of ulceration overlying the carotid
plaque. Specimens of carotid artery from pig, Rhesus monkey, and
nonatherosclerotic human (brain-dead cadaver kidney donor) were used as

normal controls. In addition, human abdominal aortas were obtained from cadaver kidney donors, atherosclerotic aortas from patients undergoing arterial reconstruction for occlusive disease or abdominal aneurysm. The tissue was subdivided into regions as follows: nonatheromatous, pre-atherosclerotic (gross evidence of lipid deposition in vessel wall), plaque, and advanced plaque (complex areas of ulceration and stenosis). All vascular specimens were quickly immersed in ice-cold 0.1 M potassium phosphate buffer, pH 7.4, and either assayed immediately or stored at -45°C.

At the time of analysis, specimens were divided into the above fractions, blotted dry, and weighed while maintaining a temperature of 0 to 4°C. The specimens were then minced and homogenized in 10 volumes of cold phosphate buffer. Homogenate protein concentrations were determined using the Bio-Rad assay. Radiolabeled PG endoperoxide H_2 (^{14}C-PGH$_2$; 15,000 cpm) was prepared from radiolabeled arachidonic acid (^{14}C-AA) as previously reported (6).

Quantitative radiochromatography as previously reported was used to study PGH$_2$ metabolism (6). Reaction mixtures contained varying concentrations of tissue homogenate protein in 100 μl of 0.1 M potassium phosphate buffer, pH 7.4, with or without 2 mM reduced GSH. The reaction was initiated by addition of the reaction mixture to a cold (0°C) Brinkman centrifuge tube containing 10 μM ^{14}C-PGH$_2$ (previously evaporated to dryness under a stream of nitrogen). The tube was vortexed immediately and incubated for 2 min at 37°C. All incubations were conducted in duplicate. The reaction was stopped and PG products extracted by addition of 400 μl of an ice-cold solution of ethyl acetate:methanol:0.2 M citric acid, pH 2.0 (15:2:1). The reaction tubes were then vortexed, centrifuged at 12,000g for 30 sec, and quickly frozen on dry ice. The upper organic layer (containing 85% to 95% of the ^{14}C-radiolabel) was spotted for thin-layer chromatography (TLC) on Analtech silica gel GHL plates; PG products were separated with the solvent system, ethyl acetate:acetic acid:hexane:water (54:12:25:60, organic phase). PG products were identified by comparison with the migration of authentic PG standards on the TLC plate. PG standards were identified by exposing the plates to iodine vapor. Radiolabeled PG products were quantitated using a Packard 7201B radiochromatogram scanner mated to a computer.

Duplicate determinations were performed at each homogenate protein
concentration for the various tissue samples.

RESULTS

The data presented in Table 1 indicate that PGI_2 synthetase activity
(as determined by the stable product of hydrolysis of PGI_2, 6-keto-$PGF_{1\alpha}$)
is present in all regions of the carotid endarterectomy specimens. There
is a gradient in 6-keto-$PGF_{1\alpha}$ formation which correlates with atheromatous
development with the least amount formed in the region of ulceration.
The data further indicate that the PGI_2 synthetase activity of the
vascular wall immediately adjacent to the area of advanced plaque
formation is similar to that determined in nonatheromatous tissue from
pig, monkey, and man. Formation of 6-keto-$PGF_{1\alpha}$ was observed in both
the intimal and subintimal fractions of nonatherosclerotic human carotid
artery. This formation, however, was decreased in the vascular segment
that had been traumatized in vivo. The activity of human carotid
arterial PGI_2 synthetase is sensitive to GSH as indicated by an increased
formation of 6-keto-$PGF_{1\alpha}$ by all tissue fractions except the area of
ulceration of the plaque. No TXA_2 formation (determined by the absence
of the stable hydrolytic product of TXA_2, TXB_2) by any of the carotid
arterial fractions was detected.

The data presented in Table 2 show that in pig, human, or monkey
carotid arterial homogenates there is no increase in PGE_2 formation
when 2 mM GSH is included in the incubation medium. A similar absence
of an effect of GSH is observed in the fraction prepared from region
of plaque (subintimal plaque, intima from stenosis and intima from
ulceration, data not shown).

The data in Table 3 indicate that 6-keto-$PGF_{1\alpha}$ formation occurred
in all areas of both the intimal and subintimal regions of abdominal
aorta. The formation of 6-keto-$PGF_{1\alpha}$ by homogenates of the intimal
and subintimal regions is similar. There is, however, a gradient in
the 6-keto-$PGF_{1\alpha}$ formation that correlates with atheromatous development.
No TXB_2 formation was detected.

The effect of GSH on PGE_2 formation is presented in Table 4. The
data indicate that there is no increase in PGE_2 formation when 2 mM
GSH is in the incubation medium.

Table 1. Carotid arterial prostacyclin synthetase activity.

Specimen (n)	6-Keto-PGF$_{1\alpha}$	
	− GSH	+ 2 mM GSH
Pig (7)	190 ± 24	272 ± 25
Monkey (6)	176 ± 27	219 ± 41
Human*		
proximal intima (7,5)	219 ± 23	255 ± 30
distal intima (8,7)	207 ± 19	254 ± 17
subintimal plaque (10,9)	126 ± 12	165 ± 12
intima from stenosis (7)	136 ± 11	165 ± 15
intima from ulcer (3,3)	60 ± 18	73 ± 19
Human**		
intima (1)	268 ± 42	330 ± 40
subintima (1)	248 ± 38	346 ± 12
Human***		
intima (1)	44 ± 4	50 ± 5
subintima (1)	77 ± 3	132 ± 7

Conditions of incubation: 10 µM PGH$_2$, 100 µg homogenate protein, 37°C, pH 7.4, 2 min.

Data are expressed as picomoles of 6-keto-PGF$_{1\alpha}$ formed per 2 min and are presented as mean ± SEM.

n = number of donors

*carotid endarterectomy donors

**nonatherosclerotic carotid arterial tissue from a beating-heart cadaver donor; data are expressed as mean ± SEM of duplicate incubations.

***nonatherosclerotic carotid artery traumatized by gun wound to neck; data are expressed as mean ± SEM of duplicate incubations.

Table 2. Carotid arterial GSH-dependent $PGH_2 \rightarrow PGE_2$ isomerase activity.

Specimen (n)	PGE₂	
	− GSH	+ 2 mM GSH
Pig (7)	141 ± 11	152 ± 15
Monkey (6)	157 ± 22	173 ± 26
Human*		
proximal intima (7,5)	164 ± 8	145 ± 8
distal intima (8,7)	174 ± 12	146 ± 8
Human**		
intima (1)	180 ± 4	138 ± 6
subintima (1)	172 ± 6	150 ± 24

Conditions of incubation: 10 µM PGH_2, 100 µg of homogenate protein, 37°C, pH 7.4, 2 min, ± 2 mM GSH

Data are expressed as picomoles of PGE_2 formed per 2 min and are presented as mean ± SEM.

n = number of donors

*carotid endarterectomy donors

**nonatherosclerotic tissue from a beating-heart cadaver donor.

Table 3. Abdominal aortic intimal and subintimal prostacyclin synthetase activity.

Specimen (n)	Homogenate protein concentration (100 µg)	
	intimal	subintimal
Nonatheromatous (4,3)	121 ± 27	130 ± 15
Pre-atherosclerotic (2,2)	123 ± 20	116 ± 8
Early plaque (2,1)	87 ± 11	111 ± 21
Advanced plaque (1)	77 ± 15	84 ± 9

Conditions of incubation: 10 µM PGH_2, 37°C, pH 7.4, 2 min

Data are expressed as picomoles of 6-keto-$PGF_{1\alpha}$ formed per 2 min and are presented as mean ± SEM.

n = number of donors

Table 4. Abdominal aortic GSH-dependent $PGH_2 \rightarrow PGE_2$ isomerase activity.

Specimen (n)	PGE_2	
	- GSH	+ 2 mM GSH
Intima		
nonatheromatous (3)	192 ± 16	154 ± 20
pre-atherosclerotic (2)	197 ± 22	205 ± 14
early plaque (2)	226 ± 18	216 ± 6
advanced plaque (1)	220 ± 3	222 ± 8
Subintima		
nonatheromatous (3)	166 ± 56	174 ± 10
pre-atherosclerotic (2)	158 ± 22	241 ± 27
early plaque (2)	156 ± 13	190 ± 7
advanced plaque (1)	154 ± 9	244 ± 8

Conditions of incubation: 10 μM PGH_2, 100 μg of homogenate protein, pH 7.4, 37°C, 2 min, ± 2 mM GSH

Data are expressed as picomoles of 6-keto-$PGF_{1\alpha}$ formed per 2 min and are presented as mean ± SEM.

n = number of donors

DISCUSSION

The data obtained in this study indicate that there is an active PGI_2 synthetase in regions of atheromatous plaque in both the carotid artery and abdominal aorta. There is, however, a gradient in the activity of this enzyme with the most advanced areas of plaque forming significantly less 6-keto-$PGF_{1\alpha}$. The grossly nonatheromatous carotid arterial intima adjacent to the area of plaque demonstrated PGI_2 synthetase activity similar to that observed in pig, Rhesus monkey, and normal human carotid artery (beating-heart cadaver donor). In addition, the human abdominal aorta also exhibited a gradient in the activity of PGI_2 synthetase with the more advanced areas of plaque forming significantly less 6-keto-$PGF_{1\alpha}$. Thus, these data demonstrate that the decrease in PGI_2 formation associated with atherosclerosis is focal (localized to areas of atherosclerotic plaque) and not a generalized condition. Decreases in PGI_2 formation localized to the area of plaque might favor platelet adhesion to the atherosclerotic plaque because it has been shown that while small concentrations of PGI_2 prevent thrombus formation, larger concentrations are required to reduce platelet adhesion (7).

Recently, FitzGerald et al. (5) reported that the urinary excretion of 2,3-dinor-6-keto-PGF$_{1\alpha}$ (a metabolite of PGI$_2$ formed in vivo) by patients with severe atherosclerosis is higher than in normal controls. These investigators suggested endogenous production of PGI$_2$ in normal control patients may be lower because of the lack of a stimulus for PGI$_2$ synthesis, and higher in atherosclerotic patients because of increased platelet-endothelial interactions. It is not known whether these increases in urinary excretion of a metabolite of PGI$_2$ are subsequent to increased vascular PGI$_2$ synthetase activity or if the source of the PGI$_2$ is another tissue. If the source is in part vascular, it is not known whether the increases in PGI$_2$ formation occur in atherosclerotic or nonatheromatous arterial regions. It is therefore premature to draw conclusions concerning focal arterial PGI$_2$ synthesis based on this study of urinary metabolites. If the decrease in PGI$_2$ formation in regions of atherosclerosis resulted in platelet adhesion, focal atheromatous progression could be stimulated by the release of platelet constituents concomitantly with stimulation of PGI$_2$ synthetase activity in the adjacent nonatheromatous arterial tissue. It is not known whether increased PGI$_2$ formation by nonatheromatous tissue could affect events occurring at the area of plaque formation. Thus, it is possible that increased urinary excretion of a PGI$_2$ metabolite could be observed even though there are focal decreases in PGI$_2$ formation subsequent to decreased PGI$_2$ synthetase activity.

There was no increase in PGE$_2$ formation when 2 mM GSH was included in the incubation medium. These data indicate that unlike the coronary artery, neither the carotid artery nor the abdominal aorta contains an active GSH-dependent PGE$_2$ isomerase (6). An inverse relationship between PGI$_2$ and PGE$_2$ formation in atherosclerosis has been previously observed in human aorta (2). These investigators proposed that atherosclerotic aortas produce significant amounts of PGE$_2$, which increase in proportion to the severity of atherosclerosis. In human carotid artery and abdominal aorta, it appears that most, if not all, PGE$_2$ formed was secondary to spontaneous hydrolysis of PGH$_2$ and not by the activity of GSH-dependent PGE$_2$ isomerase. We conclude that nonenzymatic PGE$_2$

formation is high when PGH_2 is not rapidly converted to PGI_2 by PGI_2 synthetase, and vice versa. These data indicate that the PGE_2 formed in our study resulted from the nonenzymatic hydrolysis of the unstable substrate, PGH_2.

TXA_2 formation by human carotid artery plaques has been reported (3). In our study, no TXA_2 synthetase activity (determined by identification of TXB_2, the stable hydrolysis product of TXA_2) was found in any carotid artery specimen. The protein concentrations used in this study were limited by the quantity of material and may have been too low to support levels of TXA_2 formation detectable by TLC.

SUMMARY

The present study reports that there are graduated decreases in human arterial PGI_2 synthetase activity within atherosclerotic plaque (carotid artery and abdominal aorta). The decreases are focal, as the arterial region immediately adjacent to the plaque exhibits normal PGI_2 synthetase activity. The data also indicate that both human carotid artery and human abdominal aorta lack the presence of a GSH-dependent PGE_2 isomerase for the direct conversion of PGH_2 to PGE_2.

ACKNOWLEDGMENTS

The authors wish to thank Ms. Janice Ignarro for her expert help in the preparation of the manuscript. This investigation was supported in part by National Institutes of Health grants HL29456, HL15580, HL11802, and HL18070.

REFERENCES

1. Sinzinger, H., Feigl, W., Silberbauer, K., Oppolzer, R., Winter, M. and Averswald, W. Exp. Pathol. 18:175-180, 1980.
2. Rolland, P.H., Jouve, R., Pellegrin, E., Mercier, C. and Serradimigni, A. Arteriosclerosis 4:70-78, 1984.
3. Gamache, F.W., Weksler, B.B. and Patterson, R.H. Stroke 16:8, 1985.
4. Geling, N.G., Naumov, I.S. and Antonov, A.S. Biomed. Biochem. Acta 43:281-283, 1984.
5. FitzGerald, G.A., Smith, B., Pedersen, A.K. and Brush, A.R. N. Engl. J. Med. 310:1065-1068, 1984.
6. McNamara, D.B., Hussey, J.L., Kerstein, M.D., Rosenson, R.S., Hyman, A.L. and Kadowitz, P.J. Biochem. Biophys. Res. Comm. 118: 33-39, 1984.
7. Higgs, E.A., Moncada, S., Vane, J.R., Gaen, J.P., Michel, H. and Tobelem, G. Prostaglandins 16:17-22, 1978.

15

ENDOTHELIUM DEPENDENT RELAXATION AND ATHEROSCLEROSIS

N. Sreeharan, R. Jayakody, M. Senaratne, A. Thomson and T. Kappagoda
Department of Medicine, University of Alberta, Edmonton, Alberta, Canada

In 1980, Furchgott & Zawadzki demonstrated that the endothelium of the rabbit aorta releases a factor(s) with vasodilator properties in response to acetylcholine (1). This discovery helped to explain two phenomena that had remained pharmacological "paradoxes" - (i) the potent contractile effect of acetylcholine on non-vascular smooth muscle and the concurrent vasodilator action in-vivo on most peripheral vascular beds and (ii) the inability of acetylcholine to relax isolated preparations of blood vessels in-vitro. Furchgott's group showed that the lack of relaxation to acetylcholine in helical strips of rabbit aorta (which was the standard in-vitro preparation at the time) was the result of unintentional removal of the endothelium during mounting. It was found that with care taken to avoid damage to the intima, any in-vitro preparation (whether a helical strip, a ring or a transverse strip) always relaxed to acetylcholine. Conversely, intentional removal of the intima always resulted in the loss of the relaxatory response of the preparation to acetylcholine.

The occurence of the relaxatory response in the presence of cyclooxygenase inhibitors and the demonstration of the response in the rabbit aorta, which is known to be unresponsive to prostacyclin, ruled out the possibility of a prostaglandin mediated response. The term endothelium dependent relaxatory factor (EDRF) was introduced to describe this hitherto unidentified vasodilator factor(s) (1).

Vasoactive Agents Involved in Endothelium Dependent Relaxation (EDR)

The endothelium-dependent response is not unique to acetylcholine. A number of agents have been demonstrated to induce endothelium-dependent relaxation in a variety of blood vessels and in a number of animal species. These agents include related muscarinic agonists such as methacholine and carbachol (1), the clotting factor thrombin (2), products released during platelet aggregation such as serotonin (3), ADP and ATP (4,5), mediators of local blood flow regulation such as adenosine and histamine (6), bradykinin and substance P (7), the calcium ionophore A23187 (8,9) the circulating vasoactive hormones norepinephrine (3) and vasopressin (10), arachidonic acid and other saturated and unsaturated fatty acids (11,12) and peptides including vasoactive intestinal peptide (12), calcitonin gene related peptide (13), and mellitin (14). In addition, endothelium dependent relaxation has been demonstrated, secondary to physical increments in blood flow through arteries in-situ and in-vitro (15,16).

Following the original description of EDR in the rabbit aorta, the phenomenon has been demonstrated in a wide variety of arterial preparations which include the femoral, iliac, coronary, gastric, coeliac, mesenteric, renal, splenic, saphenous, pulmonary and cerebral (12) arteries of a number of animal species (4,17-20). Studies have been reported in the dog, cat, rat, guinea pig, pig and man. Although the release of EDRF is primarily a property of arterial endothelium, it has been also documented in the femoral, saphenous, splenic and pulmonary veins of the dog to a limited number of pharmacological agents (19).

Evidence for "humoral" nature of EDRF

Evidence for the release of a humoral factor(s) from the endothelial cells in response to stimulation with acetylcholine (as well as other agonists) comes from both "transfer" and bioassay (21,22,23) experiments. The transfer experiment using the so called "sandwich mount" showed that when the intima of a strip of de-endothelialized vessel was mounted against the intima of a vascular strip with endothelium, the former regained its ability to relax to acetylcholine. In the bioassay experiments, when a segment of blood vessel with endothelium ("donor") was perfused with buffer containing acetylcholine or other agonists and the effluent passed onto a segment of blood vessel without endothelium ("recipient"), the latter demonstrated a concentration-dependent relaxation. The half life of the EDRF was calculated from the bioassay experiments by altering the transit time from the "donor" to the "recipient" and was found to vary from 6 to 80 seconds depending on the species and the experimental conditions (21,22).

Chemical Nature of EDRF

The chemical structure of EDRF remains to be elucidated. There is some evidence to suggest that it is a metabolite of arachidonic acid or another unsaturated fatty acid. Exogenous arachidonic acid (2,11,) which can be metabolised by endothelial cells is capable of eliciting endothelium dependent relaxations. However, other unsaturated and saturated fatty acids which are not metabolised by endothelial cells are capable of evoking such responses also (24). The latter observations suggest the possibility that these fatty acids are merely facilitatory in the production of EDRF.

Nevertheless, compounds which interfere with the metabolism of arachidonic acid appear to influence the phenomenon in-vitro (Fig. 1).

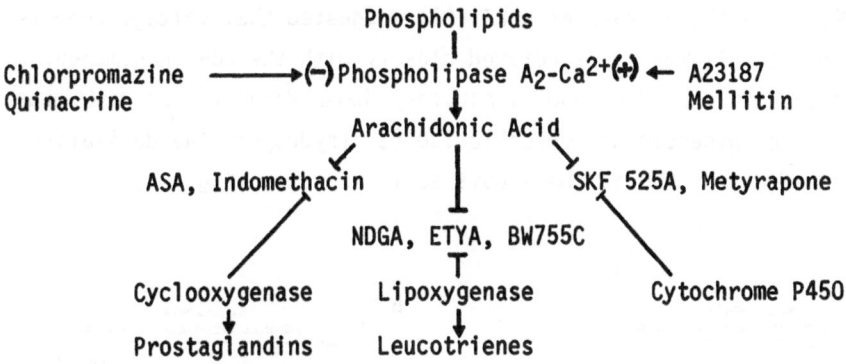

ETYA-Eicosatetraynoic Acid, NDGA-Nordihydroguaiaretic Acid
ASA-Acetylsalysilic Acid

Fig 1: Metabolism of Arachidonic Acid

For instance, inhibitors of phopholipase A_2 such as quinacrine abolish EDR, presumably by preventing the production of arachidonic acid from phospholipids. The calcium ionophore A23187 (8) and the polypeptide mellitin (found in bee venom) (14) causes EDR by activating phopholipase A_2. Inhibitors of the cyclo-oxygenases (eg. indomethacin) fail to abolish the response while inhibitors of the lipoxygenase (eg. nordihydroguaretic acid) do so (1). Thus an involvement of the products of the lipoxygenase pathway is likely, though specific blockers of the leukotrienes do not appear to have an effect on the phenomenon. Finally, Singer & Peach (9) observed that compounds which block the metabolism of arachidonic acid through the cytochrome P450 pathway abolish this response. It is emphasised that the majority of the agents found to inhibit EDR are non-specific in their action (25) and hence caution must be exercised in interpreting the findings e.g. identifying EDRF as a metabolite of these pathways.

Role of Calcium

The crucial role of calcium in the endothelium dependent relaxatory response was clearly demonstrated by the inhibition of the response in a calcium free bathing medium (9) and by the stimulation of the relaxatory response by the calcium ionophore A23187 (8). Long & Stone (26) demonstrated that calcium was necessary for the release of EDRF while Singer & Peach (9) showed that calcium channel blockers partially inhibited EDR. The observation that the calcium channel agonists Bay 68644 and (+) 202791 evoke the release of EDRF (27) suggested that voltage operated calcium channels may be associated closely with the EDR phenomenon.

However, studies from our laboratory have demonstrated that the calcium blocker nicardipine hydrochloride (a dihydropyridine derivative) is without effect on EDR in the rabbit aorta in-vitro (Fig. 2A).

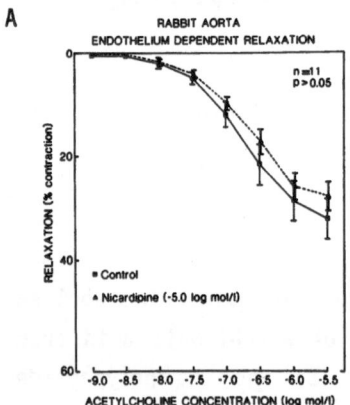 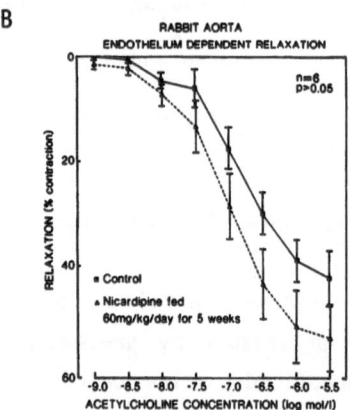

Fig. 2: Effect of nicardipine on EDR to acetylcholine in rabbit aorta A-(left); incubation in vitro. B-(right); After oral administration of nicardipine.

Further, even after the oral administration of nicardipine (60 mg/kg/day) for 5 weeks EDR was unaffected when aortic rings were examined in vitro (Fig. 2B). Finally, the role of nicardipine was investigated in a bioassay preparation (see Fig. 4 for details) in which nicardipine was applied to both the donor and the recipient tissue separately, it was found that the ability of the donor tissue to produce/release EDRF in response to acetylcholine was unaffected as was the ability of the recipient tissue to respond to it (Figure 3).

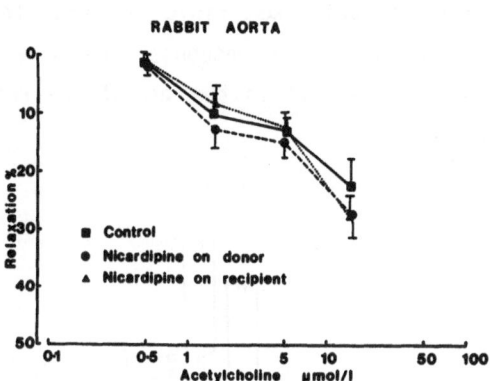

Fig. 3: Effect of nicardipine on the synthesis/release of EDRF (nicardipine on donor) and on the response to EDRF (nicardipine on recipient).

Mechanisms Involved in Formation and Release of EDRF
A. Muscarinic Receptors

The initial event in the EDR response has been considered to be an interaction of the agonist with an endothelial cell receptor. The diverse nature of the agents involved indicates that this interaction may be quite non-specific, involving differing receptors and/or pathways (28). However, it has been clearly demonstrated that the endothelial cell receptor through which acetylcholine and related agonists act is of the muscarinic type (29). This receptor is not a novel subtype and has a dissociation constant for atropine similar to other muscarinic receptors (30). This aspect of the problem was investigated using a bioassay preparation described in Fig. 4.

With the bioassay described above it is possible to investigate whether an agent which blocks the relaxation does so by inhibiting the synthesis/release of EDRF or by inhibiting the effects of the substance

(ie. chemical inactivation or interference with the relaxatory response). When acetylcholine is added to a ring of rabbit aorta with intact endothelium, it stimulates receptors on endothelial cells (muscarinic type) to release EDRF. This factor is believed to diffuse into the
underlying smooth muscle layer to mediate a relaxation. In addition,
acetylcholine acts directly on receptors on smooth muscle (muscarinic
receptors at low doses and both muscarinic and nicotinic receptors in
high doses) to mediate a contractile response. Hence when acetylcholine
produces a relaxatory response, it is the sum of the results of relaxatory and contractile forces.

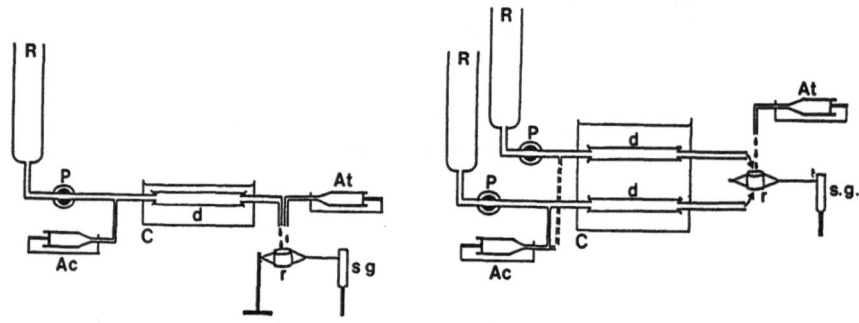

Fig. 4: Diagrammatic representation of apparatus used for experiment.
R: Reservoir for Krebs-bicarbonate buffer (maintained at 37°C) P: pump
for driving perfusate; C: tissue chamber (maintained at 37°C) d: donor
tissues; r: recipient tissue; s.g.: strain gauge for isometric recording; Ac: syringe pump for injecting acetylcholine with perfusate; At:
syringe pump for injecting atropine directly on to recipient. The donor
(d) is perfused intra-luminally and the perfusate is directed onto the
recipient (r). The apparatus on the right permits comparison between
control and atherosclerotic donor tissues.

In tissue bath experiments using rabbit aortic rings with intact
endothelium, the maximum relaxations are produced by concentrations of
acetylcholine of approximately 1.0-3.0 µmol/l. However at 10 and 100
µmol/l concentrations of acetylcholine the contractile forces overcome
the relaxatory ones. Similarly, when acetylcholine is added to a ring
without endothelium in a tissue bath, no relaxation or contraction is
seen with concentrations of approximately 1.0 µmol/l of acetylcho-

line. However at 10 and 100 μm/l concentrations of acetylcholine the
contractile responses are seen (Fig. 5).

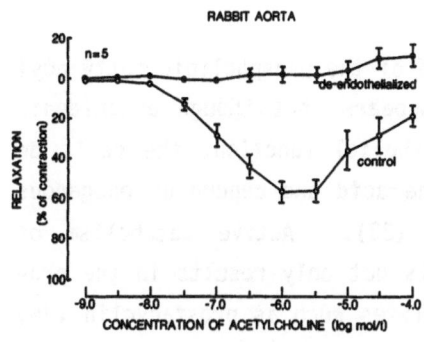

Fig. 5: Effect of Acetylcholine
on rings of rabbit aorta contrasted
with norepinephrine (1.0 μmol/1)
The control rings show relaxation
up to 1-3 μmol/1 of acetylcholine
at higher concentrations a contraction is seen.

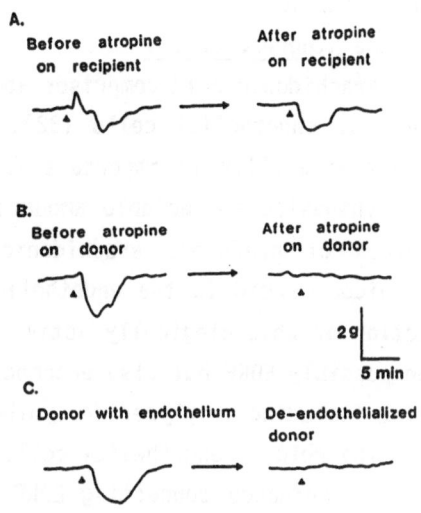

Fig. 6: Effect of atropine on
recipient (A), and donor tissue
(B) on EDR. C shows effect of
removal of endothelium in donor
tissue.

In the bioassay shown in Fig. 4, when acetylcholine is perfused
through the donor a mixture of acetylcholine and the
endothelium-dependent relaxatory factor is carried in the perfusate on
to the recipient. Since the recipient is denuded of endothelium,
acetylcholine in the perfusate will produce a contractile response and
the EDRF will produce a relaxatory response. Application of atropine to
the recipient, blocks the former effect and thereby facilitates the
demonstration of the latter (Fig. 6).

Action of EDRF on Vascular Smooth Muscle

Relaxations caused by acetylcholine or A23187 are associated with
increases in cyclic GMP in the aorta of rats and rabbits and in the bovine coronary artery(20,31). Since removal of endothelium and methylene
blue, a known inhibitor of guanylase cyclase, abolish the acetylcholine
induced accumulation of cyclic GMP (31), it has been postulated that

EDRF stimulates guanylase cyclase to produce cyclic GMP, thereby activating cyclic GMP dependent protein kinase eventually leading to dephosphorylatin of myosin light chains and to relaxation of the vascular smooth muscle.

EDR and Atherosclerosis

Arachidonic acid comprises about 10% of the phospholipid fatty acyl chain of endothelial cells (32). It appears that though arachidonic acid availability is important for endothelial function, the cells do not synthesise appreciable amounts of the acid and depend on exogenous sources of preformed arachidonic acid (33). Active metabolism of arachidonic acid in the endothelial cells not only results in the production of physiologically active metabolites such as prostacyclin (34) and possibly EDRF but also encompasses a central pathway in lipid metabolism including triglyceride synthesis (35).

The role of endothelial cells in the metabolism of arachidonic acid and the evidence connecting EDRF to its metabolic pathway has led to postulates linking this phenomenon to diseases involving blood vessels such as atherosclerosis and diabetes. In these conditions where the endothelial cells of blood vessels are altered structurally, the loss of EDR may be a concurrent functional marker (36). Endothelial damage has been demonstrated in rabbits as early as 24 hours following intravenous infusion of cholesterol oxidation derivatives (37) and within 3 weeks of cholesterol feeding (35). It has been suggested that endothelial damage occurs secondary to sub-endothelial and intimal plaques of lipid and

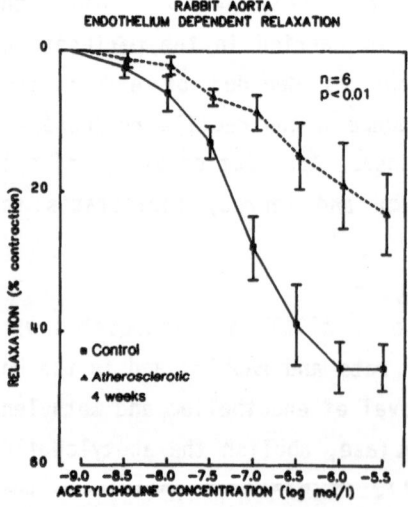

Fig. 7: Effect of feeding 2% cholesterol for 4 weeks on EDR in rabbits.

form cells (39). Progression of atherosclerosis eventually involves the media and smooth muscle cells (40).

Evidence for Impairment of EDR in Atherosclerosis

In view of its short half life (21) and the inhibitory effect of circulating haemoglobin (41) it has been suggested that EDRF is not a circulating hormone but a local one modulating vascular tone (41). Thus endothelium dependent relaxation would occur via (i) the production and release of the factor from the endothelium (ii) the diffusion of the factor through sub-endothelial (intimal) tissues and (iii) relaxation of the vascular smooth muscle in the media. Since atherosclerosis, both experimental and natural, is known to structurally affect all three of the above sites, i.e. endothelium, sub-endothelial tissues and media (40), it seems likely that atherosclerosis may lead to an impairment of EDR.

Rabbits and monkeys with experimental atherosclerosis have been used as animal models to study EDR. Increasing the dietary intake of cholesterol of rabbits (42) and monkeys (40) produces hyperlipidaemia and eventually a form of atherosclerosis, which represent human atherosclerosis in some respects. There are several studies which suggest that feeding rabbits (43,44) and monkeys (45), diets enriched with cholesterol (0.3-2.0%) resulted in the production of atherosclerosis and the loss of EDR (Fig. 7). Regression of atherosclerosis was related to a return of the phenomenon in monkeys (45) but not in rabbits.

The bioassay described in Fig. 3 was used to determine the effect of cholesterol feeding in rabbits upon the production/release of EDRF. The study was undertaken in New Zealand White rabbits. After weaning they were assigned either into an experimental group fed a diet enriched with 2% cholesterol (5799C-9, Rabbit Purified Diet, Ralston Purina Co., St. Louis, U.S.A.) or a control group which was fed a standard rabbit diet (M-0662; Masterfeeds Division, Maple Leaf Mills, London, Ontario). After 5 weeks, the animals were sacrificed and the aortas removed for the bioassay. The donor tissue was a 4 cm length of rabbit aorta and was taken from either an experimental or a control animal. The recipient was obtained from a control animal. The recipient was precontracted with norepinephrine (0.2 μmol/l) and superfused successively with fluid obtained through the donor tissues. Application of acetylcholine to the donor tissue resulted in a relaxation in the recipient. This relaxation was considerably attenuated when the perfusate was passed through an atherosclerotic donor (n=10; p<0.05). Thus, in rabbits rendered athero-sclerotic by feeding cholesterol there was an impairment in the production/release of EDRF (Fig. 8).

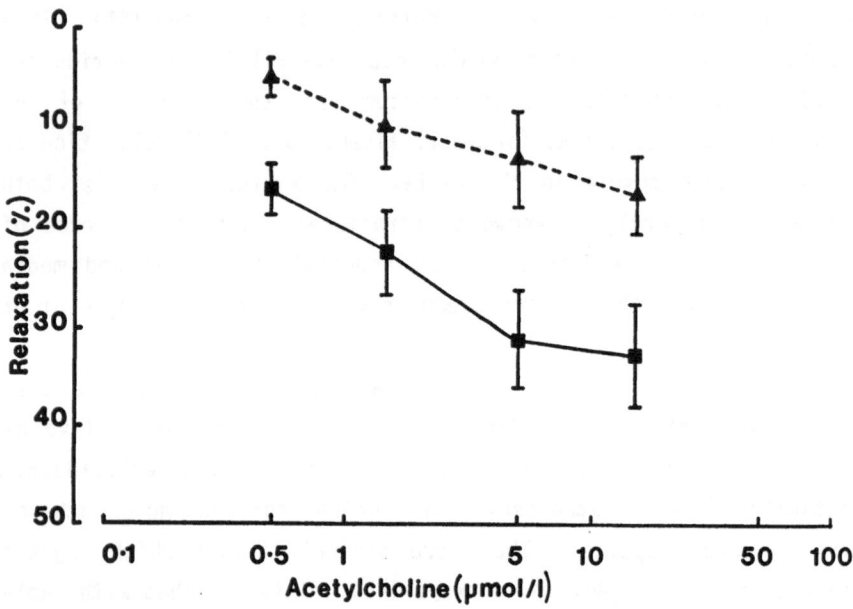

Fig. 8: Concentration-effect curves to acetylcholine in recipient aor-tic rings while infusing acetylcholine through donor aortas taken from control and cholesterol fed rabbits are shown. Ordinate: relaxation ex-pressed as a percentage of the contraction produced by norepinephrine (0.2 μmol/l). Abscissa: concentration of acetylcholine (umol/l) on a log scale. The two concentration-effect curves are significantly dif-ferent from each other (p<0.05). Mean ± standard errors of the means are shown (n=10). ▲ : atherosclerotic animals.　　　■ : control ani-mals.

The residual issue of whether there is a concurrent change in the ability of aortic smooth muscle to respond to the relaxatory factor was resolved by determing the responses in control and cholesterol fed (de-endothelialized) recipient tissues to EDRF generated by a common control donor. The relaxatory response in atherosclerotic recipients was simil-ar to that observed in control recipient (n=9; p>0.05). Thus, it could be concluded that cholesterol feeding leads to an impairment of synthesis/release of endothelium-dependent relaxation factor in rabbit aorta with no significant effect on the ability of the aorta to respond to EDRF.

The data from the studies reported here suggest that the ability of endothelial cells to mediate EDR is impaired in animals fed cholesterol and that this effect may play a role in the pathological phenomenon associated with vascular spasm.

REFERENCES

1. Furchgott, R.F. Circ. Res. 53: 557-573, 1983.
2. DeMey, J.G., Claeys, M. and Vanhoutte, P.M. J. Pharmacol. Exp. Ther. 222: 166-173, 1982.
3. Cocks, T.M. and Angus, J.A. Nature 305: 627-630, 1983.
4. DeMey, J.G. and Vanhoutte, P.M. J. Physiol. (Lond), 316: 347-355, 1981.
5. Furchgott, R.F. Trends Pharmacol. Sci. 2: 173-176, 1981.
6. Van de Vorrde, J. and Leusen, I. Arch. Int. Pharmacodyn Ther. 256(2): 329-330, 1982.
7. Chand, N. and Altura B. Science 213; 1376-1379, 1981.
8. Zawadzki, J.V., Cherry P.D. and Furchgott, R.F. Pharmacologist 22: 271, 1980.
9. Singer, H.A. and Peach M.J. Hypertension 4(Suppl II): 19-25, 1982.
10. Katusic, Z.S., Shepherd, J.T. and Vanhoutte, P.M. Circ. Res. 55: 575-579, 1984.
11. Singer, H.A. and Peach M.J. Hypertention 4(Suppl II), 19-25, 1982.
12. Davis, J.M. and Williams, K.I. Prostaglandins 27:195-202, 1984.
13. Brain S., Williams T., Tippins J., Morris H. and MacIntyre I. Nature 313:54-56, 1985.
14. Forstermann, U. and Neufang, B. Am. J. Physiol. 249(Heart Circ. Physiol. 18):H14-H19, 1985.
15. Holtz, J., Forestermann, U., Pohl, U., Giesler, M. and Bassenge, E. J. Cardiovasc. Pharmacol. 6:1161-1169, 1984.
16. Holtz, J., Pohl, U., Kellner, C. and Busse, R. Pflugers Arch. 400:R9, 1984.
17. Cherry, P.D., Furchgott, R.F., Zawadzki, J.V. and Jothianandan, D. Proc. Natl. Acad. Sci. U.S.A. 79:2106-2110, 1982.
18. Altura, B.M. and Chand, N. Br. J. Pharmacol. 74:10-11, 1981.
19. DeMey, J.G. and Vanhoutte, P.M. Circ. Res. 51:439-447, 1982.
20. Rapoport, R.M. and Murad, F. Circ. Res. 52:352-357, 1983.
21. Griffith, T.M., Edwards, D.H., Lewis, M.J., Newby, A.C. and Henderson, A.H. Nature 308:645-647, 1984.
22. Rubanyi, G.M., Lorenz, R.R. and Vanhoutte, P.M. Am. J. Physiol 249:H95-H101, 1985.
23. Kappagoda, C.T., Thomson, A.B.R., Sreeharan, N., Jayakody, R.L., and Senaratne, M.P.J. Journal of Molecular and Cellular Cardiology 18(Suppl 3):38, 1986. (Abstract)
24. Rubanyi, G.M. and Vanhoutte, P.M. Clin Res. 33:522A, 1985.
25. Feigen, L.P., Pretus, H. and Ensley, H. Blood Vessels. 23:67, 1986 (Abstract).
26. Long, C.J. and Stone, T.W. Blood Vessels, 22:205-208, 1985.

27. Rubanyi, G.M., Schwartz, A. and Vanhoutte, P.M. Fed. Proc.45(3):-426, 1986.
28. DeFeudis, F.V. Medical Hypotheses, 17:363-374, 1985.
29. Furchgott, R.F. and Zawadzki, J.V. Nature 288:373-376, 1980.
30. Furchgott, R.F. and Cherry, P.D.Zawadzki, J.V., Jothianandan, D. J. Cardiovasc. Pharmacol. 6(Suppl 2):5336-5343.
31. Rapoport, R.M. and Murad, F. J. Cyclic Nucleotide Res. 9:281-296, 1983.
32. Spector, A.A., Hoak, J.C., Fry, G.L., Denning, G.M., Stoll, L.L. and Smith, J.B. J. Clin. Invest. 65:1003-1012, 1980.
33. Spector, A.A., Kaduce, T.L., Hoak, J.C. and Fry, G.L. J. Clin. Invest. 68:1003-1011, 1981.
34. Denning, G.M., Figard, P.H., Kaduce, T.L. and Spector, A.A. J. Lipid Res. 24:993-1001, 1983.
35. Moncada, S., Gryglewski, R. and Bunting, S. and Vane, J.R. Nature, 263:663-665, 1976.
36. Rodman, N.F., Jagannathan, S.N., Jenkins, J.J. III, Rodman, J.A. and Allender, P.A. In: Scanning electron Microscopy III, SEM Inc., AMF O'Hare, 1979, p. 835-840.
37. Peng, S.K., Taylor, C.B., Hill, J.C. and Morin, R.J. Atherosclerosis, 54:121-133, 1985.
38. Goode, T.B., Davies, P.F., Reidy, M.A. and Bowyer, D.E. Atherosclerosis, 27:235-251, 1977.
39. Taylor, K., Glagov, S., Lamberti, J., Vesselinovitch, D. and Schaffner, T. In: Scanning electron Microscopy II, SEM Inc., AMF O'Hare, 1978, p. 449-457.
40. Wissler, R.W., Vesselinovitch, D., Davis, H.R., Lambert, P.H. and Bekermeier, M. In: Atherosclerosis (Ed. K.T. Lee) 454:9-22, 1985.
41. Martin, W., Villani, G.M., Jothianandan, D. and Furchgott, R.F. J. Pharm. & Exp. Therap. 232:708-716, 1985.
42. Duff, G.L., McMillan, G.C. and Ritchie, A.C. Am. J. Pathol. 33(5):845-873, 1957.
43. Jayakody, R.L., Senaratne, M.P.J., Thomson, A.B.R. and Kappagoda, C.T. Can. J. Physiol. & Pharmacol. 63:1206-1209, 1985.
44. Chappel, S.P., Griffith, T.M., Henderson, A.H. and Lewis, M.J. Br. J. Pharm.85: 266P, 1985.
45. Freiman, P.C., Mitchell, G.M., Gagnon, N.J., Armstrong, M.L., Heistad, D.D. and Harrison, D.G. Fed. Proc. 45:767,1986 (abstract).

C. METABOLIC ASPECTS OF CELL DAMAGE

16

ENERGY METABOLISM IN MYOCARDIAL ISCHEMIA AND REPERFUSION

ROBERT B. JENNINGS, KEITH A. REIMER, CHARLES STEENBERGEN, AND CHARLES E. MURRY

Department of Pathology, Box 3712, Duke University Medical Center, Durham, North Carolina 27710*

The general features of the energy metabolism of living myocytes reversibly injured by ischemia are reviewed in this paper. Most of the studies presented involve hearts subjected to very severe regional ischemia, i.e., subendocardial tissue receiving arterial collateral flows ranging between 0 and 4% of control flow. Where appropriate, results from myocardium made totally ischemic in vitro also are presented.

OVERVIEW OF THE BIOLOGY OF ACUTE MYOCARDIAL ISCHEMIA

Sudden occlusion of a major branch of a coronary artery in the open chest anesthetized dog markedly reduces arterial flow to the myocardium supplied by the occluded vessel. Collateral connections between the different coronary arteries continue to provide some flow to the ischemic region; this flow is greatest in the subepicardium and least in the subendocardium. With proximal occlusions of the circumflex artery in the open-chest anesthetized dog, subendocardial arterial flow generally ranges from 0-15% of control while subepicardial flow averages 20% but may be greater than 50% of control flow (1,2).

The general consequences of ischemia are summarized in Figure 1. When the arterial flow is depressed to the point that the supply of oxygen is deficient, aerobic metabolism is depressed and anaerobic glycolysis becomes a major source of new high energy phosphate (HEP). Furthermore, after a few seconds of significantly reduced flow, manifestations of altered cellular functions such as depressed contractile activity and electrocardiographic changes appear (3).

The depressed arterial flow of severe ischemia limits not only the entry of oxygen and substrates, but also the egress of metabolites produced in the ischemic tissue. For example the products of anaerobic glycolysis and the breakdown of creatine phosphate (CP) and the adenine nucleotide pool accumulate in the sarcoplasm and produce an intracellular osmolar load (3). The accumulation of catabolites and the fact that the supply of HEP from HEP reserves and from anaerobic glycolysis does not match the utilization of HEP by the ischemic tissue are the two major facets of the ischemic process. The imbalance in the

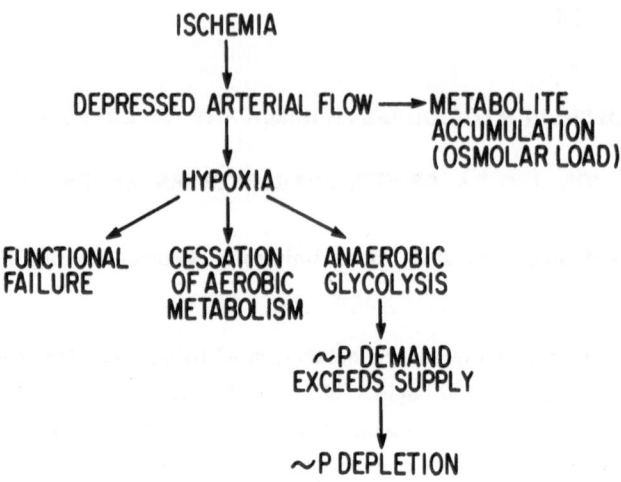

Fig. 1. The principal consequences of ischemia are shown on this diagram. Metabolites are produced intracellularly by hypoxic metabolism where they accumulate (the osmolar load) and equilibrate to a variable extent with the extracellular fluid. Since the demand of the tissue for HEP exceeds the supply, the net level of ATP falls until it is virtually zero in zones of low-flow ischemia.

supply-demand relationship causes the level of HEP in the tissue to decrease and eventually leads to the destruction of the adenine nucleotide pool (3).

The reactions which provide HEP to the severely ischemic myocytes are shown in Figure 2. The reserve supply of CP and ATP would be sufficient to support about three to four effective contractions, but, because of the rapid onset of contractile failure during ischemia, these reserves are depleted more slowly.   In the absence of oxidative phosphorylation, anaerobic glycolysis is the only significant source of new HEP. Most of the continued utilization of HEP in the ischemic tissue is believed to be energy expended in the attempt of the myocytes to contract in response to continuing electrical stimuli and to maintain cellular volume and ionic homeostasis via the activity of the Na^+/K^+ and Ca^{2+}-ATPases. In addition, other enzymatic reactions utilizing ATP can take place under ischemic conditions.   Adenyl cyclase and fatty acyl CoA synthetase are representative examples. Rough estimates of the quantitative importance of these various reactions for HEP supply are indicated (Fig. 2) by the size of the arrows (4).

MYOCARDIAL ENERGY PRODUCTION IN ISCHEMIA

The left ventricular myocardium is dependent on aerobic (mitochondrial) respiration to make sufficient energy to provide for the virtually continuous contractile activity of the heart. To appreciate the importance of aerobic respiration, it is useful to compare aerobic

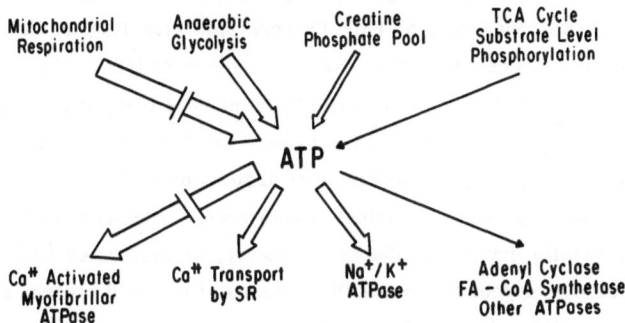

ATP PRODUCTION AND UTILIZATION
IN SEVERE ISCHEMIA

Fig. 2. The principal reactions producing and utilizing HEP in ischemic tissue are illustrated. In severe ischemia, aerobic respiration is abolished. The preexisting stores of HEP, chiefly in the form of creatine phosphate (CP) and ATP, are relatively small (Table 1). Thus, anaerobic glycolysis becomes the principal source of energy and produces about 80% of the high-energy phsophate bonds that are utilized by ischemic tissue. Energy utilization also is markedly reduced during ischemia. Cardiac contraction, which is mediated by the Ca^{2+} activated myofibrillar ATPase, consumes much of the ATP produced in aerobic myocardium. However, contraction is is severely depressed in areas of severe ischemia with the result that the affected myocardium bulges with systole. It seems likely, however, that some energy is expended early in ischemia in an unsuccessful attempt of the myocytes to contract. However, the amount is impossible to estimate with available techniques, ATP also continues to be required to remove Na^+ from the cell, to keep Ca^{2+} sequestered in the sarcoplasmic reticulum, and for a variety of other cellular processes that may continue to compete for the remaining ATP. The width of the arrows indicates the estimated quantitative importance of the various reactions. Substrate level phosphorylation of α-ketoglutarate in the mitochondria does not require O_2, but the tissue content of substrates which can be shuttled to α-ketoglutarate is small. Thus, these mechanisms do not produce a significiant quantity of new ATP. (Reproduced with permission of the publishers of ref. 4.)

and anaerobic metabolism of glucose. When sufficient O_2 is present, as many as 38 or 39μmol of HEP are produced per μmol of glucose oxidized to CO_2 and H_2O depending on whether the source of the glucose is the extracellular fluid or glycogen.(5). However, with the onset of severe ischemia, only 8-10 seconds (6) are required to utilize most of the oxygen found in the tissue as oxymyoglobin and oxyhemoglobin. Shortly thereafter, most of the creatine phosphate (CP) is utilized, phosphorylase is activated, and glycogenolysis begins. Glucose-1-phosphate enters the glycolytic pathway and three net μmoles of HEP are produced per μmole glucose-1-phosphate converted into lactate. Thus, anaerobic catabolism of glucose from glycogen produces only 8% as much ATP as could be produced from the complete mitochondrial oxidation of the same substrate. It follows that any oxygen provided by collateral flow will produce much more HEP than can be synthesized by anaerobic glycolysis. As far as myocardial energy production is concerned, the aphorism *"the oxygen from a little arterial flow goes a long way"* has much merit.

Assuming that the production of HEP by anaerobic glycolysis is tightly coupled to lactate production, one can calculate the maximum amount of HEP which can be produced using all of the glycogen of the tissue (7) plus all the glucose trapped in extracellular fluid plus substrate level phosphorylation using substrate available to the myocytes such as glutamate and αketoglutarate. (8) A maximum of 624μmoles of HEP/g dry weight (Table 1) is the total reserve of new HEP available to myocardium receiving little or no arterial flow. Another 97 μmol/g dry are available as reserves of preformed HEP. The relative contribution of anaerobic glycolysis and of the reserves of the HEP present in the ischemic myocardium, assuming that all available supplies were utilized, is summarized in Table 1. This analysis demonstrates that glycogen is the major potential source of HEP in the complete absence of O_2.

However, because anaerobic glycolysis stops before all the tissue glycogen is utilized (9), the potential HEP production shown in Table 1 never is realized. Moreover, there is an inverse relationship between lactate and ATP. in the totally ischemic myocardium (Fig. 3). Net ATP falls as anaerobic glycolysis proceeds at the slow rate characteristic of marked ischemia. Glycolysis is slowed because glyceraldehyde-3-phosphate dehydrogenase (GAPDH) is inhibited by the increased NADH and decreased pH of the tissue (10). The speed with which inhibition of the rate of HEP utilization per minute occurs is shown in Table 2 which shows that the rate of utilization during the first 1.5 minutes of ischemia is about 3 times greater than the rate observed between the fifth and tenth minute of ischemia. Note that when net tissue ATP declines to less than 1 μmol/g dry, glycolysis totally ceases (Fig. 3). Possible explanations for the cessation of anaerobic glycolysis include insufficient sarcoplasmic ATP to phosphorylate fructose-6-phosphate, severe inhibition of GAPDH, and exhaustion of supplies of substrate. The observation that tissue G-6-P is elevated markedly (7,9) at the time that glycolysis stops, suggests that substrate depletion is not responsible for the cessation of glycolysis. Moreover, only 225 μmoles of lactate are produced instead of the 400-420 μmoles potentially available from glycogen reserves.

Lactate accumulates and ATP is depleted at a higher rate in severe ischemia in vivo than in total ischemia in vitro (Fig. 3)(7,11). The difference in the rate of change probably is related to the continued electromechanical activity of heart in vivo. In fact, Lowe et al. (12), have shown that pacing the totally ischemic excised left ventricle at a rate similar to that of the open-chest anesthetized dog speeds up both ATP depletion and lactate accumulation to the levels observed in vivo.

TABLE 1. POTENTIAL SOURCES OF HEP IN MYOCARDIUM AT THE ONSET OF TOTAL ISCHEMIA

METABOLIZABLE SUBSTRATE	HEP Production in µmol/g dry
Glucose from glycogen (204 µmol G x 3 µmol HEP/µmol G)	612
Glucose of extracellular H_2O (3.5 µmol G x 2 µmol HEP /µmol G)	7
Mitochondondrial substrate level phosphorylation (Glutamate, α-ketoglutarate, etc.)	5
Total	624

RESERVES of HEP	
ATP (26 µmol g/dry x 2 µmol HEP/µmol ATP)	52
ADP (3 µmol/g dry x 1 µmol HEP/µmol ADP)	3
CP (40 µmol/g dry x 1 µmol HEP/µmol CP)	40
Other (GTP, CTP, and UTP, etc.)	2
Total	97

* An estimate of the total HEP available from all sources to totally ischemic myocardium is presented in this Table. It is based on measured levels of substrate and HEP reserves. The principal source of new HEP is anaerobic glycolysis using glucose from the 204±10 µmoles glucosyl equivalents of glycogen found in control canine left ventricle. The extracellular glucose of 3.5 µmol/g dry is based on a serum glucose of 5.5mM. Anaerobic glycolysis could contribute only 7 µmol of new HEP if all the glucose were utilized. Less than 5µmoles of glutamate and substrates convertible to succinyl CoA exist in canine left ventricle (30). The levels of "other" high energy phosphates are based on measurements made in quick frozen biopsies of canine left ventricle by Swain et al. (25).

Table 2. HIGH ENERGY PHOSPHATE UTILIZATION IN LOW-FLOW ISCHEMIA[y]

ISCHEMIA in min.	HEP UTIL. in µmol/g/dry wt./min
0 - 1.5	68.5
1.5 - 5	24.3
5 - 10	12.6
10 - 15	14.9
15 - 20	11.4
20 - 40	4.2

[y] The effect of severe ischemia on myocardial HEP utilization in the subendocardial myocardium of the circumflex bed is summarized in this Table. The lactate and ATP used in the calculation are shown together with the SEM in Fig. 3. The tissue CP ranged from 0.5 to 3.1 µmol/g dry at all intervals. All hearts had arterial collateral flows to the inner layer of 0.07 ml/min/g wet weight or less and the data at each interval is based on a minimum of 4 hearts. The sampling technique is described in detail in ref 19. HEP utilization was estimated by the equation (26-Obs ATP) x 2 + (3-Obs ADP) + (40-Obs CP). See text and ref. 7 for a description of the assumptions used in formulating this equation. After 1.5 minutes of ischemia, the amount of HEP utilized divided by 1.5 minutes yields the utilization rate per minute. Thereafter, utilization in the preceding interval of ischemia was subtracted from the measured amount of HEP utilization before normalizing to minutes.

ENERGY PRODUCTION IN RELATION TO REVERSIBLE VS. IRREVERSIBLE MYOCYTE INJURY

There is a close association between a very low ATP, cessation of anaerobic glycolysis and the presence of irreversible myocyte injury. Irreversible injury is defined by the development of cell death even though the ischemic state is eliminated by successful restoration of arterial flow. For example, after 40 minutes of ischemia, 70-80% of the severely ischemic myocytes in the posterior papillary muscle cannot be salvaged by reperfusion (11). In contrast, after 15 minutes of ischemia, the tissue is reversibly injured in the sense that restoration of arterial flow prevents the death of the damaged myocytes. Such tissue still contains 25-30% of the ATP of control myocardium and has accumulated only about 60-70% of the lactate and glucose-6-phosphate found in irreversibly injured tissue (13).

The net rate of HEP utilization, estimated from decreasing reserve supplies and from increasing lactate content (indicative of HEP production via anaerobic glycolysis) during various time intervals after the onset of ischemia is presented in Table 2. The rate of HEP utilization slows markedly after the first 90 seconds, and by 40 minutes after the onset of

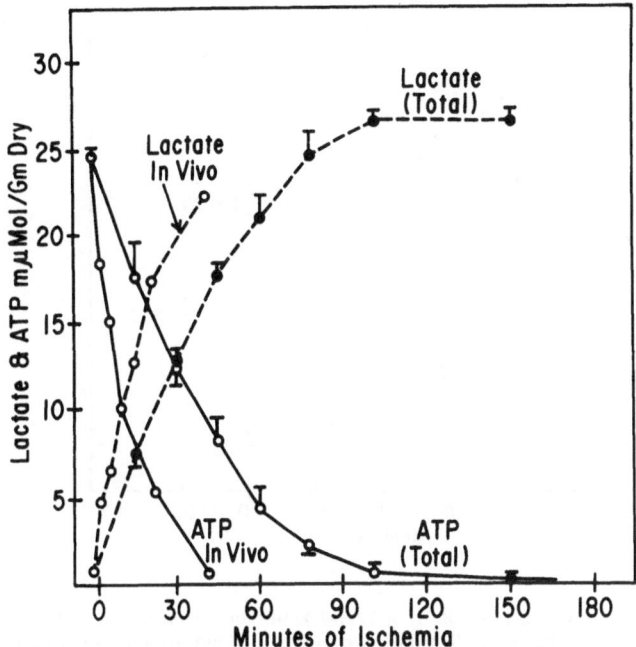

Fig. 3. The inverse relationship between the ATP and lactate of the subendocardial tissue of canine left ventricle after varying periods of total ischemia in vitro at 37° C are shown (Total). The data are from Jones et al. (9). For comparison, the ATP and lactate of severely ischemic left ventricular myocardium of the circumflex bed (in vivo) is plotted. The severe ischemia was induced by occlusion of the circumflex branch of the left coronary artery in the pentobarbital anesthetized open-chest dog heart in groups of 4-6 dogs. A different group of dogs was used for each time point on the in vivo curves. Note that even though there is no flow in the totally ischemic tissue, both ATP depletion and lactate accumulation develop much more quickly in vivo than in vitro. Most of the in vivo data is from references 4, 7, and 11.

ischemia, nearly has ceased. Thus, the irreversible state is characterized by a very low myocardial ATP and by cessation of the production and utilization of HEP (3-4).

EFFECT OF REPERFUSION WITH ARTERIAL BLOOD ON ENERGY PRODUCTION IN REVERSIBLY INJURED TISSUE

The results of reperfusion after periods of ischemia of one to 15 minutes are illustrated in Fig. 4. The most detailed studies have been done after 15 minutes of ischemia and variable periods of reperfusion (13,14). After 3 minutes of reperfusion, there is partial repletion of ATP; however, no further increase in ATP is noted after 20, 60 or even 1440 minutes (Fig. 4) of reperfusion (14). The incomplete repletion of ATP in the first three minutes is attributed to rephosphorylation of ADP and AMP which accumulated while the

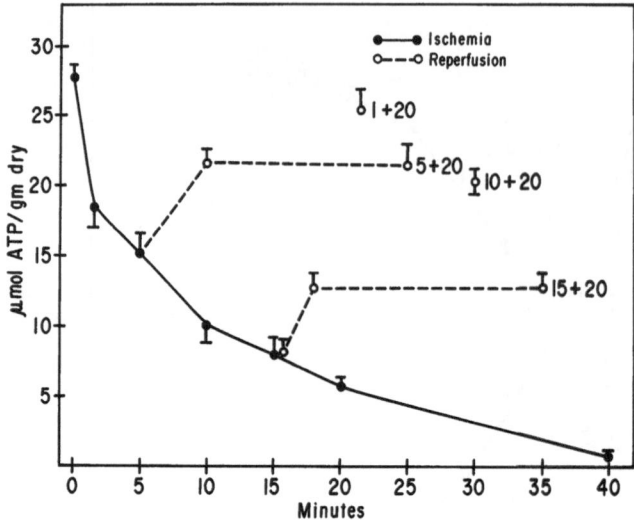

Fig. 4. The effect of varying periods of arterial reperfusion on net ATP of tissue reversibly damaged by 1,5,10, and 15 minutes of ischemia are plotted on this graph. The ATP is the mean found in 3-6 hearts at each time interval. The brackets are the standard error of the mean. The permanent ischemia data also is plotted in Fig. 3. The tissue received 20 minutes of reperfusion at each time interval and in each case showed an 8-12 μmole increase in net ATP. Most of the new ATP originated from redistribution of the nucleotides of the adenine nucleotide pool. ATP rose while tissue ADP and AMP fell.The rate at which resynthesis occurred was estimated in the 15 minute group. After 30 seconds of reperfusion, no resynthesis was not detectable but at 3 minutes after reperfusion, recharging of the adenylate pool was complete (13).

tissue was ischemic and not to de novo or salvage synthesis of adenine nucleotides (13). Resynthesis of adenine nucleotides eventually occurs, but is incomplete even four days after a 15 minute episode of ischemia (14). The slow resynthesis rate is due chiefly to the slow rate of phosphoribosyl pyrophosphate synthesis in heart (15); this molecule is rate limiting for both salvage and de novo pathways of adenine nucleotide synthesis.

It is also noteworthy that reversibly injured living myocardium salvaged by reperfusion after 15 minutes of ischemia exhibits defects in cell volume control for at least an hour and perhaps longer (13,16). Also, this tissue exhibits depressed contractility for more than 24 hours even though aerobic metabolism is functioning at the control level (18). The explanation for the loss of volume control and for the depression in contractility remains unknown.

EFFECT OF REPETITIVE BRIEF EPISODES OF ISCHEMIA AND REPERFUSION ON MYOCARDIAL ENERGY METABOLISM

Although we now believe that sarcolemmal disruption is the earliest change which is an absolute sign that cell death has occurred, it has not been possible to identify the precise series of metabolic and/or structural changes in ischemia which lead to the development of irreversible injury (3,4,11). In general terms, the deleterious effects of ischemia may be induced either by accumulation of metabolic endproducts or by depletion of HEP (Fig. 1). In hopes of differentiating the relative importance of HEP depletion vs. metabolite accumulation, we investigated the effects of repeated brief episodes of ischemia and reperfusion. Our aim was to achieve cumulative depletion of ATP and of the adenine nucleotide pool of the myocytes while frequently washing out catabolites so that the osmolar load would be reduced significantly. However, much to our surprise, cumulative ATP depletion did not develop during four successive 10 minute episodes of ischemia each separated by 20 minutes of reperfusion (19). ATP content at the end of two or even four 10 minute occlusions was no lower than after a single occlusion. Other workers have reported similar findings (20,21). Inasmuch as ATP was repleted only partially during the first and subsequent reperfusion periods, we concluded that the lack of cumulative loss of ATP during repetitive ischemic episodes indicates that the rate of ATP depletion was slower during later episodes than it was during the first episode of ischemia. Moreover, 40 cumulative minutes of ischemia caused virtually no myocyte necrosis when hearts were evaluated histologically four days after the four 10 minute episodes of ischemia. In contrast, 40 continuous minutes of ischemia caused infarcts involving 20-30% of the area at risk (2,22).

The details of the failure of ATP depletion to cumulate after 10 minutes of ischemia have been presented in a paper by Reimer and coworkers (19). These data were obtained in randomly selected open-chest anesthetized dogs subjected to one, two or four 10 minute episodes of ischemia induced by ligation of the circumflex branch of the left coronary artery. Metabolites were estimated in left ventricle which had been excised quickly and cooled for one minute in ice-cold isotonic KCl before snap freezing and lyophilizing slices of both control and damaged left ventricle. Blood flows were measured in the dry samples prior to extracting metabolites for measurement. Myocardial ATP ranged from 9.1 to 11.4 µmol/g dry weight in tissue receiving 10, 20, or 40 cumulative minutes of ischemia. Thus, no more ATP depletion was detected after four 10 minute episodes of ischemia than was found after a single 10 minute episode (Table 3). The mean arterial collateral flows in the subendocardial layer of the severely ischemic region were 0.08 ml arterial blood/minute/g wet myocardium.

The cause of the slowing in the rate of ATP depletion observed during the second or subsequent episodes of ischemia in myocardium "preconditioned" by a preceding episode of ischemia is unknown. In simplest terms, the HEP demand vs supply relationship must be altered in preconditioned myocardium. Either the demand for HEP is reduced or the amount of HEP from sources other than ATP reserves is increased, or perhaps a combination of these processes induces preconditioning. Changes in compartmentation of the adenine nucleotide pool or inhibition of degradative enzymes such as 5' nucleotidase also could be involved (19). Some of the available data on the relation between HEP production and HEP utilization during repeated episodes of ischemia is reviewed below.

One potential source of increased HEP in the preconditioned myocardium is CP. Numerous studies using instantly frozen biopsies of the zone of injury have shown that CP, after a brief episode of ischemia and reperfusion, reaches levels 25-30 µmol greater than control. This has been termed the "CP overshoot." In biopsies of myocardium reperfused after a brief period of ischemia, CP levels of 65-70 µmol/g (23-26) are usual; these levels represent phosphorylation of most of the entire creatine pool of the myocyte. A similar overshoot has been reported in superfused papillary muscle in vitro when it is paced at a slow rate (27) or in the isolated perfused heart after brief periods of ischemia or hypoxia followed by reperfusion with oxygenated media (28). Thus, myocardium entering a second brief episode of ischemia enters it with more CP and less HEP in the form of ATP and ADP than control myocardium.

The technique used for sampling the tissue for metabolites in previous studies (19) allows precise identification of ischemic tissue and measurement of the adenine nucleotide pool in tissue clearly identified to be ischemic, but yields inaccurate estimates of the CP of living myocardium. For this reason, the ventricles of three dogs subjected to 10 minutes of ischemia and 20 minutes of reperfusion were excised and frozen in isopentane at liquid nitrogen temperatures 3-4 seconds after the intraatrial injection of saturated KCl to arrest the heart. This technique demonstrated a CP overshoot in canine myocardium preconditioned by 10 minutes of ischemia; the CP increased from the 35-40µmol/g found in instantly frozen biopsies of left ventricle to 45.2±1.81 µmol CP/g dry weight (Table 3). However, the freezing technique utilized still is associated with a loss of 15-20 µmol CP from control aerobic myocardium. For this reason, we estimate that the true CP of preconditioned heart is in the range of 63-68 µmol/g dry weight (23-25).

Assuming that the CP of the tissue is 65 µmol/g dry, an extra 30 µmoles of CP is present in tissue which exhibits a net loss of 10-14 µmoles of HEP in the form of ATP Since the ADP of the preconditioned tissue is only slightly less than control and since other sources of reserve nucleotide HEP are minimal, preconditioned heart contains 16 to 20 more µmoles of HEP per gram than it would if the overshoot had not occurred. The cause of the CP overshoot is not known at present, but it may be related to an increase in the ratio of ATP/ADP and consequent increased phosphorylation of creatine.

The contribution of anaerobic glycolysis to the production and utilization of HEP can be estimated by direct measurement of lactate and reserves of HEP in myocardium receiving so little collateral flow that no significant amount of exogenous substrate and oxygen reaches the tissue, and that lactate is not washed from the tissue. Assuming that anaerobic glycolysis is coupled tightly to production of ATP, then one can estimate the quantity of HEP produced during the ischemic episode (7). In Table 4, hearts with subendocardial collateral flows of 0-2% of control were selected from the earlier study (19) and analyzed with respect to HEP utilization and metabolite levels (Table 3). The results show HEP utilization took place at the same rate during the first and second episodes of ischemia and that the rate during a fourth 10 minute of ischemia, though slightly less, was not statistically different from the rate observed during the first episode. Most of the HEP produced came from anaerobic glycolysis; the CP overshoot presumably met some of the initial demand of the tissue for HEP and slowed the onset of anaerobic glycolysis. Note that the total amount of HEP utilized in the preconditioned myocardium while it is ischemic is estimated to be much greater in 40 cumulative minutes of ischemia, i.e. 767 μmoles (208.6 + 195.9 + 176.3 + an estimated 186.1 μmol in the third episode) vs. 418.7 μmoles in 40 continuous minutes of ischemia (Table 3). Thus, more HEP utilization occurred in the preconditioned myocardium and, in the process, HEP reserves were preserved.

An increase in the amount of O_2 available early in the phase of ischemia could account for preconditioning. For example, more O_2 could be trapped in the tissue in the form of oxygenated hemoglobin and myoglobin with the result that increased ATP production, not estimatable by the methods used in Table 3, would occur. However, since reactive hyperemia has disappeared after 20 minutes of reperfusion, there is no difference in the amount of O_2 trapped in myocardium whether or not it is preconditioned. Also, an increase in the collateral flow to the preconditioned myocardium could result in greater HEP production via aerobic metabolism. However, direct measurements of flow in the tissue used for analysis showed no change between the the first and fourth episode of ischemia. Thus, increased O_2 availability is an unlikely explanation for the preconditioning effect.

Acceleration of anaerobic glycolysis during later episodes of ischemia secondary to the washout of various glycolytic inhibitors during each episode of reperfusion could account for the preconditioning effect unless supplies of glycogen become exhausted. However, there is no increase in lactate production during the second or subsequent episode of ischemia. This observation suggests that acceleration in glycolysis is not an explanation for the conditioning effect.

As noted earlier, it seems likely that the CP overshoot produced during aerobic respiration in the reperfused reversibly injured tissue is related to the decreased

TABLE 3. METABOLITES AND HIGH ENERGY PHOSPHATE UTILIZATION DURING ISCHEMIA[y]

Minutes of Ischemia (I) or Reperfusion (R)	ATP	ADP	AMP	Lactate	CP	HEP Utilization in µmol/10' Ischemic Period*	Cumulative HEP Utilization in µmol**
		in µmol/g dry					
10I	8.16	6.42	3.78	104.7	1.4	205.0	
(4)	±1.21	±1.04	±0.58	±8.33	±0.77	±7.3	
10I + 20R[yy]	20.10[d]	2.36[b]	0.32[c]	7.7[d]	45.2[d]	--	
(3)	±0.63	±.36	±.12	±2.10	±1.81	--	
10I+20R+10I	9.92	5.28	1.93[a]	87.7	1.1	198.3	403.0
(4)	±0.38	±0.40	±.30	±14.05	±0.35	±21.4	±21.4
3(10I+20R)+10I	10.50	5.32	1.56[a]	83.5	1.1	176.3	766.9
(4)	±0.63	±0.79	±0.56	±9.55	±0.22	±19.0	±19.0
40I	0.55	1.52	5.60	226.6	0.3	418.7*	
(4)	±.13	±0.14	±0.48	±11.4	±1.0	±16.8	
Non-ischemic[z]	26.06	3.88	0.39	16.1	9.1		
(9)	±0.56	±.22	±.04	±2.08	±1.09		

y   The hearts have been selected for very severe ischemia (Table 4). Metabolites were measured by the methods given in reference 13. The probability that the means are different comparing the 10I group to the other ten minute groups by a two-tailed non-paired t test is: a, $P<.05$; b, $P<.025$; c, $P<.01$; d, $P<.001$.

yy   Ventricles of the 10 + 20 group were frozen 2-4 seconds after the intraatrial injection of a saturated solution of KCl. CP of control subendocardial LV in this group was 20.9 ± 0.77. Since instantly frozen biopsies of LV contain 40 µmol CP per gm dry (29), about 19 µmoles of CP were lost from the subendocardium during excision and freezing. Thus, 64 µmoles CP are estimated to have been present in preconditioned myocardium prior to freezing, i.e., the measured 45.2 µmoles of CP plus 19 µmoles to cover the loss which occurred during freezing.

z   Control data is from nonischemic subendocardial myocardium of the anterior descending bed of hearts sampled by the techniques described in the text and in ref. 19. Frozen heart data was excluded.

*   The formula used to calculate HEP utilization in ischemic virgin myocardium after 10 or 40 minutes of ischemia is based on the data in Table 1: (26 - Obs ATP) x 2 + (3 - Obs ADP)+(40-Obs CP) = HEP Utilized During Ischemic Period. In preconditioned myocardium, the same formula was used but the ATP, ADP, and CP were changed to the levels found after 10 minutes of ischemia and 20 minutes of reperfusion (20.1 - Obs ATP) x 2 + (2.4 - Obs ADP) + (65 - Obs CP) = HEP Utilized During Ischemia. A CP of 65 was used in the calculation for the 10I + 20R + 10I and 3(10I + 20R) + 10I groups because biopsies of ischemic reperfused LV have shown this level to be present (23-25). The rate of utilization in the 10I + 20R + 10I group was indistinguishable from the virgin group (10 x 0) even if the CP of the preconditioned tissue was only 45 µmol/g dry.

**   HEP used during each 10 minute episode of ischemia was estimated by adding the mean quantity of HEP utilized in each 10 minute episode or episodes of ischemia to the calculated values observed in the 10 + 20R + 10I and 3(10I + 20R) + 10I groups. In this calculation, the HEP utilized during the third episode of ischemia is the average of the utilization during the second and fourth episode.

contractility of the preconditioned muscle (17,18) and the increased ATP/ADP ratio. Unknown is the extent to which decreased energy expenditure via contractile efforts continues to occur in preconditioned ischemic myocardium. It seems likely that some HEP is utilized via the myosin ATPase in both virgin and conditioned myocardium while it is ischemic, but no data is available as to the magnitude of this process (26).

The results of these experiments are incomplete. Much remains to be learned about the preconditioning phenomenon. Moreover, the results do not differentiate between the effects of the osmolar load vs ATP and the total adenine nucleotide depletion in inducing fatal ischemic injury. However, ongoing experiments suggest that it will be possible eventually to deplete ATP and the total adenine nucleotide pool without accumulating large quantities of endogenous metabolites.

SUMMARY

Energy production and utilization in reversibly injured myocytes has been reviewed along with a consideration of the effect of reperfusion with arterial blood on the metabolism of living tissue damaged by ischemia. Severely ischemic tissue loses ATP and the total adenine nucleotide pool quickly. ATP reaches 50% of control in 8-10 minutes. However, reperfusion after 10 minutes of ischemia results in partial repletion of ATP from ADP and AMP remaining in the tissue but the total adenine nucleotide pool of the tissue remains decreased at about 70% of control. However, such an episode of ischemia preconditions the myocardium so that no further depletion of ATP results even though the tissue is exposed to as many as three additional 10 minute episodes of ischemia; in contrast, 40 minutes of sustained ischemia depletes tissue ATP and the total adenine nucleotide pool to levels 8 and 30% of control respectively. The explanation for the slower ATP depletion during subsequent ischemic episodes remains unknown; available data suggests that the effect may be related in part to increased reserves of HEP due to a creatine phosphate overshoot in reversibly injured reperfused myocardium, and in part to slower utilization of HEP during subsequent ischemic episodes.

We are grateful for the expert technical assistance of Jean A. Wakefield, Diane Magnuson, and M.L. Hill for animal surgery, blood flow measurements, and measurment of various metabolites reported in Table 1,2, and 4.

This study was supported by National Institutes of Health Grant HL23138, K08-HL01337, and HL27416)

REFERENCES

1. Schaper, W., and Wüsten:In Pathophysiology of Myocardial Perfusion. W. Schaper, ed. Max Planck Institute for Heart Research, Elsevier/North-Holland Biomedical Press, Chapter 13, pp. 415-470, 1979.

2. Reimer, K.A. and Jennings, R.B.:Lab. Invest. 40:633-644, 1979.
3. Jennings, R.B., Reimer, K.A., and Steenbergen, C., Jr.:J. Mol. & Cell Cardiol.18:769-780, 1986
4. Jennings, R.B. and Reimer, K.A.:Am. J. Path. 102:241-255, 1981..
5. Lehninger, A.L.: Principles of Biochemistry. New York: Worth Publishers Inc., 1982, 1104 pp.
6. Jennings, R.B., Kaltenbach, J.P., Sommers, H.M., Bahr, G.F., and Wartman, W.B.:In The Etiology of Myocardial Infarction, edited by TN James and JW Keyes. Boston: Little, Brown and Co., 1963, p. 189-205.
7. Jennings, R.B., Reimer, K.A., Hill, M.L, and Mayer, S.E.:Circ. Res. 49:892-900, 1981.
8. Hochachka, P.W., Owen, T.G., Allen, J.F., and Whitlow, G.C.:Comp. Biochem. Physiol. 50B:17-22, 1975.
9. Jones, R.N., Reimer, K.A., Hill, M.L., and Jennings, R.B.: J. Mol. Cell. Cardiol. 14(Suppl 3) 123-130, 1982.
10. Neely, J.R. and Morgan, H.E.:Ann. Rev. Physiol. 36:413-459, 1974.
11. Jennings, R.B., Hawkins, H.K., Lowe, J.E., Hill, M.L., Klotman, S., and Reimer, K.A.:Am. J. Path. 92:187-214, 1978.
12. Lowe, J.E., Jennings, R.B., and Reimer, K.A.:J. Mol. Cell Cardiol. 11:1017-1031, 1979.
13. Jennings, R.B., Schaper, J., Hill, M.L., Steenbergen, C., and Reimer, K.A.:Circ. Res. 56:262-278, 1985.
14. Reimer, K.A., Hill, M.L., and Jennings, R.B.:J. Mol. Cell Card. 13:229-239, 1981.
15. Zimmer, H. and Gerlach, E.:Pflügers Archiv. 376:223-227, 1978.
16. Basuk, W.L., Reimer, K.A., Jennings, R.B.: J. Am. Coll. Cardiol. 8(Suppl A):33A-41A, 1986.
17. Braunwald, E. and Kloner, R.A.:Circulation 66:1146-1149, 1982.
18. Heyndrickx, G.R., Millard, R.W., McRitchie, R.J., Maroko, P.R. and Vatner, S.F.:J. Clin. Invest. 56:978-985, 1975.
19. Reimer, K.A., Murry C.E., Yamasawa, I., Hill, M.L., Jennings, R.B.:In press, Am. J. Physiol., Dec., 1986.
20. Swain, J.L., Sabina, R.L., Hines, J.J., Greenfield, J.C., Holmes, E.W.:Cardiovasc. Res. XVII:264-269, 1984.
21. Lange, R., Ingwall, J.S., Hale, S.L., Alker, K.J., Kloner, R.A.:Basic Res. Cardiol. 79:469-478, 1984.
22. Reimer, K.A., and Jennings, R.B.:Circ. 71:1069-1075, 1985.
23. Allison, T.B. and Holsinger, J.W.:J. Mol. Cell Cardiol. 15:151-161, 1983.
24. Schaper, J., Mulch, J., Winkler, B., and Schaper, W.:J. Mol. Cell Cardiol. 11:521-541, 5979.
25. Swain, J.L., Sabina, R.L., McHale, P.A., Greenfield, J.C. Jr., and Holmes, E.W.: Am. J. Physiol. 242 (Heart Circ. Physiol. 11):H818-H826, 1982.
26. Ichihara, K, Abiki, Y.:Am. Heart J. 108:1594, 1984.
27. Pool, P.E., Chandler, B.M., Sonnenblick, E.H., and Braunwald, E.:Circ. Res. 22:213-219, 1968.
28. Neely, J.R., Grotyohann, L.W.:Circ. Res. 55:816, 1984.
29. Dunn, R.B. and Griggs, Jr., D.M.:Circ. Res. 37:438-445, 1975.
30. Peuhkurinen, K.J., Takala, T.E.S., Nuutinen, E.M. and Hassinen, I.E.: Am. J. Physiol. 244 (Heart Circ. Physiol. 13):H281-H288, 1983.

17

THE ROLE OF BETA-ADRENOCEPTORS IN ISCHEMIA-INDUCED ACIDOSIS
IN THE ISOLATED RAT HEART : A 31-P NMR STUDY

N. LAVANCHY, J. MARTIN[*] and A. ROSSI

Laboratoire de Physiopathologie du Métabolisme Cardiaque (UA
CNRS 632) Université Scientifique, Technologique et Médicale
et [*]Groupe de Résonance Magnétique Nucléaire en Biologie et
Médecine - DRF - Centre d'Etudes Nucléaires.
GRENOBLE, FRANCE

INTRODUCTION

It has been known for a long time that ischemia of the
heart results in a decrease of the tissue pH (1,2,3). Since
glycolysis and glycogenolysis are accelerated during the
initial phase of ischemia (3,4,5,6), it is reasonable to
assume that a correlation exists between these processes and
acidification (7,8). On the basis of this assumption,
experimental protocols have been devised to examine whether
myocardial beta-adrenergic receptor stimulation plays a part
in the mechanism of ischemia-induced intracellular
acidification. Studies performed on the dog heart "in situ"
have shown that administration of beta-adrenergic blocking
drugs results in a reduction of the acidosis induced by
temporary coronary occlusion (9,10,11,12). Using 31-P NMR
spectroscopy it has also been demonstrated that propranolol
is capable of reducing the degree of acidosis developed
during total ischemia of the isolated rat heart (13,14).
However, the use of beta-adrenergic blocking agents
possessing subsidary properties has revealed that the action
of these drugs on intracellular pH could also be partly
mediated by the membrane-stabilizing property certain of
them possess (9,10,14,15). Furthermore, the strong
depressant action exerted by certain beta-adrenergic
blocking agents is probably also a contributing factor in
the action of these drugs on both energy metabolism and
intracellular acidification of the ischemic tissue. Finally,
since in clinical situations cardioselective

beta-adrenoceptor blockade is generally used, it was of interest to examine more precisely the action of beta-1-adrenoceptor blockade and/or stimulation. Experimental results obtained for the canine heart (12) suggest that myocardial acidosis during the ischemia is related to beta-1-adrenoceptor stimulation. We have shown in a previous study that reduction of ischemia-induced acidosis in the isolated rat heart could be tempered by using a selective beta-1-adrenoceptor blocking drug (acebutolol), at a concentration that did not induce any depressant action (15). Several aspects of this action suggested that the membrane-stabilizing property of the drug could be partly responsible for this effect. The present experimentation was thus designed in order to investigate comparatively the effect of the various properties of the beta-adrenoceptor antagonist. The effect of atenolol, which is a beta-1-adrenoceptor blocking agent devoid of ancillary properties, was compared with that of acebutolol which possesses mild membrane-stabilizing properties. We also utilized d-propranolol which is known to exert a strong non specific membrane-stabilizing effect associated with low beta-adrenergic antagonism, and dl-propranolol as reference.

Further beta-adrenoceptor stimulation was obtained with isoproterenol and catecholamine depletion was induced by pretreating the animals with reserpine.

Experiments were performed on the isolated rat heart rendered globally ischemic. A residual coronary flow (1% of preischemic flow) was maintained to allow the continuous perfusion of the drugs during ischemia. The 31-P NMR spectroscopy technique was used in order to be able to follow simultaneously the alteration in intracellular pH and phosphorus compound concentration respectively.

METHODS

Animals .

Hearts were excised from anaesthetized (pentobarbital 50 mg per kg b.w. i.p.) and heparinized female Wistar rats

(230-270 g). Series of rats were subjected to a pretreatment using reserpine (i.p. 0.1 mg per kg b.w. daily, 3 days successively) prior isolation of the heart.

Biochemical measurements .

These were performed on freeze-clamped "in situ" ventricles on control and reserpine-pretreated rats. Acid-soluble compounds were extracted with perchloric acid and determined as previously described (16). The glycogen content was evaluated after KOH extraction (17). All results are expressed relative to myocardial protein content in order to eliminate the effect of any change in wet weight induced by the treatment.

Perfusion conditions .

Hearts were subjected to a retrograde non-recirculatory perfusion at 37°C under a hydrostatic pressure of 9.81 kPa. They were allowed to beat spontaneously. After bubbling the medium with the O_2-CO_2 (95%-5%) gas mixture the pH of the solution at the level of the aorta was adjusted to pH 7.4 by varying the amount of $NaHCO_3$ in the fluid. The perfusion medium contained : NaCl 120 mM ; KCl 5.6 mM ; $CaCl_2$ 2.4 mM ; $MgCl_2$, 1.2 mM ; glucose 11.1 mM.

For the NMR experiments, the hearts were placed in a 15 mm diameter teflon-stoppered tube and immersed in a constant minimal volume of perfusate, the excess of which was evacuated via a peristaltic pump. The NMR tube was then placed in the bore of the magnet. Gas content and temperature of the perfusion fluid were maintained constant by using thermostatically controlled glass tubing.

Effect of drugs on the contractility of the hearts .

In a parallel series of hearts, we estimated the effect of the various drugs used on the ventricular function.

The left ventricular developed pressure (LVP : systolic pressure minus diastolic pressure) was used as indicator of the contractile function. It was monitored throughout the experiment by means of a teflon catheter (PE 160) inserted into the left ventricle via the auricle and connected to a Gould recorder via a Statham pressure

transducer. LVP changes were expressed as percentages of
the pressure developed by the 20th minute of normoxic
perfusion. The drugs were added to the perfusion fluid by
the 20th minute, the effects were measured by the 30th
minute and compared with the same variables (LVP , heart
rate, coronary flow) measured on control hearts for the same
duration (30 min) of normoxic perfusion.

Experimental protocol in NMR experiments .

After a 30 minute normoxic perfusion, each heart was
submitted to a 24 minute global low-flow ischemia (1 % of
the spontaneous pre-ischemic coronary flow) by means of a
peristaltic pump.

Each of the following drugs was fed into the perfusion
buffer throughout the entire sequence : atenolol 10^{-5}M,
dl-propranolol 10^{-5}M, d-propranolol 10^{-5}M, acebutolol 2.7 10^{-5}
M. Isoproterenol 10^{-8} M was fed into the perfusion fluid
during ischemia only. Hearts from rats pretreated with
reserpine were submitted to the same experimental procedure
but in the absence of the drugs.

NMR measurements .

31-P NMR spectra were recorded at 101.3 MHz on a Bruker
WM 250 spectrometer. The 3 minute spectra were obtained at
5000 Hz spectral width, using a 4 K data table, without
proton decoupling, by applying 45°RF pulses. A field
frequency lock, (D2O in a capillary tube), was utilized.
Each spectrum represented the average of 132 transients.

ATP, PC, Pi were calculated by integrating the areas
under the respective peaks.

Intramyocardial pH (pHi) was evaluated from the
chemical shift of the pH-dependent peak of inorganic
phosphate (Pi) relative to the creatine phosphate (PC) peak
(the latter being pH-dependent in the physiological pH
range). The calibration curve expressed in terms of chemical
shift of Pi relative to PC was plotted from the values
obtained in phosphate-buffered perchloric cardiac extract.
Taking into account the intrinsic limitations of accuracy of
both the calibration curve and the digital resolution chosen

for NMR spectroscopy, we considered each individual pH value
measurement to be accurate to within 0.05 pH unit.

Statistical procedure .

The mean values were compared using a Student's test
and, where necessary, variance analysis.

P = 0.05 was taken as the limit of significance.

RESULTS

Effect of depletion of endogenous catecholamines .

Low doses of reserpine (0.1 mg/kg daily, 3 days),
sufficient to deplete endogenous cardiac catecholamines
(18), did not significantly alter the metabolite content of
the myocardium, as shown in Table 1. Therefore, it can be
assumed that the changes induced by the drug during ischemia
of the isolated heart could reasonably be attributed solely
to the non-release of endogenous catecholamines during
ischemia and not to previous alterations in metabolite
content.

	PC micromol/g	ATP proteins	AC	glycogen mg/g proteins
Controls (28)	39.6 ± 1.1	31.4 ± 0.7	0.91 ± 0.01	26.4 ± 2.0
Reserpine (7)	39.3 ± 4.2	28.0 ± 1.5	0.90 ± 0.01	31.6 ± 2.1
P < 0.05	NS	NS	NS	NS

Table 1 Effects of reserpine treatment of the rats on
metabolite contents of the heart. Hearts were freeze-clamped
"in situ". Means ± SEM. AC = Adenylate charge (ATP + 1/2
ADP) / (ATP + ADP + AMP).

Figure 1 shows the changes in NMR spectra as observed
in control hearts compared with those observed in hearts
from reserpinized rats. The quantitative data shown in Fig.
2 reveal that, in reserpinized rat hearts, the degradation
of ATP during ischemia was less marked than that in control
hearts, while the concomitant increase in Pi was also
attenuated.

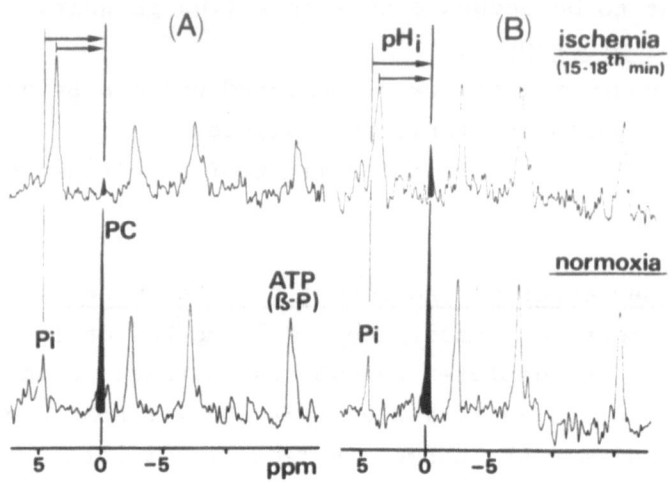

Fig. 1 31-P NMR spectra from isolated rat hearts submitted to global low-flow ischemia. Control heart (A), heart from reserpinized rat (B), Scale in part per million (ppm) with reference to the phosphocreatine frequency.

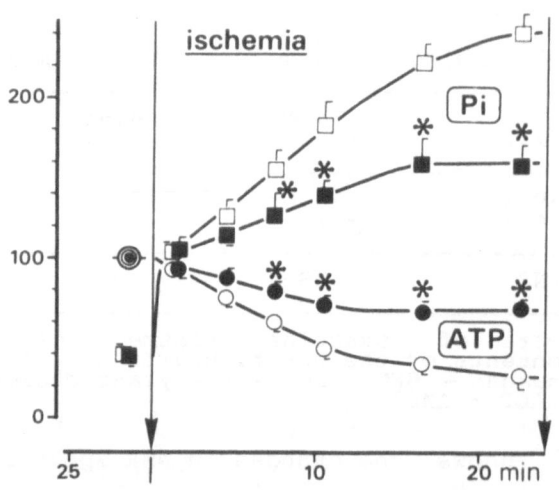

Fig. 2 Time-course changes in myocardial ATP and Pi contents during global low-flow ischemia observed by 31-P NMR spectroscopy on the isolated rat heart : reserpine-treated rats (■●, n=8) and controls (□○, n=16). ATP and Pi : percentages of the preischemic ATP value. m $\pm$ SEM. *P < 0.05 (RES vs CONT.).

The intracellular acidification developed during ischemia was also significantly attenuated by the pretreatment of the animals with reserpine (Fig. 3).

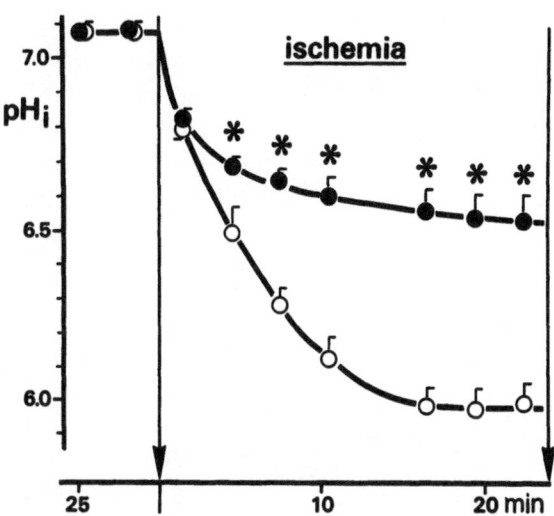

Fig. 3 Time-course changes in intracellular pH (pHi) during a 24 min global low-flow ischemia (1% of the preischemic flow, 37°C) measured by 31-P NMR spectroscopy on the isolated rat heart : comparison between hearts from reserpine-treated rats (●, n=8) and controls (○, n=16). m ± SEM. * P < 0.05.

Effects of the beta-adrenoreceptor blocking drugs .

The choice of concentration of the drugs was based on a previous work on the action of acebutolol on the ischemic isolated rat heart (16). Since significant NMR visible effects were induced by a 2.7×10^{-5}M concentration and not by one of 5.4×10^{-5}M, atenolol and dl-propranolol were used at an equipotent beta-adrenergic antagonistic concentration of 1.10^{-5}M (19).

When added to the perfusion fluid, all these drugs were able to antagonize the chronotropic effect of 10^{-8} M isoproterenol. d-Propranolol was used at the same relatively high concentration in order to examine a possible action it exerts by means of its membrane-stabilizing activity. With this dosage, d-propranolol too virtually eliminated the effect of isoproterenol 10^{-8}M.

None of the drugs displayed significant chronotropic effects on the normoxic heart (Fig. 4).

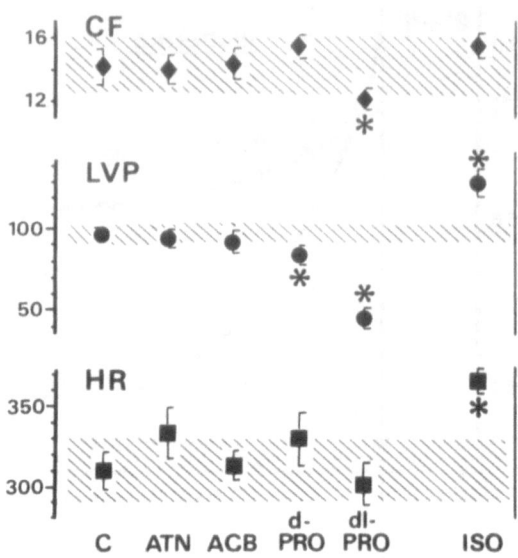

Fig. 4 Effects of drugs on heart rate (HR : beats/min), left ventricular developed pressure (LVP ; see methods) and coronary flow (CR : ml/min) in the normoxic perfused heart. Drugs were added to the buffer at the respective concentrations : atenolol 10^{-5}M (ATN), acebutolol 2.7 10^{-5}M (ACB), d-propranolol 10^{-5}M (d-PRO), dl-propranolol 10^{-5}M (dl-PRO), isoproterenol 10^{-8} M (ISO). For each index, the shaded area represents control value 2 SEM and values are m ± SEM. Different from control value * P < 0.05.

Neither atenolol nor acebutolol affected the left ventricular developed pressure (LVP) ; d-propranolol significantly reduced LVP, while dl-propranolol strongly depressed heart function.

The coronary flow of the hearts was not altered except in the presence of dl-propranolol, probably as a consequence of decreased heart activity. In addition, analysis of the 31-P NMR spectra recorded after a 25 min normoxic perfusion revealed that the depressant action of d- and dl-propranolol results in a significant increase in the PC/Pi ratio (4.4 ± 1.0, n = 6 for dl-PRO versus 2.5 ± 0.5, n = 24 for controls ; m ± S.D.).

The results presented in Fig. 5, which are obtained using the last 3 min spectrum (21st -24th min) recorded during ischemia, show clearly that all beta-adrenoreceptor antagonists exerted comparable effects. The intracellular acidification was significantly reduced and the ATP degradation was slowed down in the presence of the beta-adrenoreceptor blockers. The lower accumulation of Pi induced by the drugs was not in all cases statistically significant due to scattering in individual values.

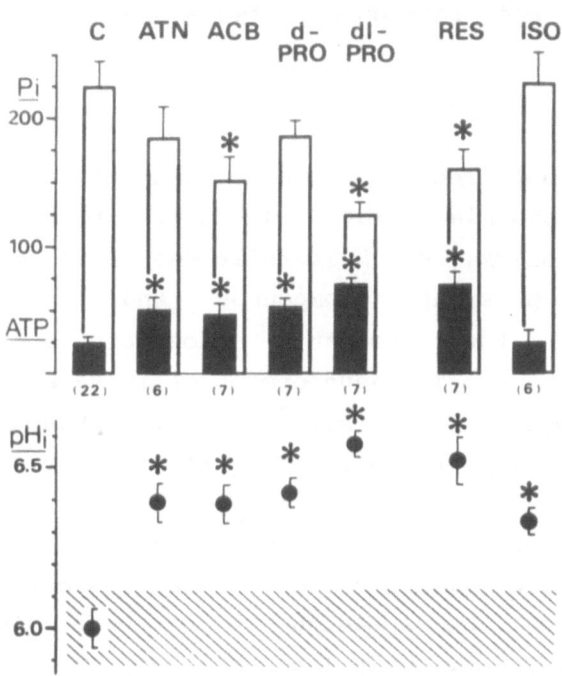

Fig. 5 Myocardial state of the isolated rat heart at the end of a 24 min low-flow ischemia (1% of the preischemic flow, 37°C), as assessed by 31-P NMR spectroscopy : effect of beta-blocking agents, isoproterenol during ischemia and reserpine-pretreatment of the rats.
Heart contents in ATP (black column) and Pi (light) are expressed in percent of the preischemic ATP content. For intracellular pH (pHi) the shaded area represents the control value ± 2 SEM. Other values are means ± SEM. Different from controls *P < 0.05.
Beta-blocking agents were added to the perfusion fluid from the beginning of the perfusion : atenolol 10^{-5}M (ATN), acebutolol 2.7 10^{-5} M (ACB), d-propranolol 10^{-5}M (d-PRO), dl-propranolol 10^{-5} M (dl-PRO). Isoproterenol 10^{-8}M was added during ischemia only (ISO). Hearts from reserpine-pretreated rats (RES).

Effect of the addition of 10^{-8} M isoproterenol during ischemia .

The data concerning the effect of isoproterenol are shown in Fig. 5. They show clearly that the ATP degradation and the Pi accumulation were not significantly different from control conditions. It is of particular interest to note that, when the beta-receptor agonist was present in the perfusion fluid during ischemia, the intracellular pH was not decreased to the same extent as in the control group. We controlled that isoproterenol 10^{-8} M did exert significant chronotropic and inotropic effects on the normoxic heart (Fig. 4).

DISCUSSION

The abrupt reduction in oxygen delivery to the cells caused by ischemia creates an immediate imbalance in the energy metabolism, which is reflected in the degradation of high-energy phosphate compounds and the simultaneous increase in the inorganic phosphate content of the myocardial tissue. The development of intracellular acidosis which accompanies the alteration in phosphate compound concentration is probably the reflect of several different mechanisms.

The stimulation of the beta-adrenoceptors by the endogenous catecholamines released at the onset of ischemia resulting in the speeding up of both glycolysis and glycogenolysis, obviously leads to the production of protons associated with lactate production (20). Moreover, the degradation of adenine nucleotides (especially ATP) together with a possible residual, though slight, mitochondrial CO_2 production contribute to the increase in proton concentration (21,22). Moreover, a possible relationship between the increase in intracellular calcium by beta-receptors stimulation and intracellular acidification is also worthy of consideration (23). Thus, the elimination of the effect of catecholamines obtained by either the complete prior depletion of the heart in catecholamines or the efficient beta 1-blockade using atenolol could provide a simple explanation of both the expected decrease of ischemia-induced intracellular acidosis and the attenuated energy imbalance in the myocardial tissue (as reflected by higher ATP and lower Pi content).

The reduction in cardiac activity induced by the cardiac depressant action of dl-propranolol 10^{-5} M, this probably independently of the beta-adrenergic antagonism (24,25), accounts for the greater effect of this drug as compared with 10^{-5}M atenolol and 2.7 10^{-5}M acebutolol which did not have any significant functional effect on the heart. Thus, in all the situations indicated above (catecholamine depletion, beta-blockade, reduction of cardiac activity), the fall-of in acidosis can be explained in terms of a reduction in proton production.

However, in the experimental model used in this study, a significant coronary flow, albeit greatly restricted, is maintained during ischemia, thereby mimicking most of the current clinical situations (26). So, a certain washing out is undoubtly maintained and, in fact, the intracellular pH reflects the state of imbalance between a speeded up proton production and a diminished (but not completely abolished) proton extrusion. It thus appears that the extent of intracellular acidification depends not only on the changes in metabolism, but must also be related to the precise conditions that create this energy imbalance (degree of residual flow). This observation provides a possible explanation of the unexpected effect of 10^{-8}M isoproterenol when added to the buffer during ischemia, i.e. similar important alterations in ATP and Pi myocardial content as in control hearts associated with significantly less intracellular acidosis than in controls. The fact that the surimposed beta-adrenergic stimulation did not induce any further degradation of ATP was also shown "in situ" on the canine heart submitted to regional ischemia (27). This result can probably be explained by assuming that the beta-adrenoreceptors are already maximally stimulated by the early release of endogenous catecholamines (28). The rapidly lower intracellular acidification developing during ischemia in the case of a perfusion with isoproterenol seems more difficult to explain. In this regard, the findings of Riegle and Clancy (29) indicating that norepinephrine markedly attenuates the changes in intracellular pH accompanying metabolic acidosis in the isolated rat heart are of interest. Our results are also consistent with the hypothesis that catecholamines are capable of reducing the intracellular proton concentration. The fact that this effect becomes significant in the presence of isoproterenol can probably be explained by the need for a higher concentration of beta-adrenoreceptor agonist than that reached in an isolated heart over the whole ischemic period as a result of the early release of endogenous catecholamines alone. These findings may also help to explain why lower pH are observed during ischemia in the isolated heart compared with that in the heart "in situ". The mechanisms by means of which catecholamines influence the pH require further studies. However it is reasonable to assume that this effect can be exerted at the level of the trans-sarcolemmal extrusion of protons. Recent studies have demonstrated that, in isolated myocardial cells, the Na^+/H^+ exchange is by far the most important mechanism ensuring the exportation of protons when the intracellular medium becomes acidotic (30,31). It can therefore be assumed that, if the Na^+/H^+ exchange remains the favoured mechanism in the isolated ischemic heart, its efficacy could be influenced by a series of trans-sarcolemmal ionic fluxes. Thus, it is possible that isoproterenol directly or indirectly acts on proton extrusion via the alterations of one or several other ionic transmembrane conductances.

Thus, a non-specific action such as the "membrane-stabilizing" activity of certain beta-blocking agents could also exert its influence on the transmembrane ionic fluxes. In a previous study, we emphasized that this property could partly explain the effect of acebutolol (16).

In conclusion , the results presented in this study suggest that the actual intracellular pH observed in the ischemic heart should not be considered solely in terms of its relationship to metabolism. Indeed, the observed evidence that isoproterenol attenuates the ischemia-induced acidosis underlines the necessity of taking into consideration the possible interaction of drugs on other mechanisms playing a part in pH regulation such as buffering or proton extrusion. Whether such interaction is directly mediated by beta-adrenoceptors or is non-specific is yet to be elucidated. In this regard, it seems possible that the membrane-stabilizing activity of certain beta-adrenoceptor antagonists comes into play in trans-sarcolemmal exchanges.

Acknowledgments : This research was supported, in part, by funds from INSERM (PRC/30068 and CRE 85.349.5 E). We are very grateful to Mrs. Dubourdeaux and Fidelis for their secretarial work. Atenolol, dl-propranolol and d-propranolol were kindly provided by ICI-Pharma (France). Acebutolol was generously supplied by SPECIA Lab. (France). Reserpine (Serpasil) was donated by CIBA-GEIGY.

REFERENCES

1. Gebert, G., Benzing, H. and Strohm, M. Pflügers Arch. 329 : 72-81, 1971.
2. Benzing, H., Gebert, G. and Strohm, M. Cardiol. 56 : 85-88, 1971/72.
3. Neely, J.R., Whitmer, J.T. and Rovetto, M.J. Circ. Res. 37 : 733-741, 1975.
4. Bing, R.J. Physiol. Rev. 45 : 171-213, 1965.
5. Williamson, J.R. Control of Energy Metabolism (Eds. B.Chance, R.W.Eastbrook and J.R.Williamson), Academic Press, New York, 1965 pp. 333-346.
6. Dobson, J.G. and Mayer, S.E. Circ. Res. 33 : 412-420, 1973.
7. Garlick, P.B., Radda, G.K. and Seeley, P.J. Biochem. J. 184 : 547-554, 1979.
8. Bailey, I.A., Radda, G.K., Seymour, A.M.L. and Williams, S.R. Biochem. Biophys. Acta 720 : 17-27, 1982.
9. Ichihara, K., Ichihara, M. and Abiko, Y. J. Pharmacol. Exp. Ther. 209 : 275-281, 1979.
10. Abiko, Y. and Sakai, K. Eur. J. Pharmacol. 64 : 239-247, 1980.
11. Izumi, T., Sakai, K. and Abiko, Y. Naunyn-Schmiedeberg's Arch. Pharmacol. 318 : 340-343, 1982.
12. Sakai, K. and Abiko, Y. J. Pharm. Exp. Ther. 232 : 810-816, 1985.
13. Pieper, G.M., Todd, G.L., Wu, S.T., Salhany, J., Clayton, F.C. and Eliot, R.S. Cardiovasc. Res. 14 : 646-653, 1980.
14. Nakazawa, M., Katano, Y., Imai, S., Matsushita, K. and Ohuchi, M.J. Cardiovasc. Pharmacol. 4 : 700-704, 1982.
15. Lavanchy, N., Martin, J. and Rossi, A. Eur. J. Pharmacol. (in press).
16. Lavanchy, N., Martin, J. and Rossi, A. Cardiovasc. Res. 18 : 571-582, 1984.
17. Lavanchy, N., Martin, J. and Rossi, A. FEBS Letters 178 : 34-38, 1984.
18. Wakade, A.R. Br. J. Pharmacol. 68 : 93-98, 1980.
19. Frishman, W. Am. Heart J. 97 : 663-670, 1979.
20. Gevers, W. J. Mol. Cell. Cardiol. 9 : 867-874, 1977.
21. Wilkie, D.R. J. Mol. Cell. Cardiol. 11 : 325-330, 1979.
22. Seelye, R.N. J. Mol. Cell. Cardiol. 12 : 1483-1486, 1980.

23. Vaughan-Jones, R.D., Lederer, W.J. and Eisner, D.A. Nature 301 : 522-524, 1983.
24. Nayler, W.G., Chipperfield, D. and Lowe, T.E. Cardiovasc. Res. 3 : 30-36, 1969.
25. Dhalla, N.S. and Lee, S.L. Br. J. Pharmac. 57 : 215-221, 1976.
26. Opie, L.H. Cir. Res. 33 : 52-74, 1976.
27. Goodlett, M., Dowling, K., Eddy, L.J. and Downey, J.M. Am. J. Physiol. 239 : H 469-H 476, 1980.
28. Wollenberger, A. and Krause, E.G. Am. J. Cardiology 22 : 349-359, 1968.
29. Riegle, K.M. and Clancy, R.L. Am. J. Physiol. 229 : 344-349, 1975.
30. Lazdunski, M., Frelin, C. and Vigne, P. J. Mol. Cell. Cardiol. 17 : 1029-1042, 1985.
31. Aickin, C.C., Ann. Rev. Physiol. 48 : 349-361, 1986.

18

PROTECTIVE AND NONPROTECTIVE EFFECTS OF DRUGS ON CARDIAC CONTRACTILE
ACTIVITY AND HIGH ENERGY PHOSPHATES DURING ANOXIA AND AFTER REOXYGENATION

M. SIESS, U. DELABAR, K. STIELER, J. LEUCHTNER, I. TEUTSCH, A. KHATTAB*,
M.B. EL HAWARY*

Department of Pharmacology, Medical Faculty, University of Tuebingen, FRG
*Department of Pharmacology, Medical School, University of Cairo, Egypt

INTRODUCTION

One important field of basic research in cardiology has been focused
during the last decade on possible cardioprotective or -nonprotective
interventions in energy metabolism or performance to improve the cardiac
cell survival during periods of anoxic or hypoxic cardioplegia and
during the critical phase of reoxygenation in cardiothoracic surgery (1, 9).
With a recently developed 'anoxia test' as a model (2, 3, 6) using superfused left guinea pig atria at rest or at a reduced anoxic contractile
work, we have studied
- a) influences on high energy phosphate levels and on the energy quotient
     (ATP/(ADP + AMP)) with precursors of AN (adenine nucleotide)-, NAD-
     and CP-synthesis (adenine, ribose, nicotinic acid, creatine),
- b) influences of drugs on contractile activity, measuring the auxotonic
     contractile work/beat and work/hr
during normoxia, anoxia and reoxygenation independent from hemodynamic
factors. In this chapter we want to give a short review about some essential
points of our findings which may be perhaps of general interest.

MATERIALS AND METHODS

are described in detail (2, 3, 4, 5, 7, 8).

RESULTS AND DISCUSSION

Protective effects on high energy phosphate levels during normoxia and anoxia

In normoxia addition of precursors (adenine 0.1 mM, ribose 0.5 - 15 mM,
nicotinic acid 0.05 mM, creatine 5 - 10 mM) increases after 5 hrs significantly AN- and NAD-, but not CP-levels to~40 % by new synthesis in
resting or beating atria (Fig. 5), (2, 4, 5, 6, 11).

During the 'anoxia test' these precursors also have saving effects on the anoxic degradation of AN- and NAD-levels even at a high beat rate (Fig. 1), if the anoxic energy yield of ATP is sufficient by anaerobic glycolysis stimulated to a maximum due to an unlimited intracellular lactate washout (2, 6).

Reduced cardiac work of left guinea pig atria by electric stimulation with a low beat rate (0.5 Hz) (Fig. 2) or standstill before anoxia has been started protects in absence of precursors AN- and NAD- but not CP-levels significantly compared with working preparations at a high beat rate.

Conclusions. Addition of the precursors adenine, ribose and nicotinic acid to cardioplegic solutions used in cardiothoracic surgery seems therefore advisable whereas creatine has no protective effect in normoxia or anoxia. Standstill before anoxia protects AN- and NAD-levels best.

Nonprotective effects on high energy phosphate levels during normoxia and anoxia

Standstill due to K^+-depolarization in NORMOXIA with increased O_2-uptake. We have seen that cardiac arrest before the start of anoxia has the best saving effect on high energy phosphates with the exception of the CP-levels. In many cardioplegic solutions, however, standstill is supported by K^+-depolarization with addition of 10 mM KCl (K_1^+) up to 60 mM KCl (K_4^+) or even higher concentrations, connected with a reduction of the temperature to 30° or 20° C of the cardioplegic solution. At 30° C we observed that these concentrations of K^+ increased the resting O_2-uptake between 8 % (K_1^+) to 100 % (K_4^+), respectively (Fig. 3, 4), (7, 8, 10). Fenn has observed this effect of K^+ 1931 on frog skeletal muscle (14). At 20° C K_1^+ and K_4^+ raise the resting O_2-uptake to the same percentage from a $\sim$20 % reduced initial value. The increased O_2-uptake is dependent on the Ca^{++}-influx through the slow Ca^{++}-channels and can be inhibited by nifedipine (10^{-6} M), if given before or at the peak of O_2-uptake 5 min after K^+-depolarization (Fig. 4). The K^+-enhanced mitochondrial activity is slightly lowered during the following 3 hrs, but remains with K_4^+ after this time far above the initial resting O_2-uptake without K^+-depolarization. Nifedipine, when added at this stage, inhibits the enhanced O_2-uptake only weakly (Fig. 3, 4).

The increased resting O_2-uptake in atria due to K^+-depolarization does not improve the high energy phosphate levels (ATP, AN, NAD, CP) or the energy quotient (Fig. 7). This could be explained by an increased energy need of ATP for the activated Na^+/K^+-pump or by an uncoupling effect. An uncoupling effect in the respiratory chain may play the most important role since the new synthesis of AN and NAD from precursors is inhibited by K_1^+ and completely stopped by K_4^+ (Fig. 5), (11). The energy quotient is here lowered highly significant indicating that in spite of the 100 % increased O_2-uptake the produced energy is insufficient for new synthesis of energy-rich phosphates (Fig. 7).

Conclusions. Concentrations above 15.9 mM KCl in cardioplegic solutions cannot be recommended for cardiac arrest in normoxia, because of the uncoupling activation of mitochondria. This can be inhibited, however, by nifedipine given simultaneously. K^+-depolarization inhibits also the new synthesis of AN and NAD from the precursors adenine, ribose and nicotinic acid.

Standstill due to K^+-depolarization in ANOXIA. During a period of 2 hrs anoxia with increased anaerobic glycolysis as only source of energy gain in resting left atria without K^+-depolarization the ATP-level is slightly reduced (-30 %) and shifted to ADP and AMP without loss of total AN. In absence and in presence of precursors the energy quotient is lowered from 7.2 to 3.1 and 6.8 to 3.6 respectively (Fig. 7), (11). These values provide an anoxic cell survival in the mean for 6 hrs in spite of a strongly degraded CP-level (-90 %). In this experiment additional protective effect of precursors in anoxia cannot be shown because the saving effect of standstill before anoxia has been started is here predominant. The survival can be proved by electric stimulation producing contractile activity as shown in the 'anoxia test' (2, 6). This anoxic reduced energy balance is deteriorated drastically by K^+-depolarization with K_4^+ to very low levels of ATP, AN, CP and NAD (Fig. 6) and a significant decrease of the energy quotient (0.5!) which cannot provide anoxic cell survival. In contrast to anoxic beating atria without K^+-depolarization precursors have here no protective effects on the energy state (Fig. 7), (11). Even a low concentration of only 15.9 mM KCl decreases the energy quotient significantly to 2.1. The same can be observed at a temperature of 20° C with K_4^+. Nifedipine (10^{-6} M), when given before, inhibits this deteriorating effect of K_4^+ on the high energy phosphate levels even on CP. The additionally deteriorating decrease of the energy quotient due to K_4^+ in anoxia is completely inhibited by nifedipine.

Conclusions. The reduced anoxic energy state which provides anoxic cardiac cell survival by increased anaerobic glycolysis for 6 hrs and more is severely deteriorated by K^+-depolarization in concentrations above 15 mM KCl to values far below anoxic cell survival. Precursors do not have here protective effects, in contrary the energy state is considerably worsened even with 15 mM KCl (K_1^+). This can be shown at 30° and 20° C.

Nifedipine inhibits the additionally deteriorating effects of K^+-depolarization on the anoxic energy state at 20° C, even on the reduced CP.

Protective and nonprotective effects of cardiotonic drugs on contractile activity during normoxia and anoxia ('anoxia test')

In left atria of guinea pigs stimulated at normoxia with 0.5 Hz the auxotonic contractile work/beat (mm x mN) will be reduced from the maximum value reached at 1.5 Hz (100 %) to~35 % due to the force-frequency relationship. In normoxia this value decreases then slowly after~2 hrs to values of~10 % of the maximum after 6 hrs ('normoxic fatigue'). During 2 hrs anoxia ('anoxia test') this normoxic reduced contractile work/beat (100 %) will be lowered to a plateau-level of 50 to 80 % of the initial normoxic value before anoxia. The anoxic contractile activity decreases then slowly and expires after 6 to 10 hrs (time to standstill = anoxic tolerance). Here all tested cardiotonic drugs (epinephrine, norepinephrine, forskolin, histamine, theophylline, caffeine, ouabain) produce transient positive inotropic actions during strict anoxia. However, the time course to standstill is considerably shortened and the anoxic 'fatigue' more expressed, presumably by an unbalance between anoxic ATP-production and increased ATP-need by the positive inotropic action: Only with the cardioglycoside ouabain a considerably and significantly increased and prolonged contractile activity can be observed (2).

In contrast, however, all investigated eicosanoids as well as bradykinine do not change the anoxic contractile work/beat, whereas in normoxia all these substances have positive inotropic effects (3, 12), presumably by an active Ca^{++}-output from cardiac mitochondria reported recently (15). The intrinsic activity on the cardiac work/beat is different: $PGE_1 > {}^17$-oxo-$PGI_2 > PGI_2 > PGE_2 > {}^2HOE$ 892 $> {}^3ZK$ 36374 $> {}^4EMD$ 42501 (Formula of number 1 - 4 s. Fig. 15). The normoxic inotropic effects decline with natural prostaglandins (10^{-5} mM) to the initial value within~1/2 hr and with the more stable analogs of PGI_2 within~2 hrs.

Reoxygenation and auxotonic contractile work

After 2 hrs anoxia reoxygenation increases suddenly the anoxic reduced contractile work with a short first overshoot of contractile work above the

NMOL / MG PROT.	CONTROL 1H NORMOXIA + 2H ANOXIA	% OF NORMOXIC CONTROL VALUE (3H)	100 μMOL/L ADENINE 500 μMOL/L RIBOSE 1H NORMOXIA + 2H ANOXIA	% OF NORMOXIC CONTROL VALUE (3H)	Δ	P
NAD⁺	2.29 ± 0.12	68 %	2.31 ± 0.25	68 %	0 %	N.S.
CP	2.13 ± 0.34	6 %	2.99 ± 0.54	8 %	+ 2 %	N.S.
ATP	5.65 ± 0.98	20 %	12.8 ± 1.56	47 %	+ 27 %	**
AN	13.06 ± 1.44	37 %	22.3 ± 2.31	64 %	+ 27 %	**

KREBS-HENSELEIT SOLUTION + 15 MMOL/L GLUCOSE (CONTROL) AND WITH ADDITION OF ADENINE AND RIBOSE, 35 °C (N = 6, X̄ ± S.E.M.), **P < 0.01

Fig. 1. <u>Anoxia-test</u>. Adenine and ribose as precursors of AN-synthesis diminish significantly the anoxic loss of ATP and total AN in spontaneously beating atria even at a high beat rate (200 b p m), but not loss of CP.

NMOL / MG PROT.	SPONTANEOUSLY BEATING ATRIA ~ 200 BEATS/MIN 1H NORMOXIA + 2H ANOXIA	% OF NORMOXIC VALUE (3H)	ELECTRICALLY DRIVEN LEFT ATRIA (0.5 Hz) ~ 30 BEATS/MIN 1H NORMOXIA + 2H ANOXIA	% OF NORMOXIC VALUE (3H)	Δ	P
NAD⁺	2.29 ± 0.12	68 %	2.7 ± 0.17	80 %	+ 12 %	N.S.
CP	2.13 ± 0.34	6 %	2.59 ± 0.96	7 %	+ 1 %	N.S.
ATP	5.65 ± 0.98	20 %	18.81 ± 0.87	68 %	+ 48 %	***
AN	13.06 ± 1.44	37 %	28.95 ± 0.73	83 %	+ 46 %	***

KREBS-HENSELEIT SOLUTION + 15 MMOL/L GLUCOSE, 35 °C, (N = 6, X̄ ± S.E.M), ***P < 0.001

Fig. 2. <u>Anoxia-test</u>. Reduction of atrial work before the beginning of anoxia preserves ATP- and AN- but not CP-levels. The best effect has standstill before anoxia (here not shown).

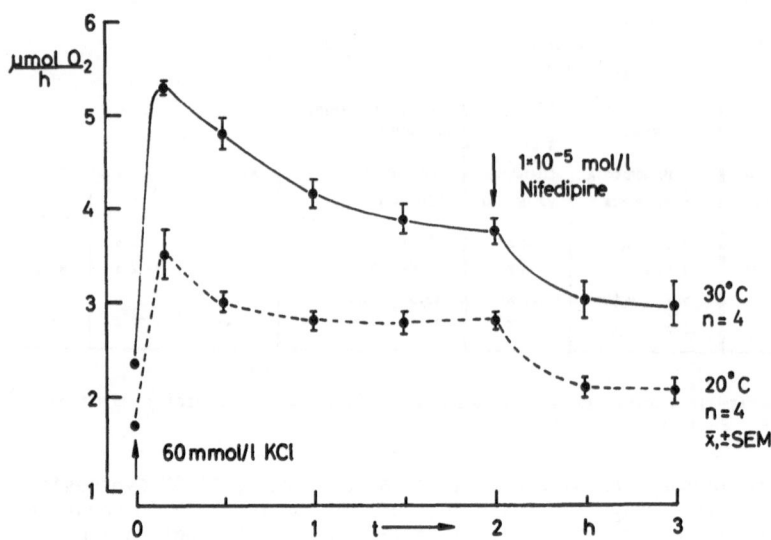

Fig. 3. <u>Similar time course of the increase of O_2-uptake in resting left atria due to 60 mM KCl at 30° and 20° C.</u> Lowering the temperature from 30° to 20° C reduces basal atrial oxygen uptake by about 20 %. Upon KCl-addition O_2-uptake initially increases to a peak value (+125 %, +105 %) and then gradually declines to a new steady-state level (+55 %, +65 %).

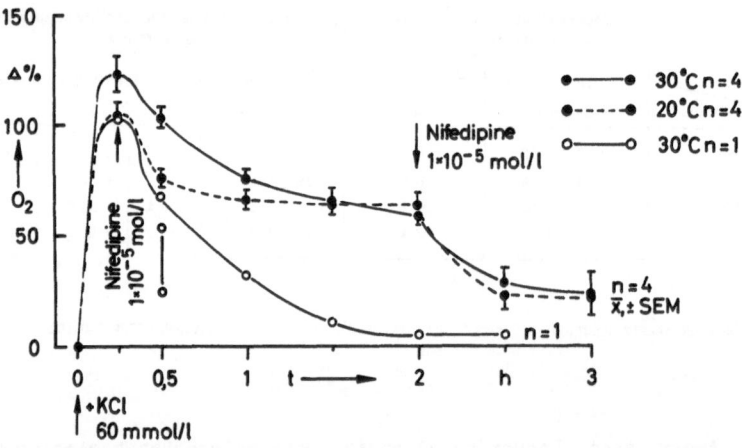

Fig. 4. <u>The inhibiting effect of nifedipine on K^+-stimulated O_2-uptake at 30° and 20° C.</u> With 60 mM KCl at each temperature an identical maximal increase of O_2-uptake of about 100 % is observed, which can be completely abolished by preincubation with nifedipine (not shown). Nifedipine given at the peak value 5 to 15 min after K^+-depolarization decreases this enhanced O_2-uptake to initial values during 1 1/2 hr, when added after 2 hrs O_2-uptake is only reduced to 25 % above the initial level (s. also Fig. 3).

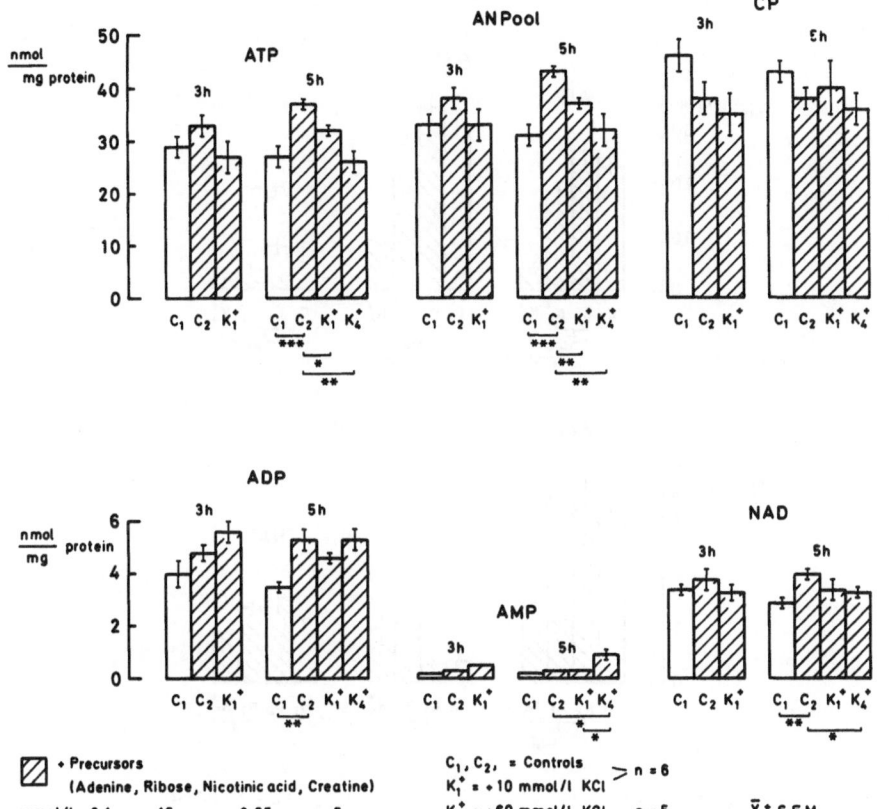

Fig. 5. AN (ATP + ADP + AMP)-, CP- and NAD-levels of resting left atria
incubated in <u>normoxia</u> without (C_1) and with (C_2) precursors, demonstrating
a significant increase (~+40 %) of AN- and NAD-levels after 5 hrs incubation.
This new synthesis is concentration-dependent inhibited by K_1^+ and K_4^+.

initial normoxic value. This is presumably due to a release of anoxic stored
Ca^{++} from mitochondria by the starting H^+-pump (Fig. 16, 17). The peak is
reached after 5 min and declines during 30 min to a plateau-level in the
range of the initial normoxic value (Fig. 8). The area under this peak
demonstrates possibly the release of endogenous Ca^{++} or a suddenly increased Ca^{++}-influx (16).

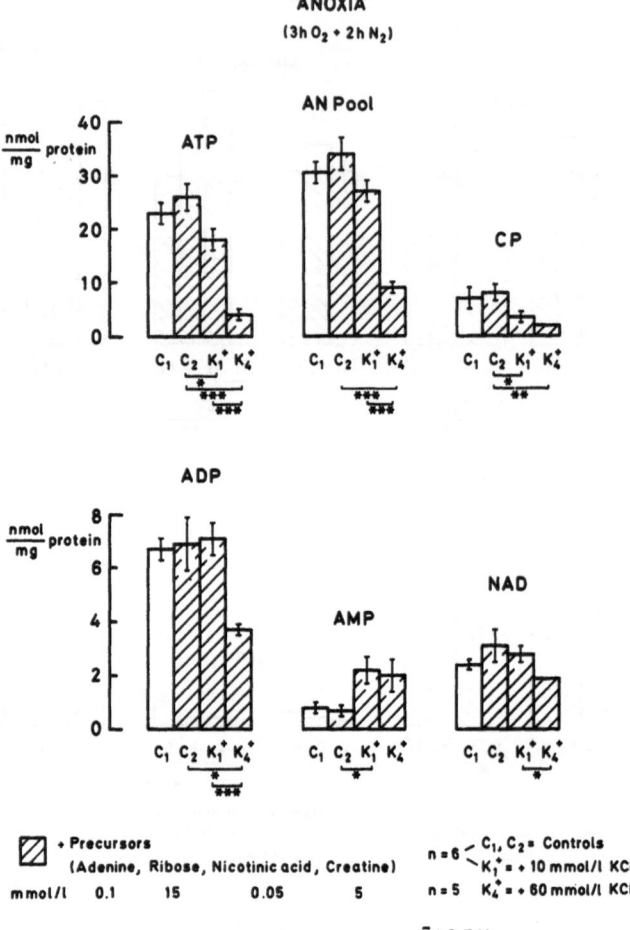

Fig. 6. AN (ATP + ADP + AMP)-, CP- and NAD-levels of resting left atria incubated in <u>anoxia</u> without (C_1) and with (C_2) precursors demonstrate a reduced energy balance, which allows by an increased anaerobic glycolysis anoxic cardiac cell survival for 6 hrs and more. K^+-depolarization with K_1^+ and even more with K_4^+ deteriorates drastically the ATP- and the total AN-levels with increase of AMP, and also the CP-levels to values far below anoxic cell survival. Also the NAD-level is lowered significantly with K_4^+ compared with K_1^+.

<u>Protective effects on the overshoot peak</u>. This peak can be inhibited by 10 mM NH_4^+ (Cl^-, acetate$^-$, aspartate$^-$) (Fig. 9) which inhibits possibly the Ca^{++}-output from the mitochondria as H^+-scavenger by entrance in the cell as NH_3, inhibiting by this way the Na^+/Ca^{++}-exchange in the mitochondrial membrane (Fig. 16, 17), (16, 20).

Nonprotective effects of the overshoot peak. All possibilities of an explanation of this peak by a sudden Ca^{++}-influx (Fig. 17) can be excluded: No inhibition of this first 'peak area' can be shown by
- slow Ca^{++}-channel-blockers: verapamil, nifedipine (Fig. 10)

		INCUBATION-TIME (HOURS)	NORMOXIA (95% O_2 + 5% CO_2)	ANOXIA (3H O_2 + 2H N_2) (95% N_2 + 5% CO_2)
WITHOUT PRECURSORS	CONTROL$_0$	0	6.7 ± 0.6	——
	CONTROL$_1$	5	7.2 ± 0.4	3.1 ± 0.3
	K_1^+	5	6.3 ± 0.3	2.6 ± 0.2
	K_4^+	5	5.9 ± 0.5	0.5 ± 0.05
WITH PRECURSORS	CONTROL$_2$	5	6.8 ± 0.5	3.6 ± 0.3
	K_1^+	5	6.7 ± 0.4	2.1 ± 0.3
	K_4^+	5	4.3 ± 0.5	0.8 ± 0.2

* $p < 0.05$ N = 6
** $p < 0.01$ C_0 N = 5
*** $p < 0.001$ WITH PRECURSORS K_4^+ N = 5

Fig. 7. The energy quotient ATP/(ADP + AMP) of resting left atria in normoxia and anoxia during depolarization with K_1^+ (10 mM KCl) and K_4^+ (60 mM KCl). In spite of the 100 % increased resting O_2-uptake due to K_4^+ the normoxic energy quotient is not enhanced, the new synthesis from precursors is inhibited and the quotient here lowered (K_4^+). The energy quotient is lowered in anoxia to values (-50 %) which provide anoxic cell survival. This value is deteriorated additionally by K_4^+ to a quotient not compatible with life (0.5). Precursors have here no protective effects, in contrary the quotient is lowered even with K_1^+.

- ß-blocker (no catecholamine output): propranolol (Fig. 11)
- Na^+-channel-blocker: tetrodotoxin (TTX)
- eicosanoids (assumed Ca^{++}-output from mitochondria)
- inhibition of Na^+/K^+-pump (no increased Na^+/Ca^{++}-exchange: ouabain)
- increase of external Ca^{++}: the peak is shifted with the same area under the peak to a higher level connected with the positive inotropic effect of Ca^{++} (Fig. 9), (16).

The 'normoxic fatigue' of contraction work/beat and the 'fatigue after reoxygenation'. The plateau-level of contractile activity after the overshoot peak remains in the range of the initial normoxic value~2 hrs (Fig. 8, 9) and declines then slowly during the 3rd and 6th hr to~50-30 %

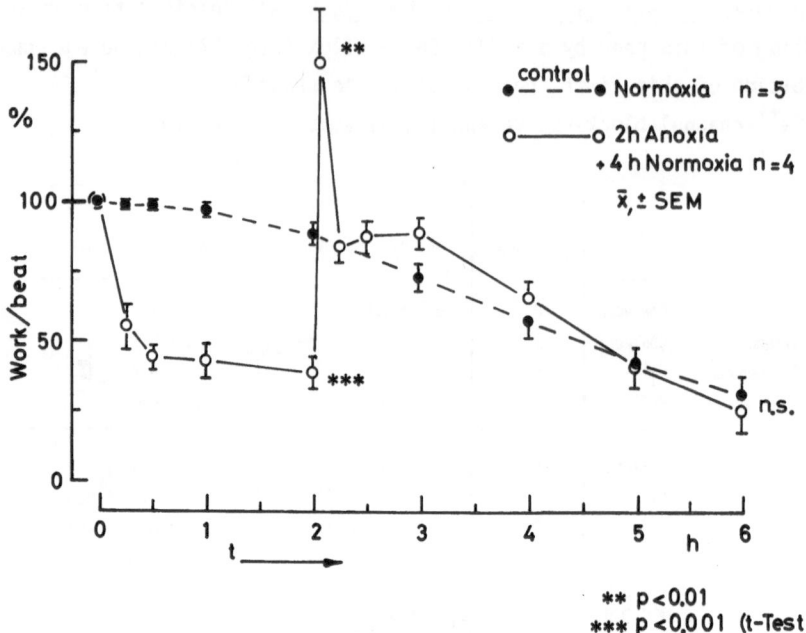

Fig. 8.
<u>Contractile work in the anoxia test (normoxia, anoxia, reoxygenation)</u>
<u>compared with the 'normoxic fatigue' of the controls.</u> (Auxotonic work/beat of
left atria, 0.5 Hz, 5 mN preload, 30° C). The reduced normoxic work/beat
(100 %) decreases in anoxia to~50 % and shows after reoxygenation a first
overshooting peak of contractile activity which declines to a plateau-level
after 30 min. From this plateau, the contractile activity decreases then
slowly to values of 50 % after 4 hrs reoxygenation ('fatigue after reoxygenation'). The normoxic control values show the same decline of contractile activity to the same degree ('normoxic fatigue'). Therefore no irreversible cell damage due to anoxia and reoxygenation can be observed, only
a functional adaptation (s. text).

of the initial normoxic value-level (100 %). The mechanism of this 'fatigue'
is unexplained. In Fig. 8 no significant difference is shown between the
'fatigue' observed after 6 hrs of normoxia and after 2 hrs of anoxia followed
by 4 hrs of normoxia (reoxygenation). Therefore an irreversible damage of
atrial cell function caused by a period of 2 hrs anoxia cannot be demonstrated. There is only an adaptive change of the contractile activity,
caused obviously by a redistribution of endogenous Ca^{++} after the start of
the H^+-pump in the mitochondria as first effect of reoxygenation (16).

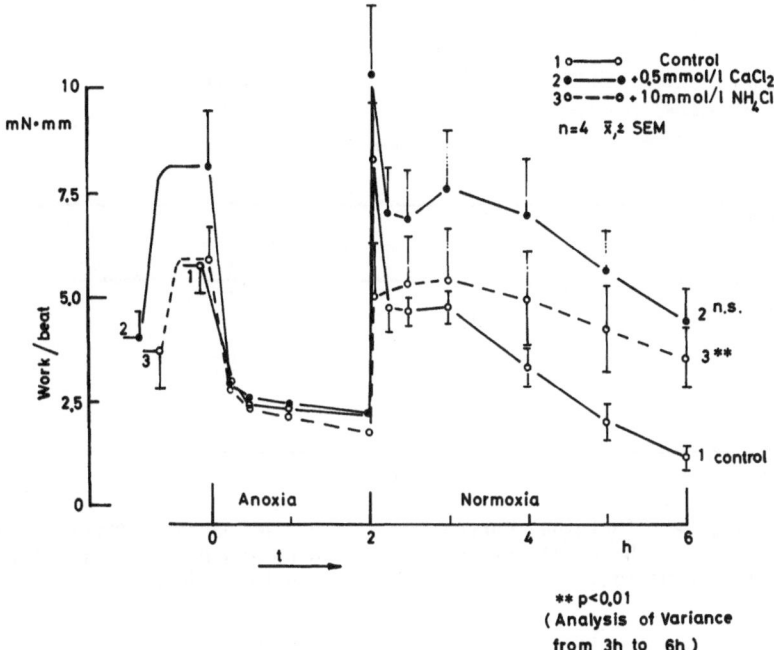

Fig. 9. <u>Contractile work in the anoxia test (s. Fig. 8)</u>. Different normoxic cardiac work by 1 (control 0 2.5 mM Ca^{++}) compared with positive inotropy by 2 (3.0 mM Ca^{++}) and 3 (2.5 mM Ca^{++} + 10 mM NH_4Cl) declining in anoxia to the same level. At reoxygenation 1 and 2 (Ca^{++}) develop the same area of the first peak shifted with 2 only to a higher level, but the slope of the 'fatigue' declines parallel. By 3 (NH_4^+) the first peak is abolished and the 'fatigue' significantly delayed.

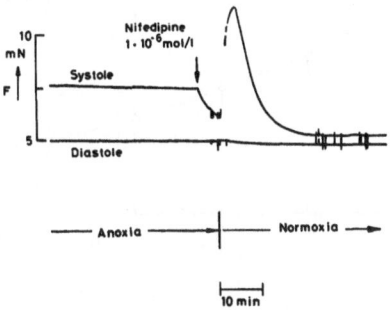

Fig. 10. <u>Reoxygenation (Original curve)</u>. Nifedipine blocking Ca^{++}-influx through the slow Ca^{++}-channels decreases anoxic and normoxic force but not the first peak after reoxygenation, proving that there is no sudden influx through these channels (s. text and Fig. 17).

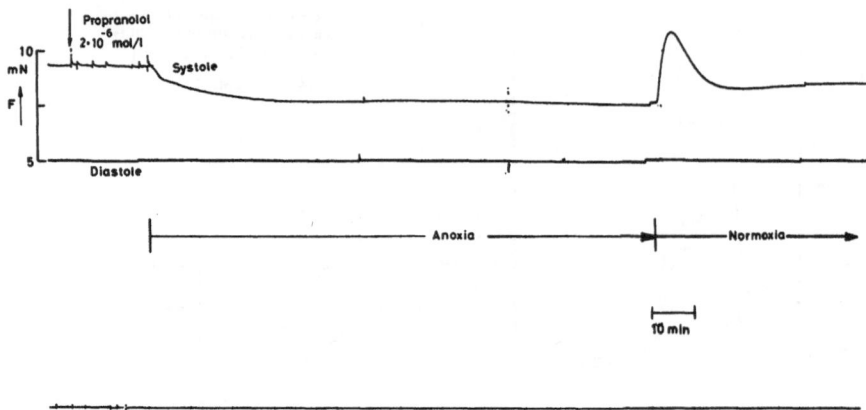

Fig. 11. <u>Anoxia test (Original curve)</u>.There is no influence of propranolol on the normoxic and the anoxic reduced force and no inhibition of the first peak after reoxygenation: catecholamine output can be excluded.

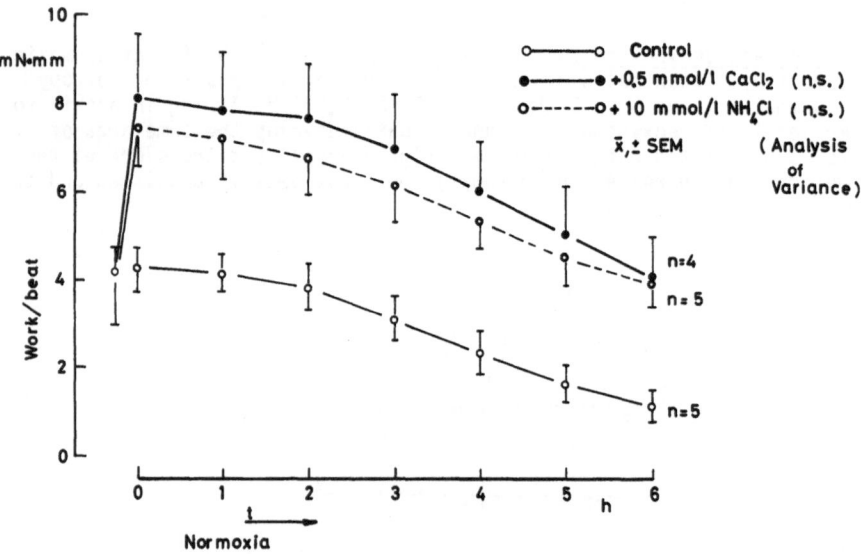

Fig. 12. <u>The 'normoxic fatigue' of contractile work</u>. The slopes of the 'normoxic fatigue' at the same positive inotropy due to 3.0 mM Ca++ and 10 mM NH₄Cl + 2.5 mM Ca++ decline from a higher level but parallel with the slope of the control (2.5 mM Ca++). The delay of 'fatigue after re-oxygenation' by NH₄Cl (Fig. 9) can here not be observed (s. text).

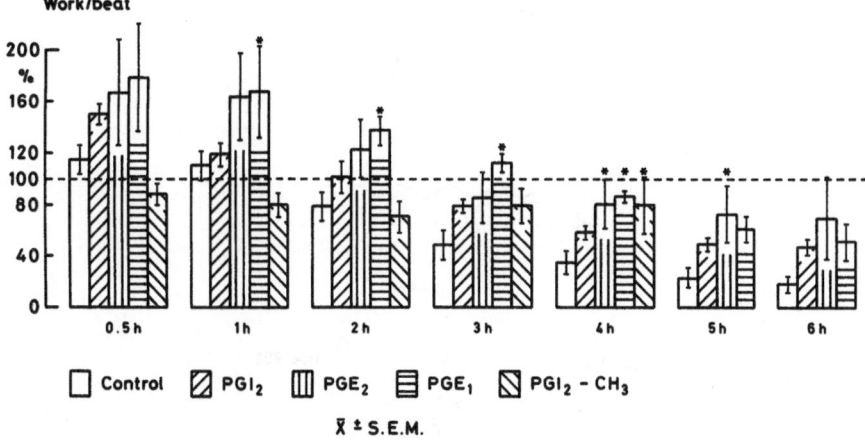

Fig. 13. <u>The 'fatigue' of contractile work during reoxygenation influenced by</u>
<u>prostaglandins (Dunnett's-test, *p < 0.05).</u> Prostaglandins (10^{-3} M) added
10 min before reoxygenation have no effects on the anoxic force. The first
peak after reoxygenation is not influenced, but the 'fatigue' delayed significantly with PGE_1, PGE_2 and methyl-PGI_2, especially after 4 hrs reoxygenation.
The normoxic inotropic actions of prostaglandins which last ~30 min cannot
be connected with this protective effect.

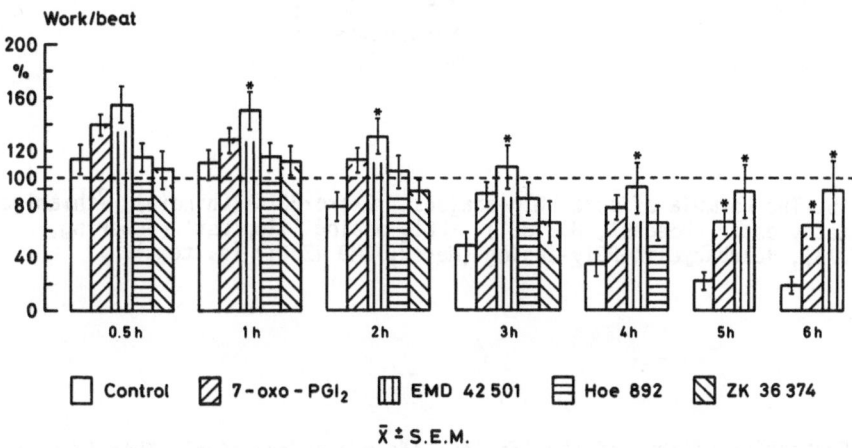

Fig. 14. <u>The 'fatigue of contractile work during reoxygenation' influenced</u>
<u>by stable PGI_2-analogs (Dunnett's-test, *p < 0.05).</u> In the same experimental
procedure as in Fig. 13 10^{-5} M 7-oxo-PGI_2 and EMD 42501 show in similar way
as prostaglandins a significant delay of 'fatigue' after 5 and 6 hrs reoxygenation. This is independent from the normoxic positive inotropic action:
EMD 42501 has here the weakest intrinsic activity and significant protective
effect on the 'fatigue' from the 1st to the 6th hr reoxygenation.

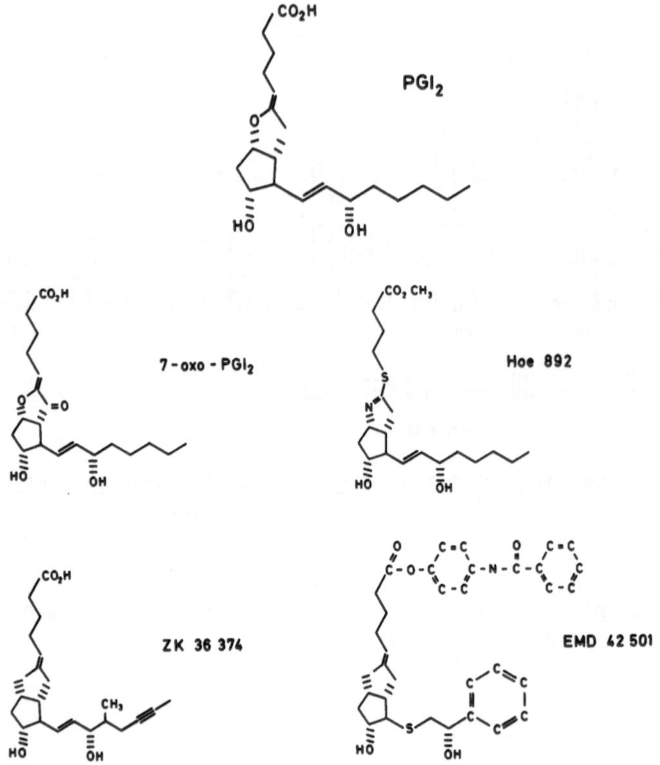

Fig. 15. The Formula of some PGI2-analogs. [1]7-oxo-PGI2 (Chinoin), [2]thiamino-
PGI2-methylester (Hoechst, HOE 891), [3]PGI2-analog 'iloprost' (Schering,
ZK 36374), [4]carbacyclin-PGI2-analog (Merck, EMD 42501) (s. text).

Protective effects of the 'fatigue after reoxygenation'. This 'fatigue'
can be delayed significantly by NH_4^+ also (16): there is a significant
delay in the decline of contractile activity after reoxygenation (Fig. 9).

The slope is significantly different from the 'fatigue after reoxygenation' without NH_4^+. The 'normoxic fatigue' during the positive inotropic effect of NH_4Cl is not influenced (Fig. 12), indicating that anoxia changes the conditions of 'fatigue' in an unknown way for protection by NH_4^+.

Eicosanoids, added 10 min before reoxygenation do not influence the first peak as mentioned above (3, 12). Eicosanoids preserve, however, the contractile activity to a later stage of the 'fatigue' during the 1st and the 6th hr of reoxygenation independent from the positive inotropic effect of these compounds (13). Significant effects could be observed with PGE_1, PGE_2, PGI_2-methylester, 7-oxo-PGI_2 and carbacyclin-PGI_2-analog (EMD 42501) (Fig. 13, 14, 15). The last compound has the weakest positive inotropic effect and the strongest protective action on the cardiac inotropy during the phase of 'fatigue'. If it could be proved that the observed 'fatigue in normoxia and after reoxygenation' is due to the high concentration of O_2 ($\sim$1.1 mM O_2 in the Krebs-Henseleit solution) and to an impairing effect on the membranes by the production 'oxygen free radicals', it could be possible that eicosanoids could act protectively as free radical scavengers in the membranes (17, 18, 19).

Nonprotective effects on the 'fatigue after reoxygenation'. Positive inotropic effects by cardiotonic drugs do not change the slope of 'fatigue' as was observed with increased external Ca^{++} (Fig. 9), epinephrine et al. Therefore, no protective effect on the 'fatigue' could be observed up to now with other cardiotonic drugs.

Conclusions. NH_4^+(Cl^-, acetate$^-$, aspartate$^-$) has protective effects on the overshoot peak after reoxygenation as well as on the slope of 'fatigue' with a significant delay of the declining contractile activity up to 6 hrs. Eicosanoids do not have a protective effect on the first overshoot peak but prevent independent from the positive inotropic activity the 'fatigue after reoxygenation' significantly. The weakest positive acting carbacyclin-PGI_2-analog (EMD 42501) has the most protective effect on this 'fatigue'.

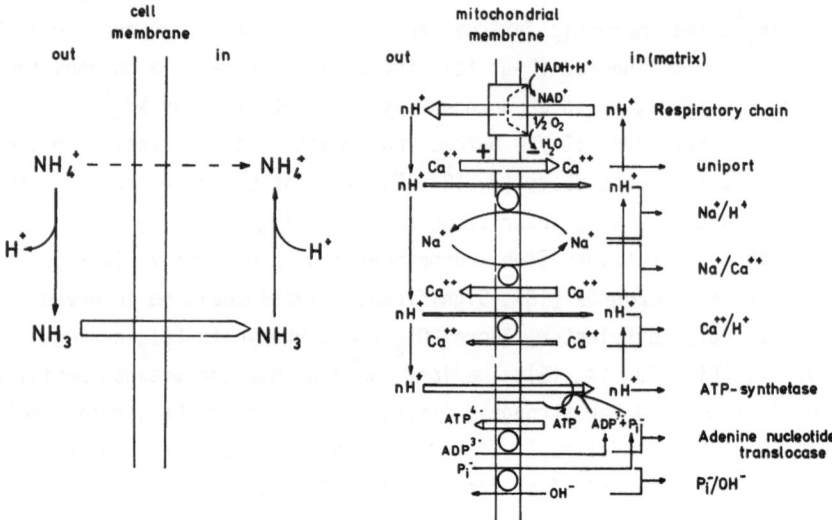

Fig. 16. Scheme of electrolyte- and ion-fluxes in the mitochondrial membrane driven by the H$^+$-pump and the effect of extracellular NH$_4^+$.

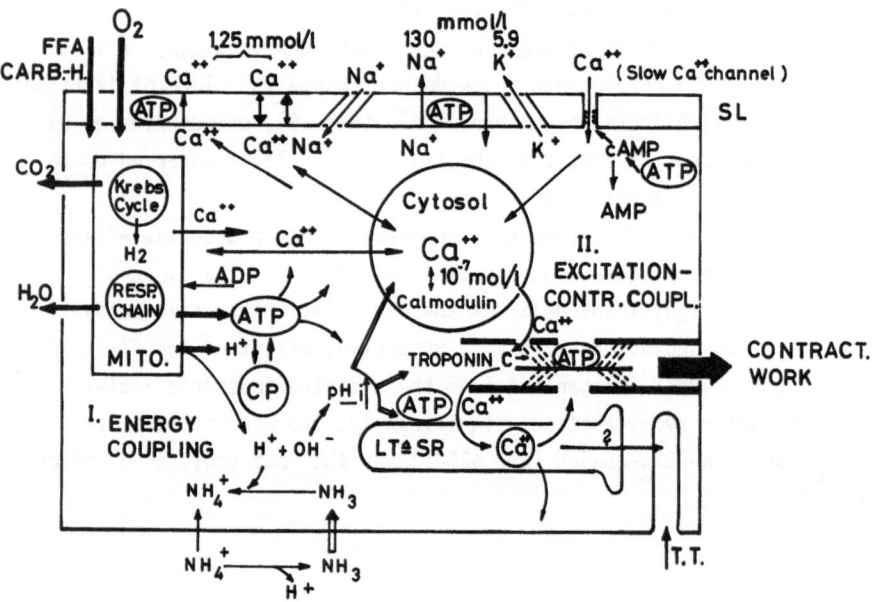

Fig. 17. Scheme of the cardiac cell as an energy-producing and -consuming system with important electrolyte- and ion-fluxes through the different membranes (s. text).

SUMMARY

A short review is given about protective and nonprotective interventions in the energy state and the contractile activity of cardiac muscle preparations to improve anoxic cardiac cell survival during anoxia and the critical phase of reoxygenation important for the composition of cardioplegic solutions used in cardiac surgery. As a model have been used superfused guinea pig atria at rest and work in a recently developed 'anoxia test' with the phases of normoxia, anoxia and reoxygenation.

During <u>normoxia a protective effect</u> on the atrial AN (ATP + ADP + AMP) and NAD-levels could be observed by addition of precursors (adenine, ribose, nicotinic acid) which increase, by new synthesis during 5 hrs incubation time, the initial values to $\sim$40 %, without change of the energy quotient (ATP/(ADP + AMP)).

<u>During anoxia</u>, these precursors inhibit significantly the anoxic degradation of ATP- and total AN-levels. The best protection of AN- and NAD-levels in anoxia could be shown by a strongly reduced atrial work or atrial standstill before anoxia has been started. The anoxic decay of CP (-90 %) cannot be saved, also no protective effects of creatine on CP-levels could be shown in normoxia and in anoxia.

<u>Nonprotective effects</u>. Standstill in <u>normoxia</u> produced by K^+-depolarization at 30° or 20° C increases the resting O_2-uptake by addition of 10 mM KCl (K_1^+) to 8 % by addition of 60 mM (K_4^+) to 100 % by an obviously uncoupling way. The K^+-induced increase of mitochondrial activity is due to Ca^{++}-influx through the slow Ca^{++}-channels and therefore dependent from external Ca^{++} and can be inhibited completely by nifedipine, when added before or during the first 5 min of K^+-depolarization. The inhibitory effect of nifedipine is lowered considerably when added after 2 hrs. A 100 % increase of resting O_2-uptake (K_4^+) is not connected with a higher energy-quotient. A new synthesis of AN and NAD from precursors is inhibited completely by K_4^+, the energy quotient here significantly lowered.

<u>Resting left atria without K^+-depolarization</u> show after <u>2 hrs anoxia</u> a lowered ATP-level (-30 %) shifted to ADP and AMP without loss of AN. NAD (-30 %) is shifted to NADH. The energy quotient is lowered in absence or presence of precursors (-56 %, -47 %), values which allow for 6 hrs and more a reduced cardiac work in spite of the decay of CP (-90 %).

K^+-depolarization decreases here additionally the energy quotient, the ATP-, the AN-, the NAD- and the CP-levels to values far below anoxic cell survival. K^+-concentrations above 15.5 mM in cardioplegic solutions and high external Ca^{++} can therefore not be recommended, even at temperatures of 20° C. However, these additional deteriorating effects of K^+ on the anoxic energy metabolism even on CP can be completely inhibited by nifedipine, if given before K^+-depolarization and anoxia have been started.

The anoxic reduced contractile activity in the 'anoxia test' lasts in the mean 6 hrs ('time to standstill') and can be prolonged only by the cardioglycoside ouabain, whereas all other cardiotonic drugs shorten the time to standstill by the positive inotropic actions during anoxia, presumably due to an unbalance between energy demand and anoxic energy supply. Eicosanoids have only in normoxia positive inotropic effects and do not change the anoxic contractile activity.

Reoxygenation increases suddenly an anoxic reduced contractile activity with a short first overshoot peak presumably due to a release of anoxic stored Ca^{++} from mitochondria by the starting H^+-pump. This peak can be inhibited completely by NH_4^+. The 'fatigue' of contractile activity during 6 hrs reoxygenation can be delayed significantly by NH_4^+, also to a higher degree with most of the investigated eicosanoids by unknown protective effects perhaps in the membranes.

ACKNOWLEDGEMENTS

These investigations have been partly supported by the Deutsche Forschungsgemeinschaft (DFG) and partly by the Dr. Karl Kuhn-Foundation. This is gratefully appreciated. We thank Ms A. Weible for her skillful assistance at the experiments and for completing tables, figures and photographs and Ms M. Weber for her excellent work to finish and type this manuscript camera-ready.

231

REFERENCES
1. Hearse, D.J., Braimbridge, M.V. and Jynge, P. Protection of the ischemic myocardium. Cardioplegia Raven Press, New York, pp. 1-440, 1981.
2. Siess, M. and Seifart, H.I. In: Advances in Myocardiology, Vol. 2, (Eds.: M. Tajuddin, B. Bhatia, H.H. Siddiqui and G. Rona), University Park Press, Baltimore, pp. 295-310, 1980.
3. Leuchtner, J. Prostanoide als Modulatoren von Funktion und Stoffwechsel der Herzmuskelzelle im Vergleich zu anderen kardiotonen Agentien. Experimentelle Untersuchungen am isolierten Herzvorhof des Meerschweinchens in Normoxie, Hypoxie und Anoxie. Naturwissenschaftliche Dissertation, Universität Tübingen, pp. 1-256, 1985.
4. Delabar, U. and Siess, M. Basic Res. Cardiol. 74, pp. 528-544, 1979.
5. Delabar, U. and Siess, M. Basic Res. Cardiol. 74, pp. 571-593, 1979.
6. Siess, M., Delabar, U. and Seifart, H.I. In: Advances in Myocardiology, Vol. 4, (Eds.: E. Chazov, V. Saks and G. Rona), Plenum Publishing Corporation, New York, pp. 287-308, 1983.
7. Siess, M. and Stieler, K. In: Methods in Studying Cardiac Membranes, Vol. 1, (Ed.: N.S. Dhalla), CRC Press Inc., pp. 87-109, 1984.
8. Siess, M. In: Cardiac Structure and Metabolism, (Eds.: K. Hosono and M. Nagano), Roppo shuppan-sha, Tokyo, pp. 1-42, 1983.
9. Siess, M. In: Pharmacological Protection of the Myocardium, (Eds.: L. Szekeres and J.Gy. Papp), Pergamon Press and Akademiai Kiado, Oxford und Budapest, pp. 67-72, 1986.
10. Stieler, K., Reich, I., Siess, M. IUPHAR 9th Internat. Congress of Pharmacology, Abstracts, No. 848 P, London, 1984.
11. Delabar, U., Stieler, K., Reich, I., Zeitler, N., Weible, A. and Siess, M. IUPHAR 9th Internat. Congress of Pharmacology, Abstracts, No. 1764 P, London, 1984.
12. Leuchtner, J., Menzel, D., Takâts, I., Szekeres, L., Siess, M. IUPHAR 9th Internat. Congress of Pharmacology, Abstracts, No. 37 P, London, 1984.
13. Leuchtner, J., Siess, M. In: J. Mol. Cell. Cardiol., Vol. 17, suppl. 3, p. 12, 1985.
14. Fenn, W.O. J. Pharmacol. Exptl. Therap. 42, pp. 81-97, 1931.
15. McNamara, D.B., Roulet, J., Gruetter, C.A., Hyman, A.L. and Kadowitz, P.J. Prostaglandins 20, pp. 311-320, 1981.
16. Stieler, K., Khattab, A., Leuchtner, J., Teutsch, I., Siess, M. N.-S. Archs. Pharmacol., 332 suppl., R 52, p. 208.
17. Lefer, A.M. and Ogletree, M.L. In: Prostaglandins in cardiovascular and renal function (Eds.: A. Scriabine et al.) Spectrum Publications, Inc., New York, pp. 175-188, 1980.
18. Stam, H. and Koster, J.F. In: Prostaglandins and other Eicosanoids in the Cardiovascular System (Ed.: K. Schroer), Karger, Basel, pp. 131-148, 1985.
19. Szekeres, L., Kotai, M., Pataricza, J., Takâts, I. and Udvary, E. Biomed. Biochim. Acta 43, 135-124, 1984.
20. Roos, A. and Boron, W.F. In: Physiological Reviews, Vol, 61, No. 2, USA, pp. 296-434, 1981.

19

MYOCARDIAL ENZYME LEAKAGE AND SUCCINIC DEHYDROGENASE
ACTIVITY OF MITOCHONDRIA CORRELATED WITH THE MORPHO-
LOGICAL CHANGES IN THE ANOXIC ISOLATED PERFUSED RAT
HEART

Jung Yeh-Chih, Wen Wen-Hu, *Han Yu-Sheng, Fu Ling-Xiong

Department of Internal Medicine, Hsin-Hua Hospital, *Department of Bio-physics, Shanghai Second Medical University,
Shanghai, CHINA

INTRODUCTION

It has been shown in the previous studies[1][2] that
in the anoxic rat myocardial cells, the mitochondria show
structural changes including its swelling, separation of the
cristae and the vacuolization, the cell membrane permeability defects demonstrated allowing the entry of lanthanum as
a tracer into the myocardial cells. When the supply of oxygen to the heart is impaired, myocardial mitochondrial function will be influenced and the cytoplasmic constituents will
leak from the anoxic myocardial cells. In the present paper,
the Langendorff isolated perfused rat heart system has been
used to study the myocardial enzyme leakage, i.e. creatine
kinase (CPK) release, and the succinic dehydrogenase (SDH)
activity of the mitochondria isolated and then to investigate their correlation with the morphological changes in the
anoxic rat myocardial cells.

MATERIALS AND METHODS

The Langendorff isolated rat heart system has been used
to set up the anoxic rat heart model by the anoxic perfusion
in which the Krebs-Hensleit medium was gased with 95% N_2-5%
CO_2 in comparison with the aerobic perfusion in which the
medium gased with 95% O_2-5% CO_2. 84 male Wistar rats with
the body weight ranging from 200 to 220 g were used as the
experimental animals in this study. The rats fast since the
night before the experimental day were operated under ether
anesthesia. After the injection of 500 u heparin through in-

ferior vena cava, the hearts were removed quickly, transferred to ice-cold perfusion buffer, and after cessation
of beating tied to the aorta cannula of the Langendorff
system for perfusion. The pH of the perfusion buffer must
be kept between 7.35-7.45, the perfusion temp. $37^{o}C$ and
the perfusion pressure at 75 cm. H_2O.

Aerobic control group: 42 experimental rats were divided
into three subgroups--15,15, and 12 rats which were aerobically perfused with 95% O_2-5% CO_2 for 20',30' and 40' respectively. The heart rate was 180-220 beats per min., and
the coronary flow greater than 12 ml/min.

Anoxic group: 42 rats were also divided into three sub-
groups--15,15 and 12 rats which were undergone anoxic perfusion with 95% N_2-5% CO_2 for 20',30' and 40' respectively.
The heart rate was maintained at 200 beats per min. by the
AXQ-1 demand pacemaker manufactured in Shanghai, with the
coronary flow rate also greater than 12 ml/min.

During perfusion, the samples were taken from the perfusate at 5',10',20',30' and 40' intervals for the determination of creatine kinase (CPK) in each experimental rat.

At the end of perfusion, the heart specimens for study were taken uniformly from the papillary muscle of the
left ventricle.

Samples for electron microscope (EM) study were fixed in
the freshly prepared 2% glutaraldehyde at pH 7.4, and post-
fixed in 1% osmium tetroxide, and then the tissues were de-
hydrated in ethanol, and embedded in Epon, finally the thin
sections studied under the Hitachi H-500 electron microscope. Samples with the size about 1 mm^3 taken were also fixed in 2% glutaraldehyde in 0.1 M cacodylate buffer with
1% La$(NO_3)_3$ at pH 7.4 for 2 hr. and then washed in buffer
with 1% La$(NO_3)_3$ two times and post-fixed in 1% osmium tetroxide with 1% La$(NO_3)_3$. After the embedding and thin-sectioning processes, the samples were studied without any
stain under EM for the observation of the distribution of
the lanthanum particles in the myocardial cells.

Separation of myocardial cell mitochondria--This method involved polytron homogenization of the heart tissue (ventricles from the experimental Wistar rat) followed by centrifugation. At the end of perfusion, the rat heart in ice-cold STM solution with 0.2498 M sucrose and 0.003 M $MgCl_2$ and Tris 0.01 M at pH 8 was finely chopped with a pair of scissors. The samples in the above solution were then polytron with KD-300 Biomixer, and then transferred to the glass homogenizer with a teflon pestle for 9 passes with the homogenizer kept in the ice-cold bath. The homogenate was then poured into the centrifuge tubes and centrifuged at 1,000 g for 12 min in the ice-cold condition. The pellet was discarded, and the supernatant containing the mitochondria was centrifuged again at 11,000 g for 40 min. Then both the supernatant and the pellet were kept. The pellet was studied in the electron microscope and confirmed to be the mitochondria morphologically and also cytochemically. All the above steps were carried out strictly at 4°C.

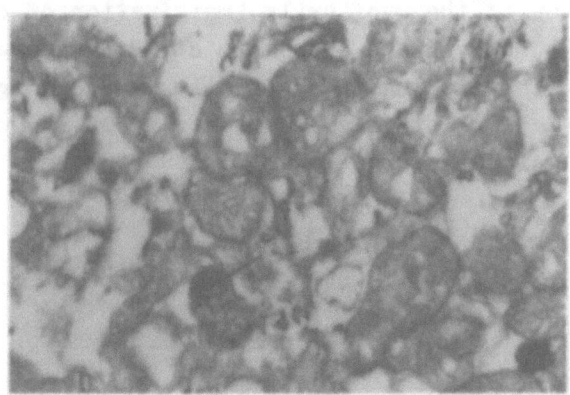

FIG.1 - The myocardial cell mitochondria separated from the rat heart tissue were identified in the electron microscope morphologically and also with succinic dehydrogenase shown cytochemically within the mitochondria (⟵———).

The succinic dehydrogenase activity of mitochondria was assayed by the spectrophotometric method with constant level of ferricyanide by recording the decrease of $Fe(CN)_6^{3+}$ absorption at 420 nm with the Hitachi model 220 double beam spectrophotometer (420 nm slit 2 nm).

$$Succinate + 2Fe(CN)_6^{3+} \longrightarrow fumarate + 2Fe(CN)_6^{2+} + 2H^+$$

The SDH activity assayed spectrophotometrically was expressed in $\triangle$ ABS/mg. protein of heart tissue/min.[3]

RESULTS

Morphological changes - In comparison to the aerobic control group, including all 3 subgroups perfused aerobically for 20',30' and 40' respectively, with normal ultrastructure of myocardial cells, i.e. normal appearance of nucleus, mitochondria, myofibrils and intercalated disc, there were significant changes in the anoxic myocardial cells. These changes were even more severe in the subgroups undergone anoxic perfusion for 30' and 40' than in the subgroup for 20'. In the 20' anoxic perfusion subgroup, there were intra-myofibrillar edema, enlarged sarcoplasmic reticulum, mild mitochondrial changes including its swelling and vacuolization. In the 30' and 40' anoxic perfusion subgroups, there were some fragmentation of the myofibrils, margination of chromatin material in the nucleus and also more striking changes in the mitochondria including the separation and disorganization of the cristae and relatively clear matrix. On the whole, all these changes were more significant in the 40' than in the 30' subgroup.

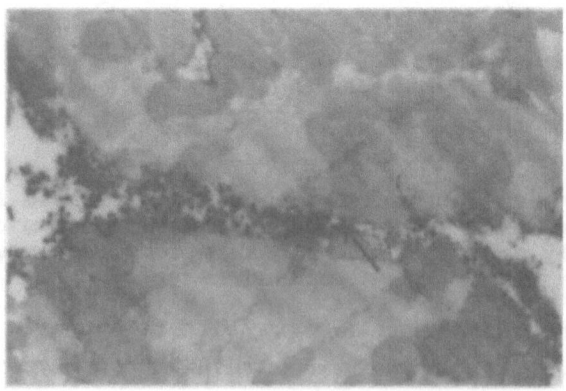

FIG.2 - In the aerobic rat heart, besides the normal ultra-

structure of myocardial cells, lanthanum (←———) was
found to be generally located extracellularly between the
myocardial cells.

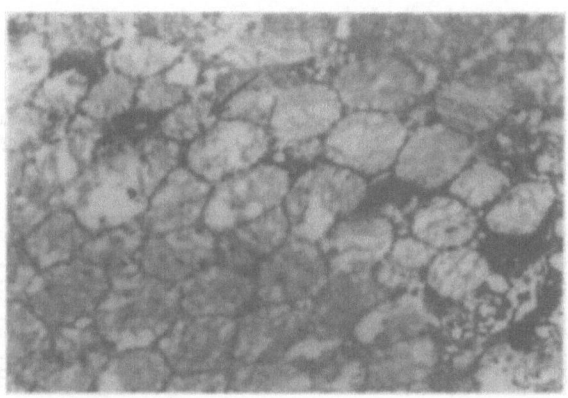

FIG.3 - In the anoxic rat heart, note the entry of lanthanum
(←———) into the myocardial cells, and also deposited within the mitochondria.

The myocardial cell membrane permeability defects demonstrated in the anoxic rat hearts with the electron-dense lanthanum
as a tracer - The lanthanum salt was used as a tracer and applied during aldehyde fixation for studying the permeability
defects. In all the aerobic control groups, lanthanum was
found to be generally concentrated to the T tubules, intercalated disc and the extracellular spaces of myocardial cells.
On the contrary, there was entry of lanthanum into the anoxic
myocardial cells in all the anoxic subgroups, more significant
in the 30' and 40' anoxic perfusion subgroups. Besides the
lanthanum particles could be seen to be deposited within the
cytoplasm, they were also clearly deposited within the mitochondria and appeared on their membranes in the latter subgroups. The entry of lanthanum into the myocardial cells was
most striking in the 40' anoxic perfusion subgroup. Thus, the
longer the anoxic perfusion period, the more severe will be
the myocardial cell membrane permeability defects happened.
Creatine kinase (CPK) release in the perfusate - The perfusate containing the coronary effluent was collected at the interval of 5',10',20',30' and 40' since perfusion for CPK de-

termination in all the aerobic control subgroups and anoxic
subgroups. It was shown from the Tab.1 and Fig.4 that CPK release was coincided with the myocardial cell membrane permeability defects demonstrated in the anoxic subgroups with the
longer anoxic perfusion period.

Tab.1 - Creatine kinase (CPK) determination (expressed in i.u.) in the perfusate containing coronary effluent collected at different intervals in
all the aerobic and anoxic groups.

Perfusion Group	5'	10'	20'	30'	40'
Aerobic Group	13.89	25.43	36.33	40.79	40.82
Anoxic Group	58.24	72.68	92.23	101.46	153.83
t Value	4.864	9.288	7.469	5.148	3.467
P Value	<0.01	<0.01	<0.01	<0.01	<0.01

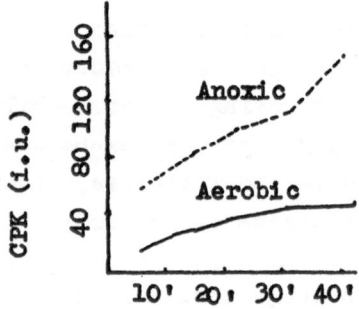

FIG.4 - CPK level in the
perfusate in aerobic
and anoxic groups.

Succinic dehydrogenase activity of the myocardial mitochondria -

Tab.2 - SDH activity of mitochondria expressed
in $\triangle$ ABS/mg protein/min in aerobic and anoxic groups

Perfusion Group	20'	30'	40'
Aerobic Group	0.0479	0.0448	0.0429
Anoxic Group	0.0288	0.0232	0.0210
t Value	2.54	4.18	3.97
P Value	< 0.05	< 0.01	< 0.01

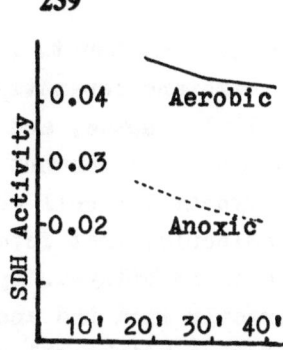

FIG.5 - SDH activity of mitochondria in aerobic and anoxic group.

It was shown clearly from Tab.2 and Fig.5 that in the aerobic control group, including the 20',30' and 40' aerobic perfusion subgroups, the SDH activity of the myocardial mitochondria was more or less stable, while in the anoxic group, including the 20',30' and 40' anoxic perfusion subgroups, the SDH activity of the mitochondria was shown to be depressed.

DISCUSSIONS

The effects of anoxia on the fine structure of the myocardial cells have been studied extensively.[1][4][5][6] The mitochondria showed striking fine structural abnormalities from the mild swelling and vacuolization to the decrease in matrix density and disruption of the mitochondrial cristae in the present study. The heart is an aerobic organ which derives the energy needed for mechanical function from the process of oxidative phosphorylation in mitochondria. Myocardial cells are almost completely dependent upon aerobic mitochondrial metabolism for their energy requirements. When tissue levels of oxygen are reduced, just as in the hypoxic or anoxic rat myocardial cells, the mitochondrial metabolism is inhibited, and the mitochondrial structural changes will be appeared. Thus, mitochondrial damage may be critical in the development of irreversible myocardial cell damage.

Besides the structural changes of the mitochondria, the myocardial cell membrane permeability was also changed due to anoxia demonstrated in anoxic isolated perfused rat heart. CPK release in the perfusate was coincided with the entry of lanthanum into the anoxic myocardial cells.[2] Thus, the sarcolemmal injury happened in the anoxic rat heart. In the myocardial cells, the sarcolemmal membrane separates the cytosol from the surrounding extracellular space, and allows for the existance of a special chemical environment within the cell. The barrier function of myocardial cell membrane is served by two sheets of lipid molecules that form a highly ordered structure, the membrane lipid bilayer. Myocardial cell membranes may be suffered directly from the anoxic injurious effect, and the leakage of myocardial cell contents including intracellular enzymes, such as creatine kinase (CPK) will be appeared in the perfusate of the anoxic isolated perfused rat heart, or in the blood of patients after acute myocardial infarction.[7][8] Creatine kinase (CPK) can be used as an enzyme marker of myocardial cell membrane permeability defect. It is possessed of the characteristics of an ideal marker enzyme, i.e. a) cardiospecificity, b) enzyme stability, c) sensitive, specific and accurate assay procedures available for the measurement of the enzyme activity and d) the enzyme exhibiting low basal plasma levels and relatively high myocardial tissue levels.[7]

As shown above, the myocardial morphological changes and cell membrane permeability defects are well established in the anoxic isolated perfused rat heart. It is interested to investigate biochemical and morphological correlates of the anoxic myocardial cells. Mitochondria are numerous in the working myocardial cells and the surface of its inner membrane makes them the major provider of ATP. In the present study, succinic dehydrogenase activity is depressed in the anoxia-induced mitochondria. This enzyme, which is a membrane-bound enzyme, has been shown by many authors[11] to be present in mitochondrial fragments. Succinic dehydrogenase activity was altered in myocardial infarction and in induced myocardial necrosis.[11] From the structural changes of the mitochondria shown morphologically and the reduced SDH activity of the mitochondria measured biochemically in the anoxic rat heart, the correlation is existed well between the structural changes and the enzyme activity. Myocardial enzyme lea-

kage due to cell membrane permeability defects and the reduced succinic dehydrogenase activity of mitochondria are correlated well with the morphological changes of the myocardial
cells in the anoxic isolated perfused rat heart. Morphological, functional and biochemical studies are the different
parameters to observe or investigate the anoxic injurious
effects on the myocardial cells.

From the clinical point of view, it is not practical to
investigate the myocardial damage in the ischemic (anoxic)
attack morphologically, because there is no indication to
perform the endomyocardial biopsy in such situation. But it
is practical and helpful to investigate the myocardial injury biochemically, i.e. to determine the creatine kinase
(CPK) and other enzymes in the blood. In the experimental
cardiology, investigation have also been undertaken in our
laboratory to study whether certain interventions including
the Chinese medicine could protect the myocardial cells from
the anoxia-induced injury through these morphological, functional and biochemical parameters. For example, methylpred-
nisolone[12] and certain Chinese medicine have been shown to
work well. After the administration of the medicines, it was
found that morphology of the anoxic injurious myocardial
cells approaching normal, the lanthanum restricted to the
extracellular space, CPK release decreased and SDH activity
of the mitochondria not so depressed. The results look en-
couraging but remain to be further investigated.

SUMMARY

The langendorff isolated perfused rat heart system has
been used to study the myocardial enzyme leakage and succinic dehydrogenase activity of mitochondria, and to investigate their correlation with the morphological changes due
to the anoxia-induced injury. 84 male Wistar rats were used
as the experimental animals, divided into the aerobic control group and the anoxic group. Besides the mitochondrial
structural changes and the myocardial cell membrane permeability defects observed, the SDH activity of mitochondria

is reduced and the CPK release increased. The morphological, functional and biochemical changes in the anoxic rat heart are correlated with each other very well.

REFERENCES

1. Jung Yeh-Chih et al, Shanghai Med J 7:33, 1984
2. Jung Yeh-Chih et al, J Mol Cell Cardiol 16(Suppl.1): 12, 1984
3. King TE, In: Methods of Enzymology Vol.10, Academic Press, New York, 1978, pp322
4. Jennings RB et al, Lab Investigation 20:548, 1969
5. Mergner WJ et al, In: Pathophysiology of Shock, Anoxia and Ischemia (Ed. Cowley RA), Wilkins, Baltimore, 1982, p.658
6. Taylor IM, J Mol Cell Cardiol 16:78, 1984
7. Hearse DJ, J Mol Med 2:185, 1977
8. Wood JM, Circulation Research 44:52, 1979
9. Williamson JR, In: Advances in Myocardiology Vol.4 (Ed. Chazov E), Plenum Med Book Co. N.Y., 1983, p.271
10. Singer TP, In: The Enzymes Vol.7 (Ed. Boyer PE), Academic Press, New York, 1963, p.383
11. Wachstein M, Am J Path 31:353, 1955
12. Jung Yeh-Chih et al, Shanghai Med J 12:712, 1985

20

HEMODYNAMIC PERFORMANCE OF ISOLATED BLOOD-PERFUSED WORKING HEARTS OF
CREATINE DEPLETED RATS IN HYPOXEMIA

B. Korecky and Y.A. Brandejs-Barry

Department of Physiology, University of Ottawa, Ottawa, Canada K1H 8M5

INTRODUCTION

Creatine phosphate (CP) has been considered an important energy
buffer maintaining high levels of adenosine triphosphate (ATP) (1). It
has also been proposed that CP shuttles energy between the mitochondria
and the sites of utilization in active tissues, particularly cardiac and
skeletal muscle (2-4). Abundant biochemical evidence has been provided
in support of the CP shuttle (5-6) however the physiological importance
of the CP shuttle could not be demonstrated (7-8). Effects of C
depletion on the function of skeletal muscles have been studied after
long-term feeding with its structural analog β-guanidinopropionate (GPA)
which inhibits normal transsarcolemmal transport of creatine.
Steady-state performance in the creatine-depleted muscles consisting
primarily of Type I fibers was not impaired, in fact their endurance
capabilities increased. In creatine-depleted muscles consisting
primarily of Type II fibers, no effect on muscle function was observed
(9).

Cardiac function has also been investigated in rats depleted of
creatine either with GPA or another structural analog,
β-guanidinobutyrate GBA (7-8). The hemodynamic performance was not
affected in the creatine-depleted hearts, when investigated using the
isolated working heart preparation perfused with a Krebs-Henseleit
solution (8). In the working heart perfused with RBC enriched perfusate
(10), the maximum performance was similar in the creatine-depleted hearts
to that of controls. However, the duration of steady state performance
was shortened, the decline of CO was faster and the number of failed
hearts increased with time as total creatine decreased. This indicates
that normal levels of CP are not essential for short term steady-state
function in normoxemia, but some minimal concentration of C and CP is
essential for long term steady-state performance.

It has also been suggested (11) that CP functions as an "energy reserve" and that the CP shuttle may be more active in hypoxia. Since in our previous experiments we did not observe any differences in the short term cardiac volume work between hearts of control and creatine-depleted rats in normoxemia, we decided to investigate the effect of decreasing arterial pO_2 on performance in the creatine-depleted heart. As in our previous experiments, creatine depletion was attained by the addition of ß-guanidinobutyrate (GBA) or ß-guanidinopropionate (GPA) to the standard diet of rats for 7 weeks. The depletion of creatine by these analogs is between 75-80% (10), therefore we postulated that with progressively increasing hypoxemia the maximum performance and submaximum steady-state performance of the isolated blood-perfused hearts of creatine-depleted rats may be reduced and/or shortened.

METHODS AND MATERIALS
Treatment of Animals

Male Sprague-Dawley rats (250-275g) were put on a diet of ground rat chow only, or containing either 2% GBA or 1% GPA. To minimize differences in body weight, animals were pair-fed as suggested by Mainwood et al. (12). Biochemical analysis of the concentrations of total myocardial creatine, GBA and GPA was done as previously described (12).

Isolated heart preparation

Rats weighing between 350 and 390 g were anaesthetized with ether and injected intravenously with 200 IU sodium heparin. After a thorocotomy, the superior and inferior venae cavae were isolated, ligated and cut, the aorta and pulmonary artery were transected and the heart was removed as described in detail (10). The heart was initially perfused with oxygenated Krebs-Henseleit in the non-working mode and then in the working mode with a RBC enriched perfusate. In our previous study (10), stored cells (3-4 weeks), preserved in citrate phosphate dextrose adenine solution (CPDA-1) were used. In the present study fresh cells (1-3 days old) were used since their P50 was 24-26 mm Hg after 3 days, which was acceptable for our experimental protocol.

The basic system was set up as before (10) but some parts of it were duplicated in order that the initial normoxemic phase could be followed by the hypoxemic phase. Therefore, additional peristaltic pump, filter, oxygenator and a large RBC perfusate reservoir were added. The two large reservoirs each containing 500 ml RBC perfusate were placed in the waterbath and maintained at 37°C. From the first large reservoir the perfusate was pumped through a Bently filter and equilibrated with 95% O_2/5% CO_2 when it passed through a hollow fiber oxygenator (Cordis Dow C-Dak 1.8). The perfusate entered the small atrial reservoir (20 ml) and returned to the first large reservoir in the waterbath through an atrial overflow outlet. From the second reservoir perfusate was pumped through a second Bently filter, then passed into an oxygenator and was equilibrated with 95% N_2/5% CO_2. The perfusate then returned into the second large reservoir and recirculated through this system until the normoxemic perfusate was replaced with the hypoxemic perfusate. This was achieved by switching a set of two-way stopcocks that allowed only one of the perfusates to enter the atrial reservoir and the heart. Since deoxygenation proceeded rather slowly, recirculation through the second circuit was begun 45 minutes before the experiment so that pO_2 of 35-40 mm Hg was obtained at the onset of the experiment.

The isolated hearts were initially perfused with normoxic perfusate and maximum cardiac output (CO) in each heart was obtained by gradually increasing the left atrial filling pressure to the values ranging between 18 and 23 cm H_2O. Once the maximum CO was obtained, the left atrial filling pressure was decreased in order to reduce the CO to 75-80% which was then referred to as the submaximum steady-state CO. Once the hearts attained submaximum steady-state CO their performance was monitored for 10 minutes at which time the normoxic perfusate was replaced with the hypoxic one. An initial increase in pO_2 (40-48 mm Hg) was observed due to the mixing of normoxic and hypoxic perfusates in the small atrial reservoir. This was followed by a gradual decrease in pO_2 due to continuous deoxygenation of the perfusate till the isolated hearts failed (failure was described as CO less than 10% of steady-state).

Samples of RBC perfusate from the aortic outflow tract and coronary sinus effluent were taken every 10 minutes throughout the experiment. Measurement of pH, pO_2 and pCO_2 were done on the IL 813 pH/Blood Gas Analyzer and oxygen content was determined using the IL 232 CO-Oximeter. Myocardial oxygen consumption (MVO_2) was calculated as a product of coronary flow times the arteriovenous oxygen difference. Cardiac efficiency was derived from the ratio of total external cardiac work produced to total energy expended. Total external cardiac work was derived from pressure (Wp) and kinetic (Wk) components.

Statistical Analysis

All data were expressed as means and standard errors of the mean and were analyzed using one-way or two-way analysis of variance. Any significant differences among the three groups were identified using the Scheffe test. Calculations of survival of the hearts in the isolated system was done using the Life Tables (13) and any significant differences were identified using the Chi-square analysis.

RESULTS

After 7 weeks on the diet, no significant differences were observed in body weights, whole heart or left ventricular weights when comparing control, GBA or GPA fed rats. The concentrations of total creatine and accumulation of GBA and GPA in the hearts of rats fed for 7 weeks are given in Table 1. Total creatine levels decreased by 78% in hearts of GBA fed rats (hGBA) and by 77% in hearts of GPA fed rats (hGPA). The concentration of GBA in the GBA-fed rats was approximately 50% lower than the concentration of GPA in GPA-fed rats, but the decline in the concentration of total creatine was similar in both groups.

	Creatine	GBA	GPA
Control	14.0 ± 1.1	—	—
GBA-fed	3.1 ± 0.9*	5.2 ± 1.2	—
GPA-fed	3.2 ± 0.5*	—	11.7 ± 1.2

Table 1: Total creatine, GBA and GPA concentrations in hearts of Control, GBA and GPA fed rats for 7 weeks. Number of animals was 5 in each group. Concentrations are expressed as mol/g of wet weight of the left ventricle (free wall and septum). Statistical significance between control and experimental groups (*p< 0.01), no significant differences betweeen GBA and GPA groups were found.

	C	GBA	GPA
n	5	5	5
Hematocrit %	26.0 ± 1.0	27 ± 1.0	26 ± 1.0
pH a	7.46 ± 0.07	7.44 ± 0.01	7.44 ± 0.01
pH v	7.44 ± 0.02	7.44 ± 0.03	7.42 ± 0.03
PO_{2a} mmHG	350 ± 51	385 ± 25	344 ± 48
PO_{2a} mmHG	34 ± 4	38 ± 3	35 ± 4
PCO_{2cs} mmHG	41 ± 6	40 ± 9	38 ± 6
PCO_{2a} mmHG	46 ± 2	43 ± 6	46 ± 4
$C O_{2cs}$ ml O_2/dl	13.2 ± 1.4	12.9 ± 1.6	13.5 ± 1.8
$C O_{2a}$ ml O_2/dl	8.8 ± 0.5	8.2 ± 1.1	9.0 ± 0.7
Hb g%	8.4 ± 0.8	9.0 ± 0.7	8.2 ± 0.6
Heart Rate/min	320 ± 20	305 ± 15	310 ± 25
Aortic Flow ml/min/g	59.2 ± 4.4	59.5 ± 5.2	53.2 ± 6.9
Coronary Flow ml/min/g	5.5 ± 2.1	5.5 ± 2.1	6.0 ± 3.2
Myocardial Oxygen Consumption ml/min/g	0.30 ± 0.1	0.27 ± 0.09	0.29 ± 0.12
Power Input mW/g	115.0 ± 10	105 ± 8	111 ± 13
Total External Power mW/g	11.4 ± 1.9	12.1 ± 2.8	10.5 ± 3.6
Efficiency %	10.1 ± 1.1	11.7 ± 1.0	9.8 ± 1.6
LVP mm Hg	129 ± 4	130 ± 4	126 ± 7
LVEDP mm Hg	6.3 ± 1.7	10.0 ± 1.9	10.4 ± 2.0
+dP/dt mmHg/sec	3750 ± 200	3985 ± 155	3280 ± 190
-dP/dt mmHg/sec	3250 ± 245	3150 ± 210	2850 ± 155

Table 2: Hemodynamic data (mean and SEM) of isolated blood perfused working heart at the end of the 10 min normoxemic period of Control, GBA and GPA rats fed for 7 weeks.
a = aortic, c.s. = coronary sinus, pO_2, PCO_2 = partial pressure of oxygen, carbon dioxide, $C O_2$ = total oxygen content, Hb = hemoglobin, LVP = peak left ventricular pressure, LVEDP = left ventricular end-diastolic pressure. The data, expressed per gram, refer to left ventricular wet weight (free wall and septum).

Table 2 shows the hemodynamic data of control, GBA and GPA groups in normoxemia. We did not observe any significant differences among the three groups in any of the parameters measured. After 10 minutes the perfusates were switched and the hearts received RBC perfusate with a starting pO_2 of 39±5 mm Hg in control group, 45±6 mm Hg in the GBA group and 45±4 mm Hg in the GPA group. The differences in pO_2 were not statistically significant. The changes observed during the hypoxemic period in the following parameters - heart rate, work input or output, efficiency and ±dP/dt among the three groups - were similar to those that occurred in CO.

The maximum steady-state cardiac output (CO) attained by 10 minutes of normoxemic perfusion was 65±5 ml/min/g in the hearts of the control fed rats (hC), 65±5 ml/min/g in the hGBA and 59±7 ml/min/g in the hGPA. No significant differences in CO were found among the three groups. When CO was expressed as percent of the initial submaximum steady state CO and related to decreasing pO_2, significant differences between the control GBA and GPA groups were observed (Figure 1).

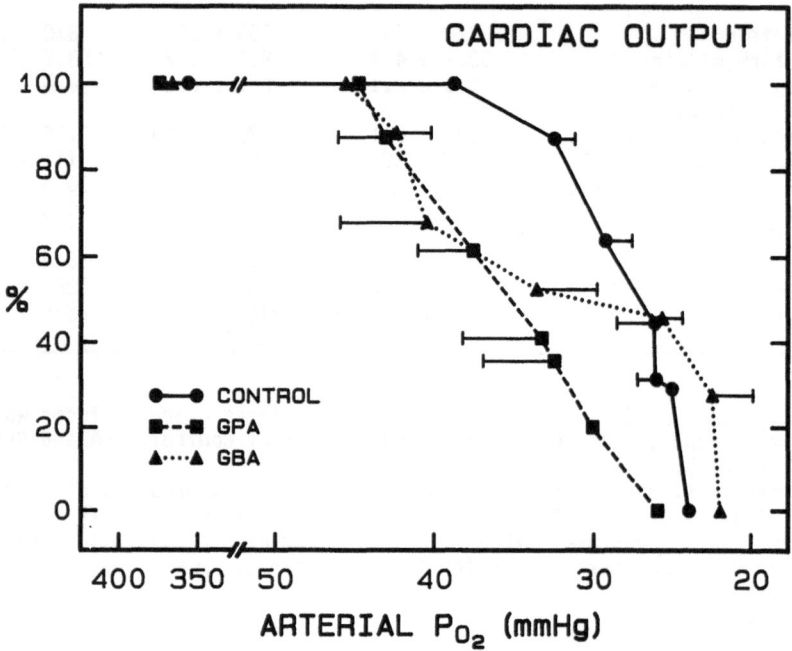

Figure 1: Effects of decreasing partial pressure of oxygen on cardiac output of control, GBA and GPA fed rats for 7 weeks. Cardiac output was expressed as a percentage of the submaximum steady-state cardiac output obtained in the first 10 minutes of normoxemic perfusion which was taken as 100%. The initial number of hearts in the group was 5.

The CO of the hGBA and hGPA began to decline (onset of decline was chosen as the point when CO decreased to 90% of the initial submaximum steady-state) at significantly higher ($p < 0.01$) pO_2 when compared to hC.

This happened at 43±2 mm Hg in both the GBA and GPA group and at 33±1 mm Hg in the control group. As the pO_2 was decreasing from 40 to 30 mm Hg the CO of hGBA and hGPA was significantly lower than that of hC. For example, at pO_2 of 33±3 mm Hg, when the CO of hC was 87%, the CO in the hGBA and hGPA declined to 52% and 40% respectively (p < 0.01).

The survival of isolated hearts as related to decreasing pO_2 is shown in Figure 2 (survival meant CO higher than 10% of the initial submaximum steady-state cardiac output).

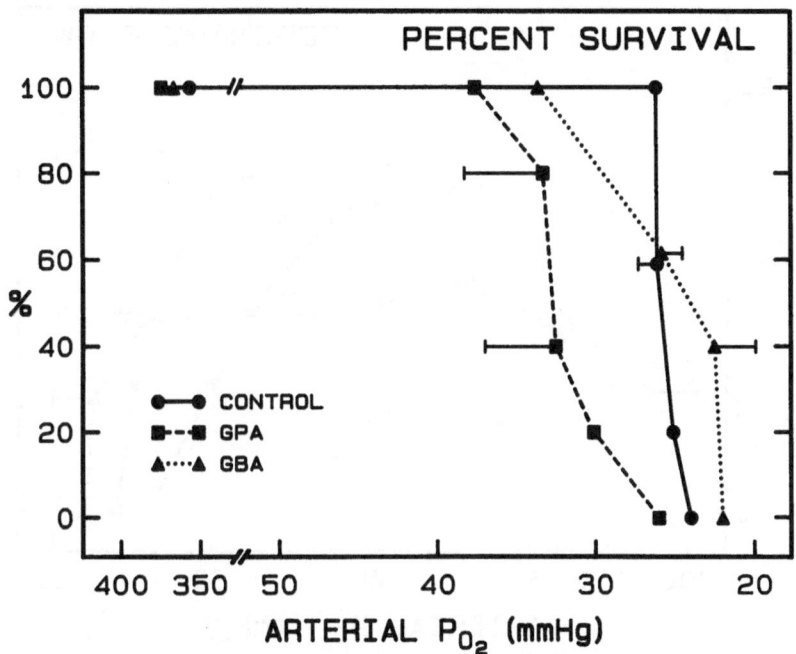

Figure 2: Percentage of surviving hearts of control, GBA and GPA rats fed for 7 weeks, whose cardiac output remained above 10% of the submaximal cardiac output obtained in normoxemia at decreasing partial pressures of oxygen. The initial number of hearts in each group was 5.

The number of hearts that survived in the GPA at pO_2 of 34±3 mm Hg was 80%, while all hearts in the control and GBA groups survived. At pO_2 of 32±4 mm Hg only 40% of hearts survived in the GPA groups (p < 0.01), while all of the hearts in the GBA and control groups survived this pO_2 value. At pO_2 of 25 mm Hg the number of surviving hearts in the GBA and control groups decreased to 60%, while all hearts in the GPA group failed.

Coronary flows in hC, hGBA and hGPA were not significantly different from each other during normoxemia (Fig. 3).

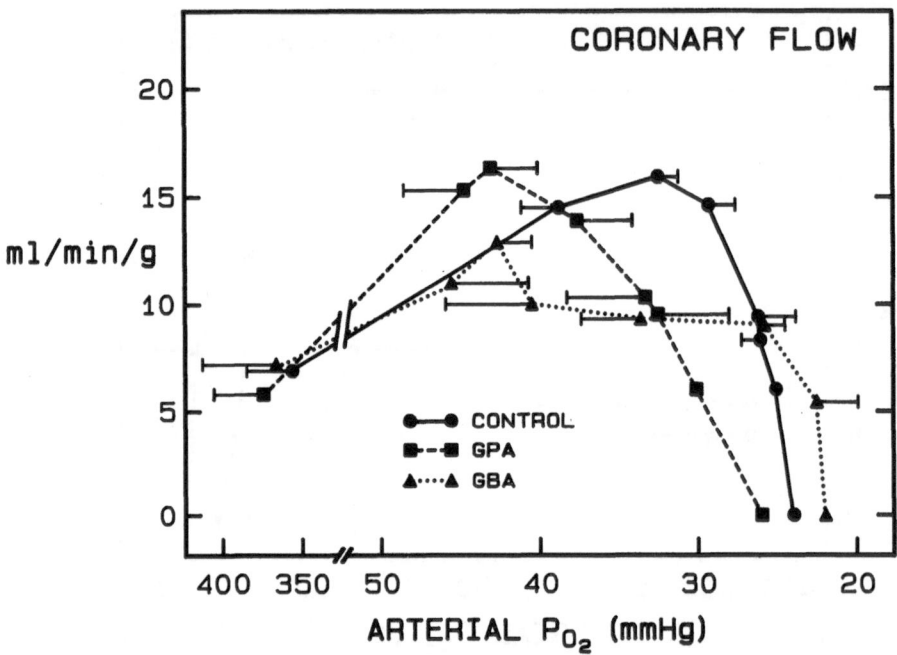

Figure 3: Effects of decreasing partial pressure of oxygen on coronary flow of control, GBA and GPA rats fed for 7 weeks. The initial number of hearts in each group was 5.

When the hearts began receiving the hypoxemic perfusate, the coronary flows increased and the maximal values reached were 15.9±1.3 and 16.3±1.2 ml/min/g in the hC and hGPA while the maximal flow reached was only 12.9±1.0 ml/min/g in the hGBA (p < 0.05). The maximum increase in coronary flow occurred at significantly lower (p < 0.05) pO_2 in the hC that is at pO_2 of 33±1 mm Hg, while in hGPA and hGBA it was at pO_2 of 43±3 mm Hg.

The left ventricular end-diastolic pressure (LVEDP) was higher in both hGBA and hGPA than in the hC in normoxemia, however the differences were not significant until the pO_2 decreased to 42±3 mm Hg (Fig. 4).

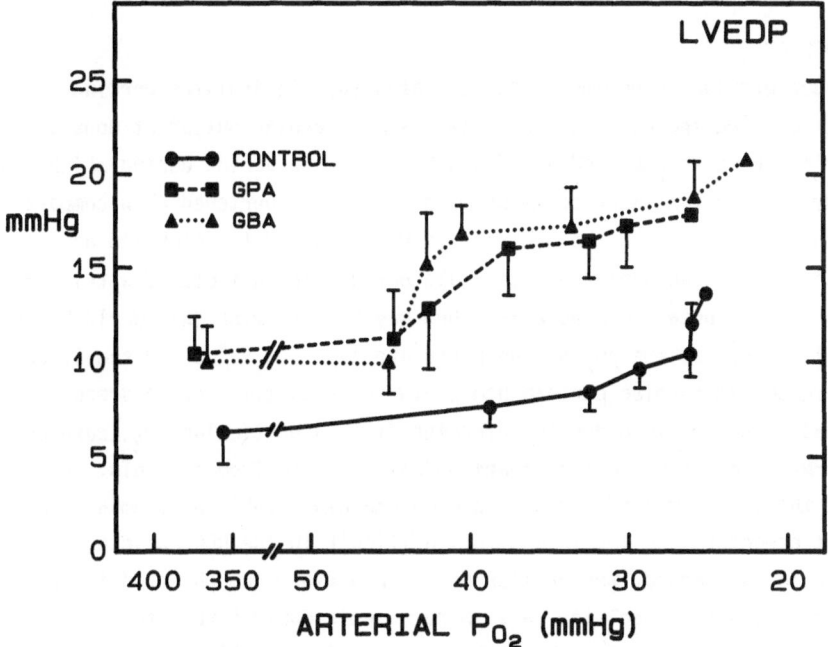

Figure 4: Effects of decreasing partial pressure of oxygen on left ventricular end-diastolic pressure in Control, GBA and GPA rats fed for 7 weeks. The initial number of hearts in each group was 5.

At this pO_2, LVEDP increased significantly (p < 0.05) in both hGBA (15.2±2.7 mm Hg) and hGPA (16.2±2.0 mm Hg) when compared to the hC (7.6±1.0 mm Hg). As the pO_2 decreased, the MVO_2 did not change significantly from the levels in Table 2 and no significant differences in MVO_2 were seen among the three groups at any time during the hypoxemic perfusion period. After the onset of failure, we did not observe any significant differences among the three groups in any of the other parameters (heart rate, work input or output, efficiency) at any instant during the time course of the experiment. The rate of tension development, dP/dt and more so, the rate of relaxation, -dP/dt, was lower in the creatine-depleted rats at pO_2 values between 40 and 30 mm Hg when compared to controls. However, the variability among the hearts in each group was too large and thus these values were not statistically significant.

DISCUSSION

Our previous experiments demonstrated that in isolated working hearts of creatine-depleted rats the maximum cardiac output at constant arterial pressure remained unchanged but the time period during which steady state volume work could be maintained was shortened when compared to control hearts. In the present study, we wanted to determine how the hearts of creatine-depleted rats would perform in an isolated working preparation exposed to hypoxemia. One way to determine this would be to stepwise decrease the pO_2 of the perfusate to a set value and see if any differences in cardiac performance would occur in time, or to decrease gradually the pO_2 in order to determine if at a particular pO_2, cardiac performance differed in the creatine-depleted rats from controls. We chose the latter method first, since maintaining stable hypoxemia at a set of predetermined levels was very difficult in the RBC enriched perfusate and second, the earlier decay in performance observed in the hearts of creatine-depleted rats in normoxemia could have interfered with the effects of hypoxemia. Upon the introduction of RBC perfusate with low and gradually decreasing pO_2, we observed that CO declined at a higher pO_2 in the creatine-depleted hearts when compared to controls. The rate at which individual hearts failed was greater in the GPA group but not so in the GBA group.

The differences in survival may be related to the following observations. In rats fed GPA, the phosphorylated GPA (GPAP) accumulates to much higher levels than the corresponding phosphorylated GBA (GBAP) in GBA fed rats. GPAP can be used by creatine kinase to a limited extent, while GBAP is not (14). In hypoxia, CP is quickly hydrolyzed and the inorganic phosphate, Pi accumulates (15). High levels of Pi have been shown to decrease the sensitivity of the myofibrils to Ca^{++}, thus decreasing maximum force development and contributing to contractile failure in hypoxia (16). Since the phosphorylated GPA can be used as a substrate for CK to a limited extent it is possible that in extreme hypoxemia it could be hydrolyzed and the Pi produced in the reaction contributed to the earlier failure observed in the GPA group.

In all three groups of hearts, the coronary flow increased to compensate for the lower oxygen tension in the perfusate. However, the increase in coronary flow in the hGBA was significantly less than the increase in hGPA. This may mean that either the myocardium of the hGBA was not as hypoxic at that time as that of the other two groups, or that the metabolites responsible for the decrease in resistance of coronary vascular bed resulting in an increase in coronary flow were not released by the tissue in the same concentrations as in hGPA.

The LVEDP was equally elevated in both hGBA and hGPA in normoxemia and has been observed by others as well (17). During hypoxemia, the LVEDP in the creatine-depleted hearts increased significantly when compared to controls. The rise in LVEDP in our experimental hearts may have been due to either an increased end-diastolic volume, or due to increased stiffness of the ventricle. We did not measure end-diastolic volume and thus we cannot rule out the possibility that the higher LVEDP was due to greater distensibility of the left ventricle in the creatine-depleted hearts. On the other hand, a rise in LVEDP may have been due to an increase in stiffness in the left ventricle that resulted from a decrease in ATP levels around the myofibrils which would lead to higher ADP levels and decreased dissociation of cross-bridges (18). Higher diastolic stiffness reflects lower distensibility of the left ventricular chamber which may impede left ventricular filling at constant filling pressures and eventually contribute to deterioration of cardiac performance.

Another consequence of decreased ATP levels is a decrease in the ATP/ADP ratio which may lead to slow down of the rate of relaxation of the myocardium. In this experiment we did observe lower rates of relaxation in both hGBA and hGPA during the hypoxemic period which progressively decreased from the rates obtained during normoxemia. In the hGBA and hGPA the creatine levels were low which in hypoxemic conditions limits CP formation not only due to the creatine deficiency, but also due to low oxidative phosphorylation. When CP levels are low, ATP is not regenerated and maintained at normal levels, the ATP/ADP ratio falls, G ATP declines and limits the uptake of Ca^{++} from the cytosol (19). This causes slowing of relaxation of the myofibrils which, at a constant filling pressure may lead to decreased end-diastolic volume and eventually to failure.

In normoxemia ATP diffuses to sites of utilization at a rate of 250 times the maximum rate of ATP utilization (20), and even though CP has a diffusion coefficient that is 30% greater than that of ATP (21), at high pO_2 levels when high energy phosphate production is not limited, the fluxes of either CP or ATP are not rate limiting for cardiac function. However, in hypoxemia less oxygen diffuses from the capillaries to various parts of the cell. Thus, oxidative phosphorylation of mitochondria may be limited to those that are in close proximity to the capillaries and the ATP produced by these mitochondria may not be able to diffuse thoughout the cell quickly enough to meet the energy demand of the cell. Therefore, in conditions where oxygen diffusion becomes a limiting factor, CP may be able to diffuse faster to the sites of utilization and regenerate ATP faster at the sites of utilization by the Lohman reaction due to its greater rate of diffusion.

When creatine concentration is reduced by about 75%, as in our experiment, the amount of CP generated by the mitochondrial oxidative phosphorylation and/or glycolysis is probably decreased. Under these conditions energy transport by the CP shuttle may become a limiting factor for turnover of energy and consequently normal ATP levels may not be maintained at the myofibrils. With normal CP levels, even at low pO_2 at which ATP production by the mitochondria is limited, ATP levels can be maintained at the myofibrils by the high CP concentrations when present. Therefore in the control hearts higher CO was maintained under hypoxemic conditions, even when pO_2 decreased from 45 to 30 mm Hg, because normal levels of CP were able to maintain the ATP/ADP ratio. However, as hypoxia progressed there was a greater reliance of glycolysis which was not able to produce a sufficient supply of ATP to maintain force development, and as metabolites accumulated, cardiac failure in these rats ensued.

We conclude, therefore, that under hypoxemic conditions, CP may become an important energy transporter, maintaining normal ATP/ADP ratio which regulates cytosolic Ca^{++} levels and mechanical function.

SUMMARY

We investigated the hemodynamic performance of the isolated blood-perfused working heart of creatine-depleted rats in hypoxemia. Rats were fed a diet containing structural analogs of creating (β-guanidinopropionate and β-guanidinobutyrate) which led to a 77% reduction in total myocardial creatine after 7 weeks of feeding. We found no differences among the three groups in the maximum cardiac output at constant arterial pressure (110 cm H_2O) and consequently in the steady state cardiac output (75% of the maximum) as well under normoxemic conditions. When this submaximum cardiac output was sustained under hypoxemic conditions, the creatine-depleted hearts began to fail at significantly higher partial pressures of oxygen when compared to control to control hearts. The percentage of hearts in the GPA group that failed at a higher partial pressure of oxygen was significantly greater when compared to the hearts of the GBA or control groups. Although coronary flow increased in response to hypoxemic conditions, the increase was significantly lower in the GBA group when compared to the control or GPA groups. A higher LVEDP was observed in creatine-depleted hearts in normoxemia and it increased in all three groups as pO_2 decreased. The rise in LVEDP can be due to increased end-diastolic volume work or to increased stiffness of the ventricle. Decreases in the ATP/ADP ratio, resulting from insufficient replenishment of ATP by CP particularly under hypoxemic conditions may have contributed to the impairment of myocardial relaxations that leads to cardiac contractile failure. We therefore conclude that in hypoxemic conditions CP may become important in energy transfer from the functioning mitochondria to the sites of utilization and maintain adequate pools of ATP.

ACKNOWLEDGEMENTS

This work was supported by the Ontario Heart and Stroke Foundation and the Medical Research Council of Canada. The authors of this study thank Mrs. Linda Jui and Mrs. Marika Masika for their skillful technical assistance.

256

1. Cain, D.F. and Davis, R.E. Biochem. Biophys. Res. Commun. 8: 361-366, 1962.
2. Bessman, S.P. and Geiger, P.J. Science 211: 448-452, 1981.
3. Jacobus, W.E. Ann. Rev. Physiol. 47: 707-725, 1985.
4. Bessman, S.P. and Carpenter, C.L. Ann. Rev. Biochem. 54: 831-862, 1985.
5. Saks, V.A., Rosenshtraukh, L.V., Smirnov, V.N. and Chazov, E.I. Can. J. Pharmacol. 56: 691-706, 1978.
6. Meyer, R.A., Brown, T.R. and Kushmerick, M.J. Biophys. J. 45: 91, 1984.
7. Jacobus, W.E. and Lehninger, A.L. J. Biol. Chem. 248: 4303-3810, 1972.
8. Shoubridge, E.A., Jeffry, F.M.H., Heogh, J.M., Radda, G.K. and Seymore, A.M.L. Biochim. Piophys. Acta. 846: 25-32, 1985.
9. Petrofsky, J.S. and Fitch, C.D. Pflugers Arch. 384: 123-129, 1980.
10. Brandejs-Barry, Y.A. and Korecky, B. Devel. Cardiovasc. Med. 1986, in press.
11. Ingwall, J.S., Kobayashi, K. and Bittl, J.A. Biomed. J. 41: 1a, 1983.
12. Mainwood, G.W., Alward, M. and Eiselt, B. Can. J. Physiol. Pharmacol. 60: 114-119, 1982.
13. Fleiss, J.L., Dunner, D.L., Stallone, F. and Feinne, R.R. Arch. Gen. Psych. 33: 189-196, 1976.
14. Fitch, C.D. and Chevli, R. Metabolism 29: 686-690, 1980.
15. Allen, D.G., Morris, P.G. and Orachard, C.H. J. Physiol. 343: 58-59p, 1983.
16. Kentish, J. J. Physiol. 370: 585-604, 1986.
17. Saks, V.A., Kupriyanov, V.N. and Smirnov, V.N. Proc. Int. Union Physiol. Sci. 16: 66, 1986.
18. Mainwood G., Alward, M. and Eiselt, B. Can. J. Physiol. Pharmacol. 120-127, 1982.
19. Hasselbach, W. and Oetliker, H. Ann. Rev. Physiol. 45: 325-339, 1983.
20. Jacobus, W. Biochim. Biophys. Res. Commun. 133: 1035-1041, 1985.
21. Mainwood, G.W. and Rakusan, K. Can. J. Physiol. Pharmacol. 60: 98-102, 1982.

PHOSPHORUS NUCLEAR MAGNETIC RESONANCE MEASUREMENTS OF INTRACELLULAR pH IN
ISOLATED RABBIT HEART DURING THE CALCIUM PARADOX

T.J.C. RUIGROK[12], J.H. KIRKELS[2], C.J.A. VAN ECHTELD[2], C. BORST[1] and F.L.
MEIJLER[12]

[1]Department of Cardiology, University Hospital, Catharijnesingel 101, 3511 GV
Utrecht, The Netherlands, and [2]Interuniversity Cardiology Institute of The
Netherlands

INTRODUCTION

In 1883 Ringer [1] reported that contraction of an isolated frog heart
rapidly ceased when calcium was removed from the extracellular fluid. Similar
experiments with isolated rat hearts were performed by Zimmerman and Hülsmann
[2]. During perfusion with a calcium-free solution contraction of the heart
ceased while electrical activity was maintained. They reported: "Returning to
a normal perfusate after more than 2 min resulted in the disappearance of the
electrocardiogram, and, after the heart had contracted a few times, these
contractions passed off completely and contractile activity was not restored.
The heart lost its colour and acquired a pale and mottled appearance. This
phenomenon, whereby the heart maintained its red colour and electrical activity
when the perfusion medium was changed from normal to calcium-free, but lost
these properties on return to normal, we called the calcium paradox." The calcium paradox has been demonstrated in rat, mouse, guinea-pig, rabbit and dog
heart [3,4], in superfused strips of the human heart [5], and also in the frog
heart [6] although the amphibian heart is more resistant to the calcium paradox
than the mammalian heart.

The calcium paradox is characterized by an excessive influx of calcium
into the cells [7], which may be divided into an early, relatively small gain
in cytosolic calcium, and a subsequent, massive influx [8]. Evidence has been
provided that the slow channels and the Na^+-Ca^{++} exchange mechanism are involved in the primary gain in tissue calcium once calcium is readmitted to the
perfusion fluid. The protective effect of calcium antagonists on the calcium
paradox has been the subject of controversy [9]. From recent publications,
however, it is clear that in a submaximal or mild form of the calcium paradox
calcium antagonists may be protective [10,11]. Thus it is reasonable to assume
that one of the routes of calcium entry during the calcium paradox is through

the slow channels. That calcium entry also occurs through the Na^+-Ca^{++} exchange mechanism, can be concluded from studies in which the extent of the calcium paradox was modified by changing the extracellular sodium concentration during the calcium-free or reperfusion period [12,13]. It should be noted, however, that the specific activity of the Na^+-Ca^{++} exchange mechanism as such is not affected by calcium depletion of the heart [14]. Other factors that may be responsible for the primary gain in calcium are the sodium-potassium and calcium pumps of the sarcolemma, and the calcium pump of the sarcoplasmic reticulum, whose activities are decreased by calcium-free perfusion [14-16].

The raised cytosolic calcium may then trigger a number of events, including energy-dependent accumulation of calcium and phosphate by mitochondria [17] and activation of various ATPases [18], contracture-mediated disruption of intercalated disc junctions [19], vesiculation of the sarcolemma and severe aggregation of intramembrane particles [20], loss of cytosolic constituents [2], and a secondary uncontrolled entry of calcium [8]. The precise sequence of these events and their relative importance still have to be elucidated. Hydrolysis of ATP and accumulation of calcium by mitochondria with deposition of insoluble calcium phosphate, are proton-generating processes [21,22]. Hence, it has been suggested that cytosolic acidification with a consequent stimulation of cytosolic and lysosomal (phospho)lipases, is an important factor in the origin of the calcium paradox [17,18]. In the present study phosphorus nuclear magnetic resonance (^{31}P NMR) spectroscopy was used to investigate the course of intracellular pH during the calcium paradox in isolated perfused rabbit heart.

MATERIALS AND METHODS

Isolated rabbit hearts were perfused at 37°C by the method of Langendorff [23] at a constant pressure of 80 cm H_2O. The standard perfusion fluid had the following composition (mmol/l): NaCl, 124.0; KCl, 4.7; $MgCl_2$, 1.0; $NaHCO_3$, 24.0; Na_2HPO_4, 0.5; $CaCl_2$, 1.3; glucose, 11.0. During calcium-free perfusion, calcium was omitted from the standard perfusion fluid and no correction was made for the small change in osmolarity. The perfusion fluids were equilibrated with 95% O_2 and 5% CO_2, and the resulting pH was 7.4 at 37°C. The perfusion sequence was: 10 min control perfusion with standard perfusate, 10 min calcium-free perfusion, and 5 min reperfusion with standard perfusate.

^{31}P NMR spectra were recorded on a Bruker MSL 200 spectrometer equipped with a wide bore (150 mm) 4.7 Tesla superconducting magnet, using a pulse

repetition rate of 2.32 s and a pulse angle of 90°. Accumulated free induction decays were obtained from 6 or 128 transients on submerged rabbit hearts in a total volume of 55 ml in a 30 mm tube and exponentially multiplied, resulting in a line broadening of 20 Hz and 10 Hz, respectively. Zero ppm was assigned to the resonance position of creatine phosphate at pH 7.0. Intracellular pH was measured from the chemical shift of the intracellular inorganic phosphate (P_i) peak, using a titration curve obtained from a solution containing 10 mmol/l ATP, 10 mmol/l creatine phosphate, 10 mmol/l P_i, 10 mmol/l NADPH, 10 mmol/l glucose-6P, and 10 mmol/l $MgCl_2$. Results are expressed as mean ± S.D. of six experiments.

RESULTS AND DISCUSSION

Fig. 1 shows a typical ^{31}P NMR spectrum during control perfusion. In all hearts intracellular pH, which was calculated from the position of the intra-

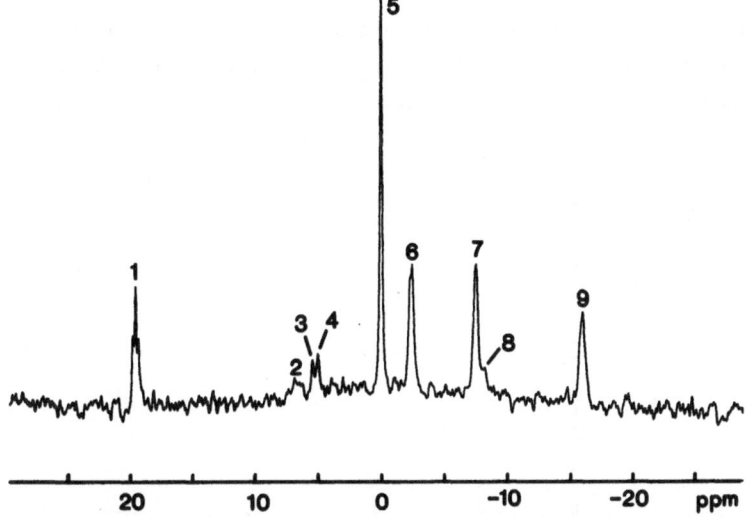

Fig. 1. ^{31}P NMR spectrum of a rabbit heart obtained from 128 scans, and taken between 5 and 10 min of control perfusion with standard perfusate. Resonances are assigned as follows:
    1: methylene diphosphonate (external reference compound)
    2: phospho-monoesters
    3: extracellular P_i
    4: intracellular P_i
    5: creatine phosphate
    6: γ phosphate of ATP
    7: α phosphate of ATP
    8: NAD(H)
    9: β phosphate of ATP

cellular P_i peak, amounted to 7.1. In some hearts the intracellular P_i peak was absent in the spectrum that was taken during the subsequent calcium-free perfusion (Fig. 2). This is most likely a result of incorporation of P_i into high-energy phosphates, since myocardial creatine phosphate and ATP levels increase during calcium-free perfusion [24]. When the intracellular P_i peak was present, intracellular pH was calculated to be 7.1. Upon reperfusion with calcium-containing solution there was a sudden and severe decline of intra-cellular creatine phosphate and ATP levels. In the heart that was used for Fig. 3, intracellular pH varied from 7.1 to 6.9 between zero and 80 s of reper-fusion. After approximately 1.5 min of reperfusion the intracellular P_i peak, and also the high-energy phosphate peaks, were no longer perceptible. Mean intracellular pH values of all hearts amounted to 7.1 ± 0.1 (0–20 s); 7.1 ± 0.1 (40–60 s); 7.0 ± 0.1 (80–100 s).

These results demonstrate that there was no appreciable fall of intra-cellular pH when the hearts were reperfused with calcium-containing solution. It is true that pH data were obtained only during the first 100 s of reper-fusion, i.e. the period that the intracellular P_i peak was perceptible. It should be noted, however, that the calcium paradox damage develops so rapidly

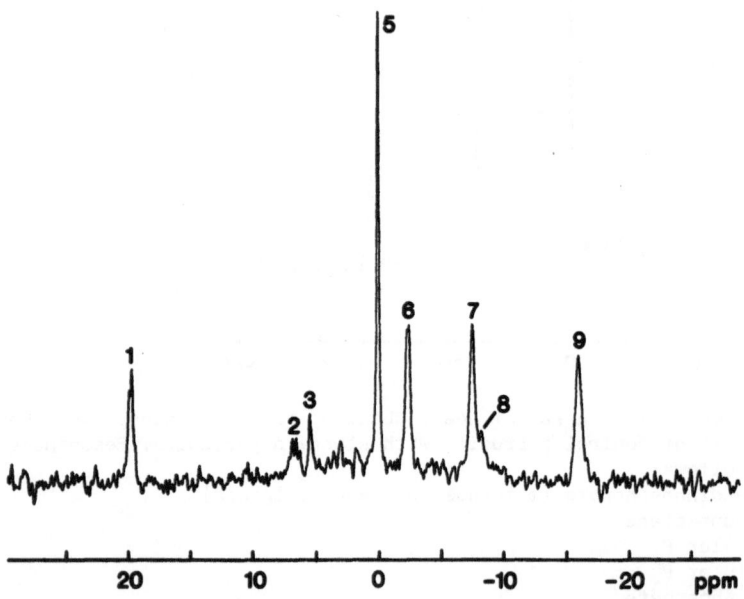

Fig. 2. ^{31}P NMR spectrum of a rabbit heart obtained from 128 scans, and taken between 5 and 10 min of calcium-free perfusion. Numbered peaks: see legend to Fig. 1.

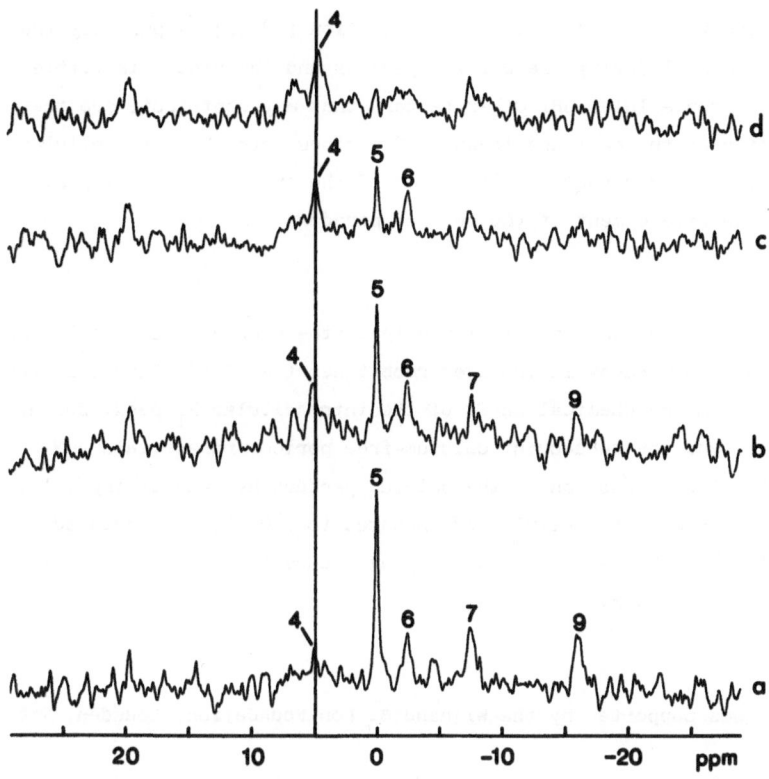

Fig. 3. ^{31}P NMR spectra of a rabbit heart obtained from 6 scans, and taken between 0–20 s (a), 20–40 s (b), 40–60 s (c) and 60–80 s (d) of reperfusion with calcium-containing solution. Numbered peaks: see legend to Fig. 1. Intra-cellular pH was measured from the chemical shift of the intracellular P_i peak, and amounted to 7.1 (a), 7.2 (b), 7.0 (c) and 6.9 (d). The vertical line indicates the position of the P_i peak at pH 7.0.

that the release of intracellular components such as enzymes, which is one of the characteristics of the calcium paradox, is maximal between 60 and 90 s of reperfusion [25]. Fig. 3 clearly shows that there is an almost simultaneous disappearance of the high-energy phosphate peaks and the P_i peak during the calcium paradox. This is in contrast with the situation during ischemia, where creatine phosphate and particularly ATP levels decline more gradually and the P_i peak shows a marked increase [26]. Leakage through the disrupted sarcolemma [20] into the extracellular space, and uptake by mitochondria together with calcium may be responsible for the rapid disappearance of P_i from the cytosol during the calcium paradox.

As mentioned in the introduction, both breakdown of ATP and accumulation of calcium by mitochondria are proton-generating processes. However, breakdown of creatine phosphate is a proton-consuming reaction [18,22]. Apparently these opposite effects cancel during the calcium paradox and the result is little or no change in intracellular pH. Other factors that may contribute are the buffering capacity of the cell and leakage of protons into the extracellular space. It can be concluded that acidification of the cytosol does not play a causal role in the development of the calcium paradox.

SUMMARY

^{31}P NMR spectroscopy was used to investigate the course of intracellular pH during the calcium paradox in isolated rabbit heart at 37°C. Intracellular pH was measured from the chemical shift of the intracellular P_i peak. During control perfusion and the subsequent calcium-free period intracellular pH amounted to 7.1. After induction of the calcium paradox by readmitting calcium to the perfusion fluid, intracellular pH amounted to 7.0. It is concluded that acidification of the cytosol does not play a causal role in the development of the calcium paradox.

ACKNOWLEDGEMENT

This study was supported by the Wijnand M. Pon Foundation, Leusden, The Netherlands.

REFERENCES

1. Ringer, S. J. Physiol. 4: 29–42, 1883.
2. Zimmerman, A.N.E. and Hülsmann, W.C. Nature 211: 646–647, 1966.
3. Hearse, D.J., Humphrey, S.M., Boink, A.B.T.J. and Ruigrok, T.J.C. Eur. J. Cardiol. 7: 241–256, 1978.
4. Zimmerman, A.N.E., Daems, W., Hülsmann, W.C., Snijder, J., Wisse, E. and Durrer, D. Cardiovasc. Res. 1: 201–209, 1967.
5. Lomský, M., Ekroth, R. and Poupa, O. Eur. Heart J. 4 (Suppl. H): 139–142, 1983.
6. Ruigrok, T.J.C., Slade, A.M. and Poole-Wilson, P.A. Eur. Heart J. 4 (Suppl. H): 89–96, 1983.
7. Alto, L.E. and Dhalla, N.S. Am. J. Physiol. 237: H713–H719, 1979.
8. Nayler, W.G., Elz, J.S., Perry, S.E. and Daly, M.J. Eur. Heart J. 4 (Suppl. H): 29–41, 1983.
9. Ruigrok, T.J.C. In: Control and Manipulation of Calcium Movement (Ed. J.R. Parratt), Raven Press, New York, 1985, pp. 341–365.
10. Meno, H., Kanaide, H. and Nakamura, M. J. Pharmacol. Exp. Ther. 228: 220–224, 1984.
11. Ohhara, H., Kanaide, H. and Nakamura, M. J. Mol. Cell. Cardiol. 14: 13–20, 1982.
12. Dhalla, N.S., Alto, L.E. and Singal, P.K. Eur. Heart J. 4 (Suppl. H): 51–56, 1983.
13. Nayler, W.G., Perry, S.E., Elz, J.S. and Daly, M.J. Circ. Res. 55: 227–237, 1984.

14. Lamers, J.M.J., Stinis, J.T. and Ruigrok, T.J.C. Circ. Res. 54: 217–226, 1984.
15. Lamers, J.M.J. and Ruigrok, T.J.C. Eur. Heart J. 4 (Suppl. H): 73–79, 1983.
16. Preuner, J. Basic Res. Cardiol. 80 (Suppl. 2), 19–24, 1985.
17. Ruigrok, T.J.C., Boink, A.B.T.J., Spies, F., Blok, F.J., Maas, A.H.J. and Zimmerman, A.N.E. J. Mol. Cell. Cardiol. 10: 991–1002, 1978.
18. Grinwald, P.M. and Nayler, W.G. J. Mol. Cell. Cardiol. 13: 867–880, 1981.
19. Ganote, C.E. and Nayler, W.G. J. Mol. Cell. Cardiol. 17: 733–745, 1985.
20. Post, J.A., Nievelstein, P.F.E.M., Leunissen-Bijvelt, J., Verkleij, A.J. and Ruigrok, T.J.C. J. Mol. Cell. Cardiol. 17: 265–273, 1985.
21. Brierley, G.P., Murer, E. and Bachmann, E. Arch. Biochem. Biophys. 105: 89–102, 1964.
22. Gevers, W. J. Mol. Cell. Cardiol. 9: 867–874, 1977.
23. Langendorff, O. Pfluegers Arch. 61: 291–332, 1895.
24. Boink, A.B.T.J., Ruigrok, T.J.C., Maas, A.H.J. and Zimmerman, A.N.E. J. Mol. Cell. Cardiol. 8: 973–979, 1976.
25. Ruigrok, T.J.C., Boink, A.B.T.J., Slade, A., Zimmerman, A.N.E., Meijler, F.L. and Nayler, W.G. Am. J. Pathol. 98: 769–790, 1980.
26. Ruigrok, T.J.C., Van Echteld, C.J.A., De Kruijff, B., Borst, C. and Meijler, F.L. Eur. Heart J. 4 (Suppl. C): 109–113, 1983.

22

HYPERCONTRACTURE OF ISOLATED ADULT RAT HEART MYOCYTES:
MULTIPLE CAUSES AND A COMMON MECHANISM

R. A. ALTSCHULD, M. R. LAMBERT, AND G. P. BRIERLEY

Departments of Physiological Chemistry and Medicine
The Ohio State University Medical Center, Columbus, Ohio 43210

INTRODUCTION

The hypercontracture of adult rat ventricular myocytes is an
indication of severe and irreversible damage. Normally rectangular and
striated myocytes are converted into grossly disorganized round forms
as the consequence of an excessive and seemingly uncontrolled
shortening of the myofibrils. Under the light microscope,
hypercontracture can often be seen to occur after multiple spontaneous
cycles of contraction and partial but incomplete relaxation that
gradually reduce the overall length of each myocyte. In the final
stages, the myofibrils appear to fuse into a nearly amorphous central
mass, and the mitochondria and fragments of the sarcoplasmic reticulum
are extruded into large superficial blebs of cytosol (see 1 for typical
micrographs).

The morphology and ultrastructure of hypercontracted isolated
myocytes are highly reminiscent of contraction band necrosis in the
whole heart. Contraction bands develop at the periphery of a
myocardial infarction, in reperfused ischemic tissue, and after
exposure to toxic agents (see 2 for a review). The oxygen paradox and
the calcium paradox in isolated perfused hearts replicate many key
features of in vivo contraction band necrosis, including the massive
release of cytosolic enzymes and other soluble proteins (3-5). An in
vitro ischemia-reperfusion model has also been developed and shown to
exhibit respiration-dependent contraction band formation similar to
that of the oxygen paradox (6).

The hypercontracture of isolated and unattached myocytes differs
from contraction band formation in whole hearts in that a loss of
cytosolic components need not occur. Hypercontracted myocytes continue
to exclude trypan blue and retain such enzymes as lactic dehydrogenase
and creatine phosphokinase and, in some cases, levels of ATP comparable

to those of normally elongated myocytes (7). In the absence of
intercellular attachments, hypercontracture produces only an internal
rearrangement of structural components. The same process occurring in
attached muscle cells might be expected to produce physical stresses on
the cell membranes of sufficient force to cause physical damage.
However, the fragmentation of the sarcolemma could be the primary event
leading to the development of contraction bands in at least some forms
of irreversible whole heart damage.

Previous studies from this laboratory have described a variety of
conditions that will produce the hypercontracture of intact or
digitonin-permeabilized isolated myocytes (1, 7-9, 12). The present
communication summarizes this work and discusses the common underlying
mechanism for the excessive shortening of the myofibrils that leads to
the development of <u>in situ</u> contraction bands or the rounding up of
isolated myocytes.

RESULTS AND DISCUSSION
Calcium tolerance of isolated myocytes

The preparation of isolated adult rat heart myocytes requires a
period of calcium depletion to loosen intercellular attachments along
the fascia and macula adherens junctions of the intercalated disks.
After the cells are isolated, the readmission of physiologic amounts of
extracellular calcium can cause a variable fraction of the viable "rod-
shaped" myocytes to hypercontract (10). The number of these calcium
intolerant myocytes is increased by washing and storing the cells at
low temperatures (0-5°C), a condition that increases intracellular
Na^+, depletes K^+, and increases the rate and extent of labeling
when the myocytes are challenged with mM $^{45}Ca^{2+}$. If the
sodium-loaded myocytes are allowed a period of metabolic activity at
more physiologic temperatures, Na^+/K^+ ratios gradually decline and
there is a parallel increase in the number of calcium tolerant myocytes
(7). Calcium tolerance can be improved further by the gradual
readmission of calcium; extracellular calcium reduces the monovalent
cation permeability of the sarcolemma, and the myocytes extrude
additional Na^+ and decrease Na^+/K^+ to normal whole heart values
(11). In the presence of ouabain, normal monovalent cation gradients
are not restored, the cells remain sodium loaded, and all hypercontract

in the presence of mM Ca^{2+} (7). The hypercontracture associated
with calcium intolerance appears to result from excessive calcium
intake via the electrogenic Na/Ca exchange transporter and possibly the
voltage-gated slow channels of the sarcolemma (7,8,12), and not an
irreversible change in passive permeability to calcium.

Cytosolic free Ca^{2+} and hypercontracture

Isolated myocytes accumulate the fluorescent Ca^{2+} probe, quin2,
when incubated with its tetraacetoxymethyl ester. Quin2 has a
relatively high affinity for Ca^{2+} and thus can be used both to report
and to manipulate the cytosolic pCa of isolated myocytes (12). With
sodium loaded myocytes, high concentrations of intracellular quin2 (1-4
mM) inhibit hypercontracture and decrease the maximum cytosolic free
Ca^{2+} produced when the cells are challenged with 1 mM $CaCl_2$. The
effects of quin2 are concentration-dependent, and when the values of
free Ca^{2+} are extrapolated to zero quin2, a mean cytosolic free
Ca^{2+} of approximately 1 µM can be predicted to produce complete
hypercontracture in a population of myocytes. When free Ca^{2+}
reported by quin2 is 400 nM, 50% of the cells hypercontract, while the
Ca^{2+} of suspensions of elongated and calcium tolerant myocytes is in
the 150-200 nM range (12).

Interestingly, the peak free Ca^{2+} reported by quin2
fluorescence in electrically stimulated calcium-tolerant myocytes
incubated with isoproterenol was found to exceed 400 nM, but this
concentration was present only for a fraction of a second and declined
to the resting value fairly rapidly (13). It may be that a normal but
unabated activation of the contractile apparatus, in the absence of an
imposed resting tension, can produce hypercontracture in untethered
myocytes. Calcium overloads can also cause cycles of calcium-induced
calcium release and reaccumulation by the sarcoplasmic reticulum (14),
and the spontaneous contractile activity observed in sodium-loaded
myocytes can be attributed to this reaction (1). Vigorous and rapid
spontaneous contractions often precede hypercontracture.

The precise Ca^{2+} required for hypercontracture or spontaneous
contractile activity cannot be determined with a heterogeneous
population of quin2-loaded myocytes. Quin2 fluorescence becomes quite
insensitive to intracellular free Ca^{2+} in excess of 1 µM, so the

contribution of cells containing high levels of Ca^{2+} will be missed
by this reagent. Moreover, the effects of cytosolic free Ca^{2+} on the
myofibrils are modulated by the concentration of $MgATP^{2-}$ and by other
variables.

Reoxygenation-induced hypercontracture

Myocytes incubated anaerobically without glucose lose ATP and
total adenine nucleotides as a function of time (9,15). The lost
adenine nucleotides can be accounted for by an increase in cellular IMP
and extracellular adenosine and inosine. A small amount of
hypoxanthine may also be produced, but this probably can be attributed
to slight contamination of the myocytes by endothelial cells or other
cell types rich in nucleoside phosphorylase. The activity of this
enzyme in the myocytes per se seems to be negligible (15).

Between 15 and 45 minutes of anoxia, there is an increase in the
number of myocytes that appear to be in anoxic or rigor contracture
(9,16). These cells retain well aligned sarcomeres and an orderly
arrangement of intracellular structural elements, but sarcomere lengths
are greatly reduced, and many of the myocytes assume a nearly square
shape (see Fig. 1, ref. 9). Abrupt anoxic contractures of individual
myocytes can be readily observed under the light microscope and
recently were recorded on videotape (17). Such transitions can be
observed only under strictly anoxic conditions or in myocytes poisoned
with a respiratory inhibitor; with hypoxia there appears to be a
continuum of sarcomere lengths that decrease gradually as a function of
time (18).

The increase in the number of myocytes in anoxic contracture
closely parallels the loss of ATP from the cell population, and it has
been proposed that an abrupt anoxic contracture occurs when an
individual myocyte exhausts its glycogen stores and ATP production
ceases (16). After 45 minutes, when nearly all of the myocytes are in
contracture, the reintroduction of glucose does not lead to the
production of lactic acid, presumably because of insufficient ATP for
the hexokinase and phosphofructokinase reactions. Whole cell ATP is
less than 1 nmole/mg biuret protein, and disruption of the sarcolemma
with low levels of digitonin does not significantly alter cellular ATP
content (15). These data indicate that residual ATP is contained in

the mitochondrial matrix, and for all practical purposes, the cytosolic compartment of an anoxic myocyte is devoid of ATP after 45 minutes.

With continued anaerobiosis, there is a gradual increase in the number of rectangular and striated myocytes that stain with trypan blue and release cytosol enzymes. The non-viable myocytes have extensively fragmented cell membranes, and the mitochondria contain numerous myelin figures and amorphous densities. However, the sarcomeres are well-aligned, with no evidence of hypercontracture (19).

If anoxic, ATP-depleted myocytes are reaerated prior to the loss of cell membrane integrity, ATP and total adenine nucleotides increase at the expense of the IMP pool, and the ability to produce lactic acid from added glucose during a subsequent period of anoxia is restored (15). Reoxygenation also causes a variable fraction of the cell population to hypercontract (9). By tracking the response of individual myocytes to anoxia and reoxygenation, Stern et al. (17) established that myocytes in anoxic contracture for less than 10 minutes relax and regain the ability to contract with electrical stimulation, whereas those in the square form for more than 20 minutes hypercontract in response to reoxygenation.

The number of myocytes that hypercontract during reoxygenation is decreased when the incubation is carried out in a nominally calcium-free medium (20 μM total Ca^{2+} by atomic absorption analysis), but this response is not wholly dependent on Ca^{2+}, since the inclusion of 0.1 mM EGTA further reduces but does not abolish reoxygenation-induced hypercontracture (9). In addition, when myocytes are incubated anaerobically with 5 mM iodoacetate to inhibit ATP production from stored glycogen, ATP falls to a barely detectable value within 15 minutes, and reoxygenation in a nominally Ca^{2+}-free medium supplemented with 1.0 mM EGTA causes more than 90% of the viable myocytes to hypercontract (20). In the iodoacetate-poisoned myocytes, reoxygenation produces a very slight rebound in cellular ATP, the total adenine nucleotide pool does not increase, and IMP is degraded to inosine. A significant resynthesis of cystolic ATP can be inferred, however, from a decline in Na/K ratios and a rebound in phosphocreatine.

Reoxygenation-induced hypercontracture is abolished both by inhibitors and uncouplers of oxidative phosphorylation, indicating that, in the absence of glycolytic activity, mitochondrial ATP production is essential for the overcontraction of the myofibrils. However, it has recently been shown that the gradual increase in rounded myocytes that occurs during prolonged incubations in the presence of calcium and glucose is not eliminated by anaerobiosis or respiratory inhibition with 3 mM amytal (21). ATP, whether produced by oxidative phosphorylation or anaerobic glycolysis, can support hypercontracture.

Sarcolemmal damage and hypercontracture

After the many experimental manipulations needed to disperse an intact heart into individual myocytes, prior to the washing steps used to remove debris and non-muscle cells, and prior to the readmission of calcium, we invariably observe a number of rounded myocytes that stain with trypan blue. On the other hand, in these preparations, non-viable rod-shaped myocytes are extremely rare. The non-viable round cells could arise from dislocations in energy metabolism or calcium distribution similar to those described in the previous sections, but primary damage to the sarcolemma, as for example when the gap or nexus junctions of adjacent cells are cleaved, is also a strong possibility.

Digitonin at low concentration (16 µg/mg myocyte protein) selectively disrupts the sarcolemmae of isolated myocytes, but has no discernable effect on the mitochondria, sarcoplasmic reticulum, or myofibrils (1). Digitonin is commonly used to produce chemically skinned cells for studies of compartmentalization or subcellular function (1, 15), and digitonin lysis can also be useful for defining the possible consequences of physical membrane damage in intact, elongated myocytes.

The digitonin lysis of intact respiring myocytes suspended in a medium containing 1-2 mM Ca^{2+} produces a nearly instantaneous hypercontracture of the entire cell population. An identical response is observed for myocytes suspended in a nominally Ca^{2+}-free medium containing approximately 20 µM total contaminant Ca^{2+}. The addition of chelator (0.1-1.0 mM EGTA) to the Ca^{2+}-poor buffer slows the hypercontracture of lysed myocytes, but after 5-10 minutes at room temperature, all of the cells assume a rounded shape. Since free Ca^+ in the presence of chelator is well below the 150-200 nM of rod-shaped calcium-tolerant myocytes, factors other than elevated free Ca^{2+} must be capable of producing hypercontracture.

Myocytes that are treated with rotenone to inhibit NADH-linked mitochondrial electron transport do not hypercontract in a Ca^{2+}-poor medium following digitonin lysis. In the absence of a calcium chelator, the addition of succinate, a respiratory substrate that bypasses the rotenone block, causes all of the lysed cells to hypercontract within seconds. With EGTA present, this process is again slowed but not abolished. However, if the lysed cells are first washed several times to remove liberated cytosolic components or are incubated with crude apyrase to degrade liberated ATP and ADP, succinate addition has no effect on morphology. Finally, if the digitonin-lysed elongated myocytes are extracted with 1% Triton X-100 to dissolve the mitochondria and other membranous structures (see Fig. 3 of ref. 20 for a micrograph of a Triton-extracted myocyte) the addition of succinate has no effect, and the removal of liberated cytosolic components is unnecessary for the elimination of hypercontracture. With adventitious Ca^{2+} chelated by 1.0 mM EGTA, incubation of the elongated and striated detergent-insoluble ghosts with 10 μM Mg-ATP causes hypercontracture of the entire population in 3-5 minutes at room temperature.

Effects of pCa and pMgATP on digitonin-lysed myocytes

It is apparent from the experiments with intact and digitonin-lysed myocytes that hypercontracture can be produced either by an excess of free Ca^{2+} or a paucity of ATP, but it will not occur in the complete absence of high energy phosphate. To characterize this phenomenon in more quantitative terms, elongated digitonin-lysed myocytes were incubated in precisely defined buffers of known pCa (-log M Ca^{2+}) and pMgATP (-log M $MgATP^{2-}$) for exactly 3 minutes at 30°C and the numbers of rectangular and round forms counted (see ref. 1 for complete experimental details). At a pMgATP of 4, all of the lysed myocytes hypercontracted regardless of the pCa. This response was observed even in a nominally Ca^{2+}-free buffer supplemented with 1.0 mM EGTA, and in which the computed pCa and that reported by a calcium selective electrode exceeded 8.0 (less than 10 nM Ca^{2+}). As pMgATP was increased (concentration decreased) the number of rounded forms decreased, and in the absence of added ATP, the number of hypercontracted cells did not differ from that observed prior to the addition of rotenone and digitonin. The response to these exceedingly low concentrations of ATP was unaffected by pCa, but was shifted to higher pMgATP by succinate. The presence of the respiratory substrate also retarded the depletion of ATP in these protocols. The Ca^{2+}-independent hypercontracture of digitonin-lysed myocytes at very low Mg-ATP can be equated with Ca^{2+}-independent actomyosin ATPase activity, in which the formation of rigor bonds between actin and myosin produces a conformational change similar to that which occurs when Ca^{2+} binds to troponin in the presence of physiologic concentrations of ATP (22).

Higher concentrations of ATP inhibited hypercontracture at low Ca^{2+} but were without effect in the presence of high Ca^{2+}. Multiple families of curves were generated by titrating pMgATP in the presence of various controlled pCa's (see Fig. 12, ref. 1 for an example). Figure 1 summarizes the pMgATP and pCa at which 50% of the chemically skinned myocytes exhibited a Ca^{2+}-dependent hypercontracture (i.e., added $MgATP^{2-}$ greater than 0.1 mM). At an ATP similar to that of the cytosolic compartment in normal aerobic cells (10mM), half of the cells became rounded in 3 minutes at a free Ca^{2+} of 1 µM. Because hypercontracture is a time dependent and obviously heterogeneous phenomenon at the intermediate values of pCa and pMgATP shown in Figure 1, the data are not inconsistent with the observation that nearly all intact myocytes hypercontract after a 10 min incubation when the mean free Ca^{2+} reported by quin2 fluorescence remains at 1 µM. With 2-3 mM ATP, levels comparable to those found in myocytes reoxygenated after 45 minutes of anoxia, half of the cells hypercontracted at or below a free Ca^{2+} of 200 nM, which is within the range reported by quin2 fluorescence for the cytosol of resting elongated calcium tolerant myocytes (12, 13).

According to the data of Figure 1, there need not be an increase in the resting cytosol free Ca^{2+} to produce hypercontracture under conditions where ATP is continuously produced from a depleted pool of adenine nucleotides. Conversely, it is obvious that a physiologic concentration of cytosolic ATP is not incompatible with hypercontracture if Ca^{2+} influx via Na/Ca exchange and other

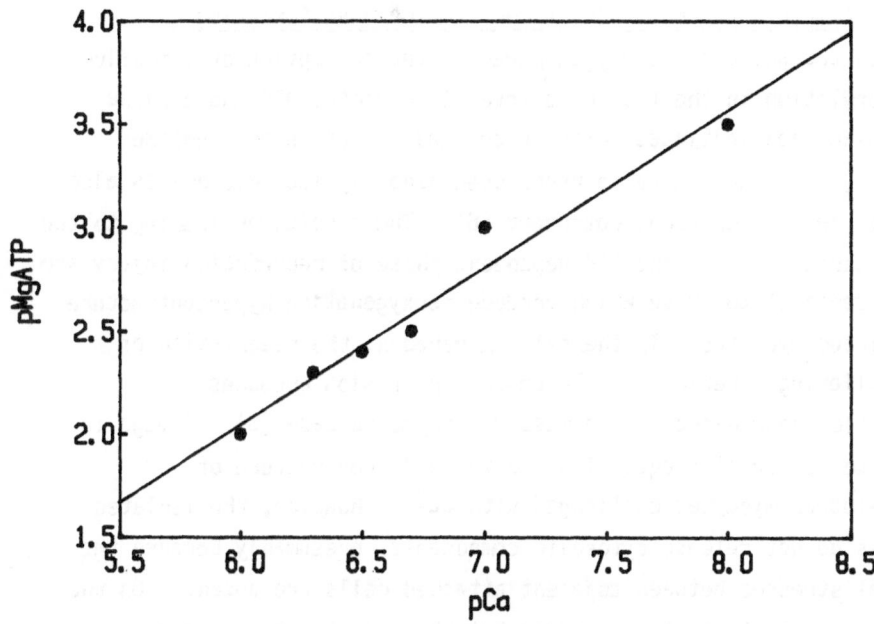

Fig. 1. pCa and pMgATP associated with the hypercontracture of 50%
of digitonin-lysed myocytes after 3 minutes at 30°C, pH 7.20.
In the region above the regression line, nearly all of the cells are
in the disorganized round form. When values for pMgATP and pCa fall
below the line, the myocytes are normally elongated. (Replotted from
data of ref. 1.)

physiologically relevant pathways overwhelms the relaxation process and
the free Ca^{2+} of the cytosol cannot be brought below 1 μM. Finally,
if the sarcolemma of a respiring myocyte is physically or chemically
disrupted, the pCa of the myofilament space equilibrates with that of
the extracellular medium. In most experimental protocols, this Ca^{2+}
is sufficient to produce hypercontracture in the presence of ATP.
Disruption of the sarcolemma also causes the loss of cytosolic ATP, but
a residual small pool of adenine nucleotides can support
hypercontracture if ATP is continuously replenished by oxidative
phosphorylation. If mitochondrial ATP production is blocked by an
inhibitor or uncoupler of oxidative phosphorylation, however, trapped

ATP is consumed and the loss of soluble enzymes and cofactors precludes glycolytic resynthesis of ATP. Under these conditions, there is insufficient residual ATP to support a full hypercontracture.

Hypercontracture and whole heart contraction band formation

In the whole heart oxygen paradox, the resumption of oxidative phosphorylation in the face of a severely depleted ATP and adenine nucleotide pool initiates contraction band formation and enzyme release (23). The damage to reperfused globally ischemic hearts also involves an ATP-dependent component (6). The conditions leading to the oxygen paradox and to the ATP-dependent phase of reperfusion injury are thus identical to those which produce reoxygenation hypercontracture in isolated myocytes. In the calcium paradox, the readmission of Ca^{2+} following a period of calcium-free perfusion produces contraction band necrosis and massive enzyme release (3). Damage in this case is formally equivalent to the hypercontracture of sodium-loaded myocytes challenged with Ca^{2+}. However, the isolated myocytes do not release cytosolic components, presumably because the physical stresses between adjacent attached cells are absent. On the other hand, digitonin lysis causes both hypercontracture and a loss of cytosolic enzymes and metabolites to the suspending medium. Hypercontracture in the intact heart could conceivably be the result and not the cause of irreversible membrane damage. This seems to be the case in calcium free perfused hearts challenged with caffeine (24), and it has been suggested that physical membrane damage may precede full hypercontracture in the classical calcium paradox (25). The situation with respect to the oxygen paradox and reperfusion damage is probably more complex. Under these conditions, dislocations in energy metabolism and possibly calcium homeostasis, when combined with a weakening of the sarcolemma and/or its attachments, may conspire to produce contraction band necrosis when mitochondrial ATP production resumes.

SUMMARY

The hypercontracture of isolated adult rat heart myocytes is the cellular equivalent of contraction band necrosis. This form of irreversible damage results from an uncontrolled shortening of the myofibrils which fuses the thick and thin filaments into a disorganized mass and expels interfibrillar mitochondria into clear areas of cytosol. Hypercontracture can result from such seemingly dissimilar phenomena as a calcium overload, the resumption of oxidative phosphorylation in the face of a severely depleted adenine nucleotide pool, and the chemical or physical disruption of the sarcolemma of a respiring ventricular muscle cell. Studies of chemically-skinned and detergent-extracted isolated adult rat heart myocytes established that hypercontracture is an ATP-dependent process that occurs in the presence of elevated free Ca^{2+}, abnormally low concentrations of ATP, or intermediate levels of each. Dislocations in the concentrations of Ca^{2+} and ATP bathing the myofibrils are adequate to explain the contraction band necrosis associated with the oxygen paradox, the calcium paradox, and reperfusion damage, and the calcium intolerance and the reoxygenation-induced hypercontracture of isolated myocytes.

ACKNOWLEDGEMENTS

The studies were supported by grants-in-aid from the Central Ohio Heart Chapter, Inc. We wish to thank Dr. R.S. Vander Heide, Northwestern University Medical School, for helpful discussions of this topic.

REFERENCES

1. Altschuld, R.A., Wenger, W.C., Lamka, K.G., Kindig, O.R., Capen, C.C., Mizuhira, V., Vander Heide, R.S., and Brierley, G.P. J. Biol. Chem. 260: 14325-14334, 1985.
2. Ganote, C.E. J. Mol. Cell. Cardiol. 15: 67-73, 1983.
3. Zimmerman, A.N.E., and Hulsman, W.C. Nature 211: 646-647, 1966.
4. Hearse, D.J., Humphrey, S.M., and Chain, E.B. J. Mol. Cell. Cardiol. 5: 395-407, 1973.
5. Ganote, C.E., Seabra-Gomes, R., Nayler, W.G., and Jennings, R.B. Am. J. Pathol. 80: 419-450, 1975.
6. Ganote, C.E. and Humphrey, S.M. Am. J. Pathol. 120: 129-145, 1985.
7. Altschuld, R.A., Gibb, L., Ansel, A., Hohl, C., Kruger, F.A., and Brierley, G.P. J. Mol. Cell Cardiol. 12: 1383-1395, 1980.
8. Altschuld, R.A., Hostetler, J.R., and Brierley, G.P. Circ. Res. 49: 307-316, 1981.
9. Hohl, C.M., Ansel, A., Altschuld, R.A., and Brierley, G.P. Am. J. Physiol. 242: H1022-H1030, 1982.
10. Powell, T. and Twist, V.W. Biochem. Biophys. Res. Commu. 72: 327-333, 1976.
11. Hohl, C.M., Altschuld, R.A., and Brierley, G.P. Arch. Biochem. Biophys. 221: 197-205, 1983.

12. Lambert, M.R., Johnson, J.D., Lamka, K.G., Brierley, G.P., and Altschuld, R.A. Arch. Biochem. Biophys. 245: 426-435, 1986.
13. Thomas, A.P., Selak, M., and Williamson, J.R. J. Mol. Cell. Cardiol. 18: 541-545, 1986.
14. Fabiato, A. Basic. Res. Cardiol. 80 (suppl.): 83-87 , 1985.
15. Geisbuhler, T., Altschuld, R.A., Trewyn, R.W., Ansel, A.Z., Lamka, K., and Brierley, G.P. Circ. Res. 54, 536-546, 1982.
16. Haworth, R.A., Hunter, D.R., and Berkoff, H.A. Circ. Res. 49: 1119-1128, 1981.
17. Stern, M.D., Chien, A.M., Capogrossi, M.C., Pelto, D.J., and Lakatta, E.G. Circ. Res. 56: 899-903, 1985.
18. Piper, H.M., Schwartz, P., Spahr, R. Hutter, J.F., Spieckermann, P.G. Pflugers Arch. 410: 71-76.
19. Wenger, W.C., Murphy, M.P., Kindig, O.R., Capen, C.C., Brierley, G.P., and Altschuld, R.A. Life Sci. 37, 1697-1704, 1985.
20. Brierley, G.P., Hohl, C.M., and Altschuld, R.A. In: Myocardial Injury (Ed. J.J. Spitzer), Plenum, N.Y., 1983, pp. 231-248.
21. Vander Heide, R.S., Angelo, J.P., Altschuld, R.A., and Ganote, C.E. Am. J. Pathol., 1986, in press.
22. Moss, R.L., and Haworth, R.A. Biophys. J. 45: 733-742, 1984.
23. Ganote, C.E., McGarr, J., Liu, S.Y., and Kaltenbach, J.P. J. Mol. Cell. Cardiol. 12: 387-408, 1980.
24. Vander Heide, R.S. and Ganote, C.E. Am. J. Pathol. 118: 55-65, 1985.
25. Vander Heide, R.S., Altschuld, R.A., Lamka, K.G., and Ganote, C.E. Am. J. Pathol. 123: 351-364, 1986.

23

MECHANICAL RESTITUTION AND INOTROPIC RESERVE OF THE RAT HEART FOLLOWING HETEROTHERMAL GLOBAL ISCHEMIA

J.S. JUGGI AND P. BRAVENY

Department of Physiology, Faculty of Medicine, Kuwait Universtiy, Kuwait (A. Gulf)

INTRODUCTION

The efficacy of low temperature on the post-ischemic recovery of the heart activity was studied using the technique of heterothermal irrigation of the ventricles. During one hour lasting no-flow ischemia, the cavity of one ventricle was irrigated with 37°C non-oxygenated Krebs-Henseleit (KH) buffer, the other with 20°C KH. During the reperfusion period, the intraventricular pressures were simultaneously recorded by inserted balloons and compared with the post-ischemic data. Ventricular end diastolic pressure was kept constant for all protocols of study. Control and reperfusion temperature was 34°C. In protocol 'A', right ventricle (RV) irrigation temperature was kept at 37°C and the left ventricle (LV) at 20°C. In protocol 'B', the temperature gradient was reversed. This technique produced a temperature gradient of 7-10°C between RV and LV.

Our previous study (1) showed that after 15 minutes of reperfusion, the isovolumic contractions of the spontaneously beating perfused rat hearts were significantly more depressed in the ventricle which was irrigated at 37°C during ischemia.

In the present preliminary report, we investigated other parameters of functional recovery which would allow more insight into the mechanism of low temperature preservation.

INOTROPIC RESERVE:

When the basic frequency of the heart is increased, the maximal isometric force increases in a stepwise fashion and reaches a higher level of steady state (positive staircase or Bowditch effect; 2). When

the higher stimulation frequency is switched back to the steady state
frequency, the built up inotropism becomes evident in the first beat
(post - stimulation potentiation or Woodworth phenomenon; 3), and
thereby it gradually attains the steady state level ('negative
staircase'). The capacity of the cardiac muscle to build-up inotropism
has been attributed to the modifications of calcium entry and extrusion
through the sarcolemma (4). Pre- and post-ischemic inotropic reserve
of the heart was, therefore, quantified by the technique of
post-stimulation potentiation.

To produce complete heart block, the atria were removed and septum
cut at the A.V. node level. The heart was stimulated at a basal rate
of 2.5/sec. The inotropic reserve to a train of rapid stimulation (15
impulses at 5/sec) was recorded before and after ischemic arrest.
Post-stimulation potentiation was expressed as the increment of
pressure of the first beat after stimulation and separately as the sum
of increments of pressures of the second through fifth post-stimulation
beat. The results (Table 1) showed that the inotropic reserve was
significantly less affected in the ventricle which underwent the
ischemic period at 20°C as compared to the ventricle at 37°C. The
first and the subsequent beats showed identical depression following
ischemic arrest at 37°C.

Table I. Ventricular Inotropic Reserve
(Normalized mean values for 5 experiments)

	Protocol A		Protocol B	
	RV Ischemia 37°C	LV Ischemia 20°C	RV Ischemia 20°C	LV Ischemia 37°C
P, Beat I (% SS Control)	18	51	40	21
P, Beat 2-5 (% SS Control)	19	42	33	19

P, Ventricular developed pressure; SS, Steady State.

MECHANICAL RESTITUTION:

The amount of activator calcium available to the myofilaments is a function of the interval between beats(5,6).   The resulting force-

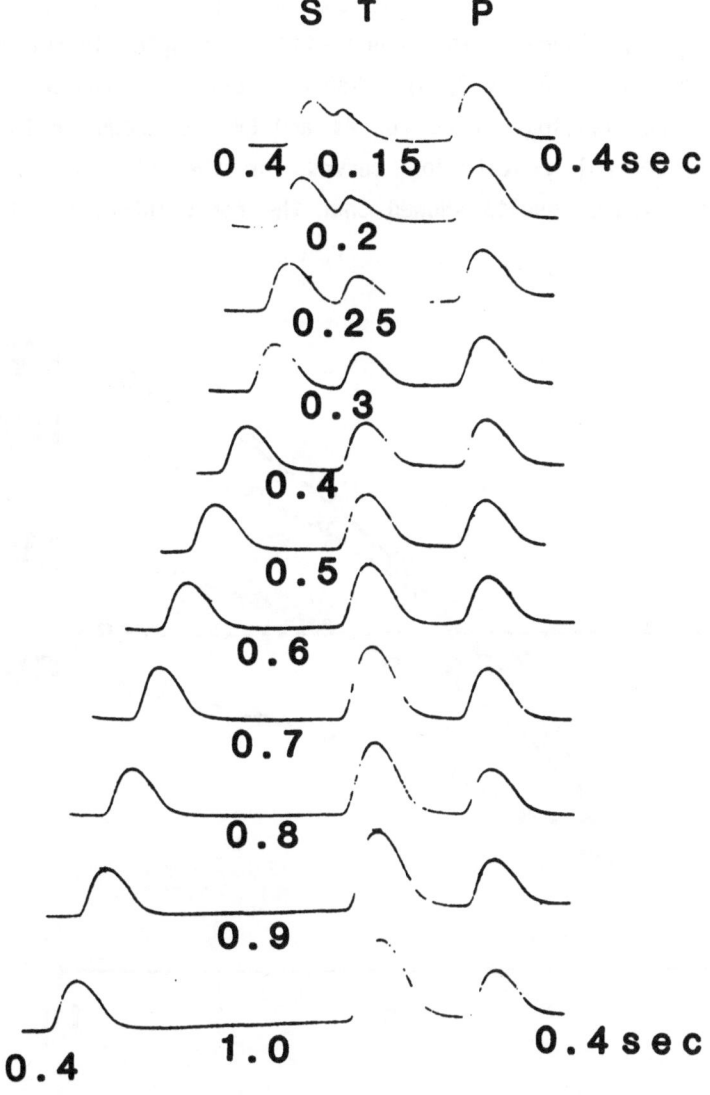

Fig. 1.   The effect of change of interval between steady state beats on the test (T) and potentiated (P) contractions.   Control rat heart, perfused at 34°C.   Steady state (S) = 0.4 sec, right ventricle pressure recordings.

interval relationship has been studied by plotting the mechanical restitution curves (7). The contractile strength of the test beat is plotted as a function of time interval between a steady state stimulus and a subsequent test stimulus (Fig. 1). When the test interval is short, the test beat is of low contractile strength; as the test interval is prolonged, the contractile strength increases in a monoexponential manner (8,9,10). Representative pre and post-ischemic mechanical restitution curves for RV and LV are shown in Fig. 2 and Fig. 3. Control restitution curves for the RV and the LV were identical. These results showed that the force-interval relationship

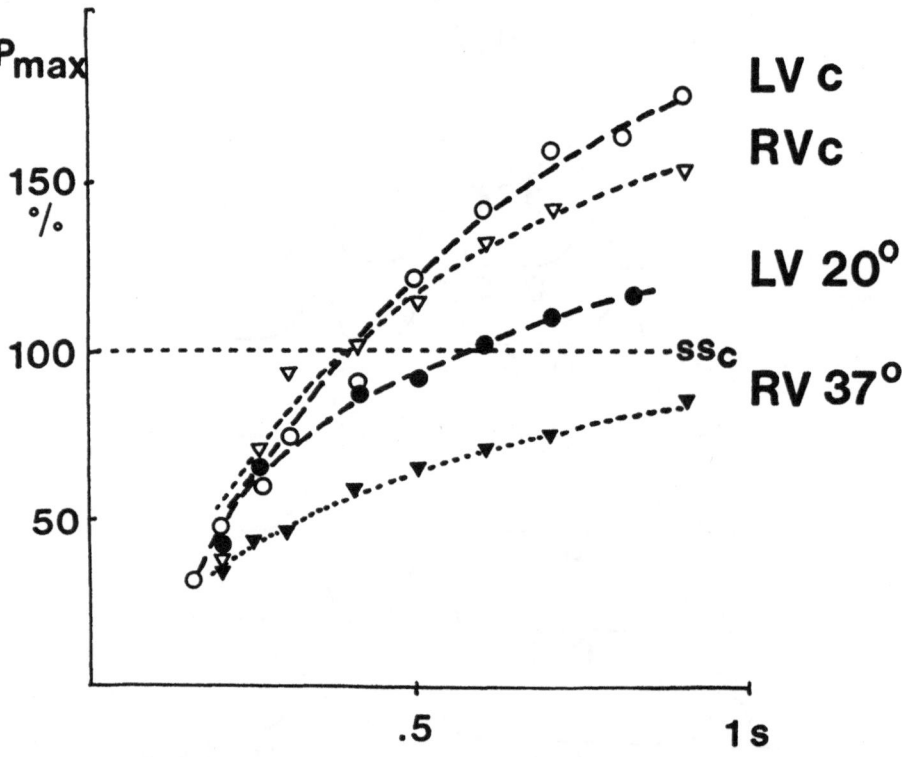

Fig. 2.   Mechanical restitution curves for the RV and LV.   Protocol A, normalized intraventricular pressure plotted as a function of test beat interval.   Steady State (SS) = 0.4 sec.

for the RV and LV of the rat heart was similar despite differences in their anatomical shape and mass, supporting the earlier conclusions of Burkhoff et al. (11), for the canine heart. The restitution process was more depressed in the ventricle which underwent ischemia at 37°C as compared with the other ventricle at 20°C. These data indicate that either the cellular level of activating calcium is reduced or else the sensitivity of myofilaments to calcium is altered.

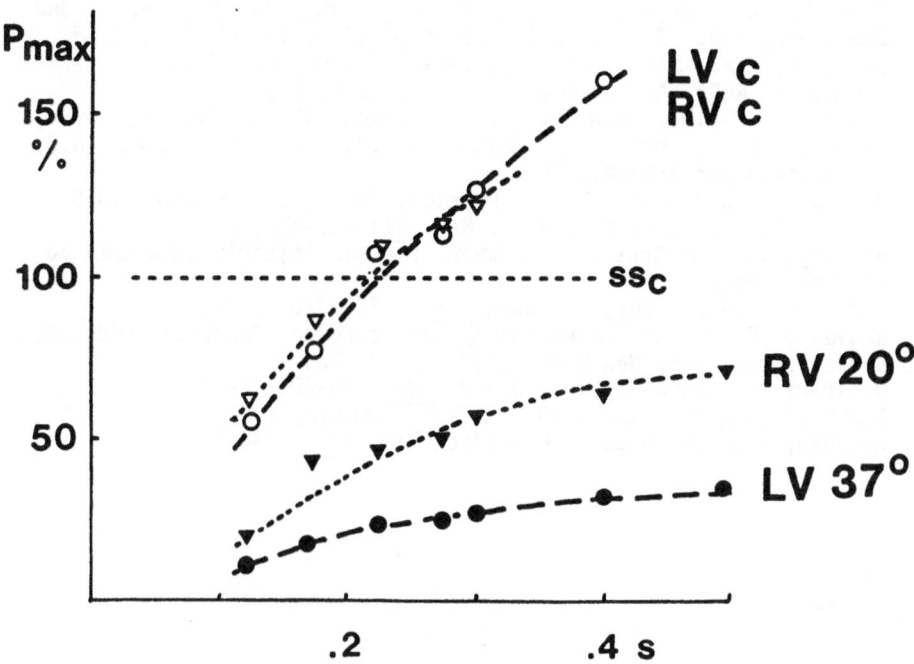

Fig. 3.   Mechancial restitution curves for the RV and LV. Protocol B, normalized intraventricular pressure plotted as a function of test beat interval. Steady State (SS) = 0.25 sec.

SUMMARY:

By exposing the RV and LV of the perfused rat heart to different temperatures (20°C, 37°C) during one hour lasting no-flow ischemia, the protective effect of hypothermia could be invariably proved in the same heart. Post-ischemic reperfusion loss of cellular calcium control may be minimized by maintaining adequate hypothermia during ischemic arrest.

Supported by Kuwait University MYO11 research grant.

REFERENCES:
1. Mognieh, L., Juggi, J. S., Braveny, P., Yousof, A.M. and Shuhaiber, H.J. J. Mol. Cell. Cardiol. 18 (suppl I): 139, 1986.
2. Bowditch, H.P. Ber. sachs Ges. (AKad.) Wiss, 652, 1871.
3. Woodworth, R.S. Am. J. Physiol. 8: 213-249, 1902.
4. Anderson, P.A.W., Manring, A., Serwer, G.A., Benson, D.W., Edwards, S.B., Armstrong, B.E., Sterba, R.J. and Floyd, R.D. Circulation 60: 334-348, 1979.
5. Braveny, P. and Kruta, V. J. Physiol. Paris, 50: 192-194, 1958.
6. Cranefield, F. Bull N.Y. Acad. Med. 41: 419-427, 1965.
7. Braveny, P. and Kruta, V. Arch. Intern. Physiol. Biochem. 66: 633-652, 1958.
8. Kruta, V. and Braveny, P. Nature 187: 327-328, 1960.
9. Braveny, P. In: Pharmacology of cardiac function (Ed. O. Krayer),MacMillon, New York, 1963, pp. 73-76.
10. Wohlfart, B. Acta Physiol. Scand, 106: 395-409, 1979.
11. Burkhoff, D., Yue, D.T., Franz, M.R., Hunter, W.C., Sunagawa, K., Maugham, W.L. and Sagawa, K. Circ. Res. 54: 468-473, 1984.

D. CALCIUM ANTAGONISTS AND MYOCARDIAL ISCHEMIA

24

CALCIUM ANTAGONISM AND THE ISCHEMIC MYOCARDIUM

W.G. NAYLER, W.J. STURROCK and S. PANAGIOTOPOULOS.

Department of Medicine, University of Melbourne, Austin Hospital, Heidelberg, Victoria, 3084, Australia.

INTRODUCTION

This paper does not attempt to provide a comprehensive overview of the Ca^{2+} antagonists, or of their use in the management of ischemic heart disease, since detailed reviews are already available (1-4). Instead the paper describes the results of some experiments we have recently undertaken to further explore the protection these drugs provide for the ischemic and reperfused hearts.

Irrespective of its cause - persistent and severe coronary artery spasm, embolism, plaque rupture or platelet aggregation - a sustained and severe reduction in coronary blood flow disturbs the metabolic (Fig. 1) and mechanical functioning of the heart (5,6).

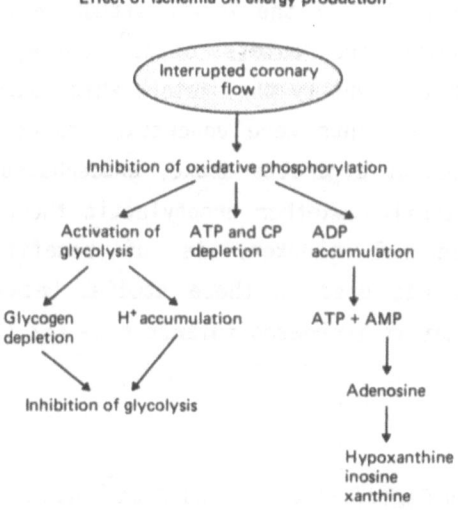

Fig. 1. Schematic representation of the metabolic consequences of an inadequate coronary blood flow.

Within one or two beats active tension development begins to decline (7), and metabolic by-products accumulate. Within 15 min the tissue reserves of adenosine triphosphate (ATP) and creatine phosphate (CP) are exhausted. The heart responds to this challenge by switching to anaerobic glycolysis. This is an inefficient method of producing ATP. Moreover the glycogen stores are of limited capacity and the protons which are generated inhibit further glycolysis. After only a few minutes of ischemia the changes caused by inadequate perfusion are reversible, so that the restoration of adequate coronary perfusion ultimately results in complete recovery. Reperfusion under these circumstances, therefore, is beneficial because without reperfusion the damage caused by inadequate coronary perfusion at this stage would have progressed until all the tissue in the affected area was irreversibly, and hence lethally injured. Reperfusion itself, however, can provoke injury because it can precipitate a massive and uncontrolled gain in Ca^{2+} which in turn signals cell death and tissue necrosis (8,9). Controversy exists as to whether the uncontrolled gain in Ca^{2+} which occurs under these conditions actually triggers the cascade of events that results in cell death (10), or whether the uncontrolled Ca^{2+} gain is simply an expression of pre-existing lethal injury that was sustained during the ischemic episode (11). If the former situation applies then it is important to establish the route(s) of Ca^{2+} entry, to devise ways of controlling it and to identify the factors which exacerbate it.

The following experiments were undertaken to establish whether nicotine - a component of cigarette smoke, exacerbates post-ischemic Ca^{2+} gain and to determine whether prophylactic therapy with a Ca^{2+} antagonist (slow channel blocker) is of benefit under these conditions. Nicotine was used in these studies because two recent reports have shown that it increases infarct size (12,13).

METHODS

Effect of Nicotine on Reperfusion - Induced Ca^{2+} Gain

Adult female Sprague Dawley rats (150-200g) maintained on a standard diet were used for these experiments.

Perfusion

The rats were lightly anesthetized with a diethylether - O_2 mixture and heparinized (200 I.U.). The hearts were excised, immersed in ice-cold Krebs-Henseleit (K-H) buffer for 2 min and then perfused in the non-recirculating Langendorff mode at 37°C as previously described (14). Coronary flow was maintained at 10-12 ml/min, using a Watson Marlow flow inducer .

Perfusion Buffers

These were prepared in distilled water. The K-H buffer contained, in mmol/l: NaCl, 119.0; $NaHCO_3$, 25.0; KCl, 4.6; KH_2PO_4, 1.2; $MgSO_4$, 1.2; $CaCl_2$, 1.3; and glucose, 11.0. Nicotine was added when required, to provide a final concentration of 0.15 µg/ml. The plasma of cigarette smokers has been shown to contain approximately 0.15 µg nicotine/ml (15). The perfusion buffers were gassed with 95% O_2 + 5% CO_2, (pH 7.4) and maintained at 37°C.

Perfusion Sequence

Some of the hearts were perfused with Krebs-Henseleit buffer throughout the duration of the experiment. Others were made globally ischemic at 37°C for either 30 or 60 min and then reperfused. In some instances nicotine was introduced 15 min before making the hearts ischemic. On other occasions it was introduced 15 min before the hearts were made ischemic and maintained throughout reperfusion. At the end of the perfusion sequence the hearts were assayed for tissue Ca^{2+} (16), 'reflow area' (17) and norepinephrine content (18).

Pretreatment with Ca^{2+} Antagonists

Having established that adding nicotine to the perfusion buffer causes an increase in the amount of Ca^{2+} accumulated upon reperfusion other experiments were undertaken to establish whether pretreatment with Ca^{2+} antagonists attenuate this gain. The drugs used were anipamil, which is a newly developed, long-acting derivative of verapamil (19) and verapamil.   When anipamil-treated rats were required they were injected subcutaneously (s.c.) for three days with 20 mg/kg anipamil on a once daily basis.   Five hrs after the last injection the rats were sacrificed and their hearts perfused as described above, with and without nicotine.   Preliminary studies confirmed that this regime of anipamil pretreatment reduces the blood pressure of spontaneously hypertensive rats (p<0.01).   Anipamil was also shown to displace specifically bound [^{3}H] verapamil (Dillon, unpublished results).

Other experiments were included here, using verapamil as the Ca^{2+} antagonist of choice.   In these experiments verapamil was added to the perfusion buffer to provide a final concentration of $1x10^{-6}M$. The drug was added 15 min before making the hearts ischemic and was retained throughout reperfusion. Nicotine (0.15 µg/ml) was present throughout.

Mechanical Function Studies

When required, peak developed (systolic) tension was monitored by means of a Narco-F-60 Biosystems myograph (Houston, Texas) attached to the left ventricular apex (16). The output from the myograph was displayed on a Narco Biosystems Physiograph MK IV recorder (Narco-Biosystems, Houston, Texas) and calibrated in gram tension.

Nicotine and Left Ventricular Norepinephrine

Throughout these experiments some of the hearts were assayed for left ventricular norepinephrine.   The method has been described in detail elsewhere and involves perchloric acid treatment followed by alumina extraction, with the eluate from the alumina column being subjected to high performance liquid chromatography with electrochemical detection (18).   Dihydroxybenzylamine was used as the internal standard.

Statistical Analysis

The results were analysed by Student's 't' test, or one-way analysis of variance, and expressed as mean ± SEM of at least six experiments. p<0.05 was accepted as the limit of significance.

RESULTS

Effect of nicotine on post-ischemic Ca^{2+} gain

Fig. 2 shows that adding nicotine to the coronary perfusate of aerobically perfused hearts to provide a final concentration of 0.15 µg/ml failed to cause any increase in their tissue Ca^{2+}.

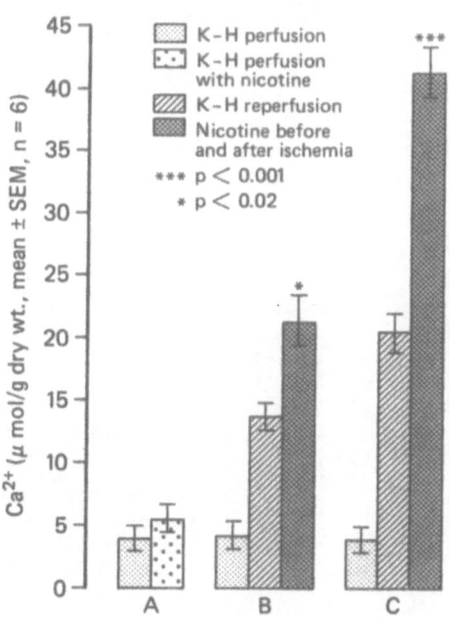

Effect of 0.15µg/ml nicotine on tissue Ca^{2+} (A) during aerobic perfusion, and during reperfusion after (B) 30 minutes, and (C) 60 minutes of ischemia.

Fig. 2. Effect of 0.15 µg/ml nicotine on tissue Ca^{2+}. Tests of significance relate to the increase in Ca^{2+} gain due to the presence of nicotine, relative to the K-H reperfused hearts.

Figure 2 also shows that reperfusing control hearts after 30 or 60 min of global ischemia with K-H buffer causes a significant (p<0.001) gain in tissue Ca^{2+}, and that this gain is further enhanced if nicotine (0.15 µg/ml) is included in the perfusion buffer. This exacerbating effect of nicotine on post-ischemic Ca^{2+} gain was more pronounced after 60 than after 30 min of ischemia (Fig. 2). Moreover it was not an effect which could be accounted for in terms of an altered 'reflow area' (Fig. 3), the area of reflow obtained upon reperfusion with K-H buffer after 60 minutes of ischemia being approximately the same as that obtained upon reperfusion in the presence of nicotine (0.15 µg/ml).

These results establish, therefore, that a concentration of nicotine equivalent to that present in the plasma of cigarette smokers exacerbates Ca^{2+} gain during post-ischemic reperfusion without altering the 'reflow area'.

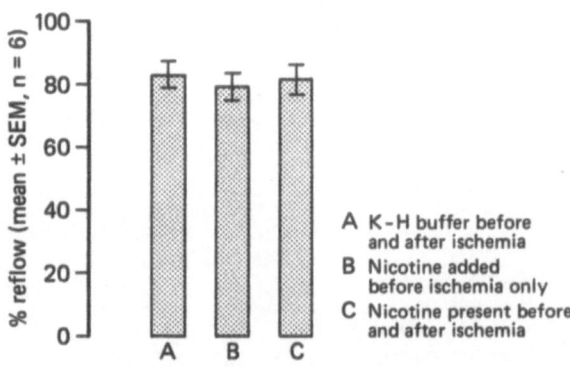

Effect of 0.15 µg/ml nicotine on reflow area after 60 minutes of ischemia.

A K-H buffer before and after ischemia
B Nicotine added before ischemia only
C Nicotine present before and after ischemia

Fig. 3. Effect of 0.15 µg/ml nicotine on the proportion of the ventricles which were reperfused after 60 min of global ischemia at 37°C. Note that 0.15 µg/ml nicotine had no effect.

One possible explanation for these findings could be that nicotine has exacerbated the spontaneous release of norepinephrine that occurs during the ischemia-reperfusion cycle (18). Fig. 4 shows that such an explanation is untenable. Thus the addition of 0.15 µg/ml nicotine to the perfusion buffer of aeobically perfused hearts failed to promote a release of endogenous norepinephrine. Moreover, although 60 min of ischemia followed by 15 min of reperfusion promoted a loss of endogenous ventricular norepinephrine, (Fig. 4) adding 0.15 µg/ml nicotine so that it was present before the ischemic episode as well as upon reperfusion neither enhanced nor attenuated this release. Hence, although 0.15 µg/ml nicotine increases the amount of Ca^{2+} that accumulates during post-ischemic reperfusion, this effect cannot be attributed to an effect of nicotine on ischemia-reperfusion induced displacement of endogenous norepinephrine.

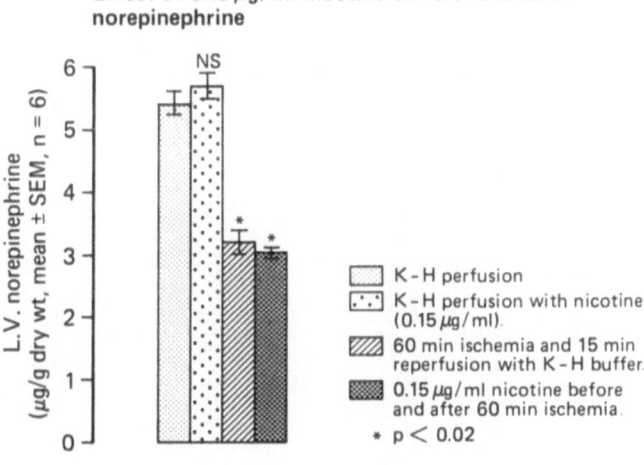

Effect of 0.15 µg/ml nicotine on left ventricular norepinephrine

Fig. 4. Effect of 60 min ischemia and reperfusion, with and without 0.15 µg/ml nicotine on ventricular norepinephrine. Tests of significance relate to the effect of ischemia and reperfusion with and without nicotine.

Effect of 0.15 µg/ml nicotine on heart rate and ventricular active tension generation

To exclude the possibility of the effect of nicotine on reperfusion-induced Ca^{2+} overload being due to an altered heart rate or force of contraction, these parameters were measured in hearts perfused with K-H buffer containing 0.15 µg/ml nicotine. Under the experimental conditions which applied here adding 0.15 µg/ml nicotine to the coronary circulation of isolated, aerobically-perfused, spontaneously beating rat hearts failed to promote any significant change in either heart rate or force of contraction.

Effect of verapamil on the nicotine (0.15 µg/ml)-induced exacerbation of post-ischemic Ca^{2+} gain

Pretreatment with Ca^{2+} antagonists reduces post-ischemic Ca^{2+} gain (20). Figure 5 confirms this fact. In addition it shows that pretreatment with $1 \times 10^{-6}M$ verapamil attenuates the exacerbation of post-ischemic Ca^{2+} gain caused by the presence of 0.15 µg/ml nicotine.

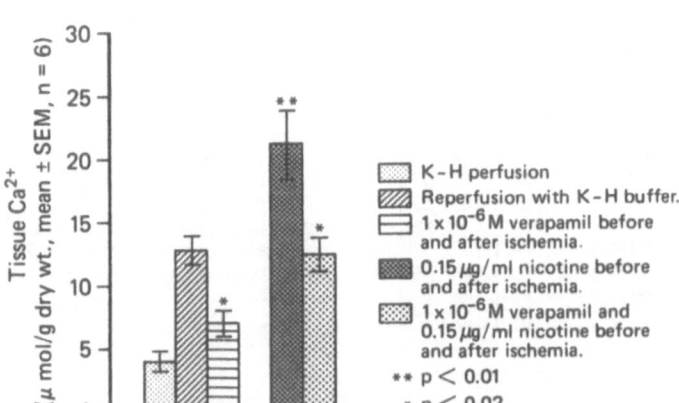

Effect of verapamil on the nicotine-induced exacerbation of reperfusion-induced Ca^{2+} gain

K-H perfusion
Reperfusion with K-H buffer.
$1 \times 10^{-6}M$ verapamil before and after ischemia.
0.15 µg/ml nicotine before and after ischemia.
$1 \times 10^{-6}M$ verapamil and 0.15 µg/ml nicotine before and after ischemia.
** p < 0.01
* p < 0.02

Fig. 5. Effect of adding $1 \times 10^{-6}M$ verapamil to the perfusion buffer before and after isolated hearts were made ischemic for 30 min, with and without nicotine.

One possible explanation for this attenuating effect of verapamil pretreatment, is that some of the excess Ca^{2+} gain that occurs
during post-ischemic reperfusion involves excess Ca^{2+} entry through
the slow channels. Other explanations are possible, however. For
example verapamil has an energy sparing effect (21), and it slows the
loss of purine precursors (22). There may be other explanations however, because as we have reported here, pretreatment with verapamil
depletes the cardiac stores of norepinephrine. Some typical results
are listed in figure 6. These results were obtained during a series
of experiments in which three strains of sex - and age-matched rats -
Sprague Dawley (SD), WKY (Wistar Kyoto), and spontaneously hypertensive (SHR) rats were given verapamil (50 mg/kg/day) orally for 6
wks. This provided a mean plasma level of approximately 100 ng/ml

Hence prolonged therapy with verapamil depletes the cardiac
reserves of norepinephrine (Fig. 6). However whether this contributes to the ability of verapamil to protect against the reperfusion-
induced gain in Ca^{2+} is unknown.

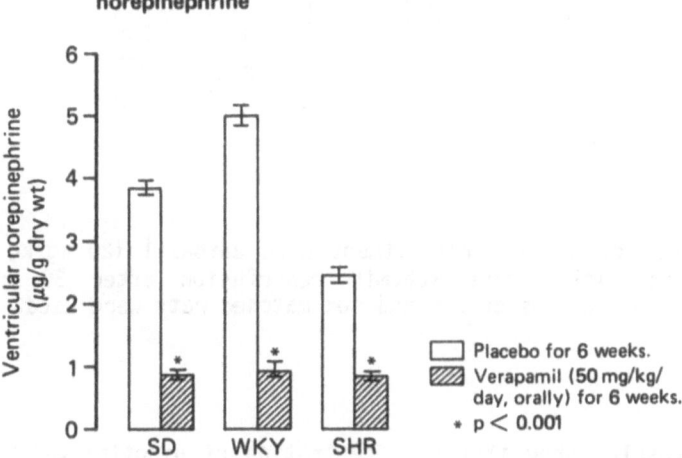

Effect of chronic verapamil therapy on ventricular norepinephrine

Placebo for 6 weeks.
Verapamil (50 mg/kg/ day, orally) for 6 weeks.
* p < 0.001

Fig. 6. Effect of 6 wks pretreatment with verapamil to provide a
plasma level of 100 ng/ml in left ventricular norepinephrine in
hearts isolated from Sprague Dawley (SD), Wistar Kyoto (WKY) and
spontaneously hypertensive (SHR) rats. The rats were age and sex
matched.

294

Effect of the long-acting Ca^{2+} antagonist, anipamil, on post-ischemic Ca^{2+} gain

Anipamil is a verapamil derivative, with a relatively long half-life. Figure 7 shows that pretreating rats with 20 mg/kg anipamil subcutaneously for three days attenuates the gain in Ca^{2+} that occurs during post-ischemic reperfusion after 30 min of global ischemia at 37°C.

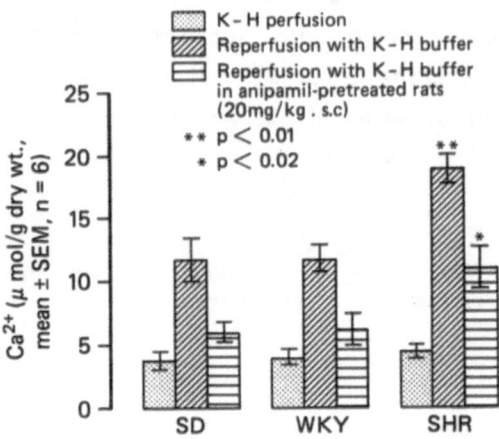

Fig. 7. Effect of 3 days pretreatment with anipamil (20 mg/kg s.c.) on Ca^{2+} gain during post-ischemic reperfusion after 30 min of ischemia. Three strains of age and sex matched rats were used.

DISCUSSION

These results show that a concentration of nicotine which could be found in the plasma of cigarette smokers, exacerbates post-ischemic Ca^{2+} overload. This effect of nicotine could not be accounted for in terms of an artifact due to an altered area of reflow, nor could it be explained in terms of an early exhaustion of

the endogenous energy reserves due to an effect of nicotine on heart
rate or force of contraction. An effect on the release of endogenous
norepinephrine has also been excluded. However, the fact that pretreatment with the Ca^{2+} antagonist - verapamil - attenuated this
effect of nicotine is of interest, because it could provide an
approach to the therapeutic management of the effect of cigarette
smoking on infarct size (12.13). Cigarette smoking increases infarct
size (12,13) and previous investigations have shown that an uncontrolled gain in Ca^{2+} signals the death of cardiac myocytes (8,9). The
present investigations show that the Ca^{2+} antagonists can reduce
post-ischemic Ca^{2+} overload, provided that they are used prophylacti-
cally, and that at therapeutic dose levels, they reduce the exacerbation of post-ischemic Ca^{2+} gain caused by plasma levels of nicotine
equivalent to that found in the plasma of smokers. There are several
reasons why Ca^{2+} antagonists should exert such a protective role.
They include (Fig. 8) an effect on energy preservation, and the loss
of purine precursors, as well as a possible effect on one of the
routes of Ca^{2+} entry.

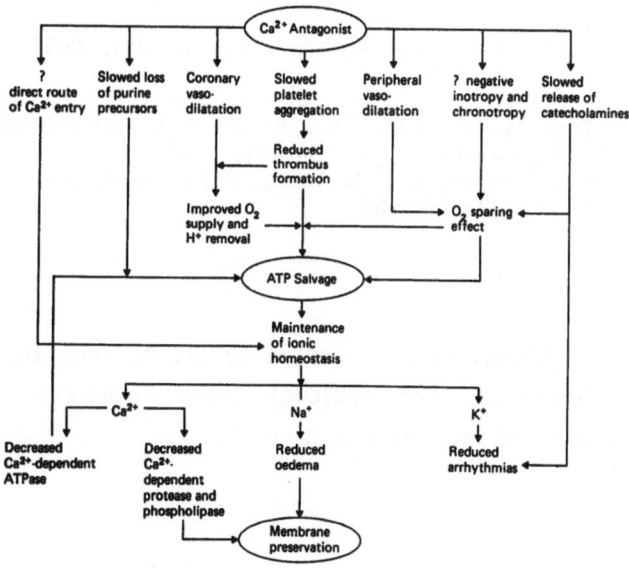

Fig. 8. Schematic representation of the possible mechanisms involved
in the protective effect of Ca^{2+} antagonist therapy.

REFERENCES

1. Nayler, W.G. and Horowitz, J.D. Pharmacol. Therap 20: 203-262, 1983.
2. Henry, P.D. Am. J. Cardiol. 46: 1047-1058, 1980.
3. Saini, R.V. In: Cardiovascular Pharmacology (Ed.M. Antonaccio), Raven Press, 2nd Ed, New York, 1984, pp415-452.
4. Opie, L.H. Pharmacol. Therap. 25: 271-291, 1984.
5. Braasch, W., Gudbjarnason, S., Puri, P.S., Ravens, K.G. and Bing, R.J. Circ. Res. 23: 429-438, 1968.
6. Hearse, D.J. J. Mol. Cell. Cardiol. 9: 605-630, 1977.
7. Poole-Wilson, P.A., Harding, D.P., Bourdillon, P.D.V. and Tones, M.A. J. Mol. Cell. Cardiol. 16: 175-187, 1984.
8. Nayler, W.G. Am. J. Pathol. 102: 262-270, 1980.
9. Jennings, R.B. and Reimer, K.A. Am. J. Pathol. 102:241-255, 1981.
10. Nayler, W.G. and Elz, J.S. Circulation: In Press, 1986.
11. Jennings, R.B. In: Calcium Antagonists and Cardiovascular Disease (Ed. L. Opie), Raven Press, New York, 1984 p85-96.
12. Masden, R.R. and Flowers, N.C. Am. Heart. J. 99: 242-248, 1980.
13. Sridharan, M.R., Flowers, N.C., Hand, R.C., Hand, J.W. and Horan, L.G. Am. J. Cardiol. 55: 1407-1411, 1985.
14. Nayler, W.G., Perry, S.E. and Daly, M.J. J. Mol. Cell. Cardiol. 15: 735-747, 1983.
15. Isaac, P.F. and Rand, M.J. Eur. J. Pharmacol. 8: 269-275, 1969.
16. Nayler, W.G., Perry, S.E., Elz, J.S. and Daly, M.J. Circ. Res. 55: 227-237, 1984.
17. Humphrey, S.M., Gavin, J.B. and Herdson, P.B. J. Mol. Cell. Cardiol. 12: 1397-1406, 1980.
18. Nayler, W.G. and Sturrock, W.J. J. Cardiovasc. Pharmacol. 7: 581-587, 1985.
19. Raschack, M., Kapp, W. and Heimann, E. J. Mol. Cell. Cardiol. 16: Suppl 2, No 168, 1984.
20. Nayler, W.G. Eur. Heart. J. 4: Suppl C, 33-41, 1983.
21. Lange, R., Ingwall, J., Hale, S., Alker, K.J., Braunwald, E. and Kloner, R.A. Circulation. 70: 734-741, 1984.
22. de Jong, J.W., Harmsen, E., de Tombe, P.P. and Keijzer, E. Eur. J. Pharmacol. 81: 89-96, 1982.

ACKNOWLEDGMENT

These investigations were supported by grants from the Tobacco Foundation of Australia, the National Heart Foundation and the National Health and Medical Research Council.

25

BIOCHEMICAL AND ULTRASTRUCTURAL ALTERATIONS IN CARDIAC
MEMBRANES DURING ISCHAEMIA-REPERFUSION: PROTECTION BY A
CALCIUM ENTRY BLOCKER

J.M.J. Lamers[a], C.E. Essed[b], J.A. Post[c], A.J. Verkleij[c],
F.J. ten Cate[d], W.J. van der Giessen[d] and P.D. Verdouw[d]

Departments of Biochemistry I[a], Anatomy I[b] and Thoraxcentre[d],
Erasmus University Rotterdam, and Institute of Molecular
Biology[c], State University of Utrecht, The Netherlands

INTRODUCTION

The possibility of protecting myocardial cells from the
damaging effects of ischaemia-reperfusion has received considerable attention in recent years. The rationale for the
use of Ca^{2+} entry blockers is that they directly interfere
with processes leading to Ca^{2+} overload and which are involved
in the production of irreversible injury. Although these
drugs have diverse chemical structures, they prevent Ca^{2+}
influx through the sarcolemma by blockade of voltage-dependent
Ca^{2+} channels (1, 2). By this mechanism Ca^{2+} entry blockers
e.g. inhibit platelet activation, suppress calcinosis of
atheromatous plaques, reduce arterial blood pressure, relieve
coronary spasm, improve myocardial O_2 balance by a lowered
O_2 demand (negative inotropism and chronotropism) and increase
O_2 supply by coronary vasodilation. Because of these multiple
effects on platelets, heart and systemic circulation it is
difficult to ascertain the mechanism(s) of cardioprotection
during ischemia-reperfusion in vivo.

During the past ten years it has become increasingly
evident that development of Ca^{2+} overload of the myocardium
plays an important role in causing tissue injury during
ischaemia and, in particular, reperfusion (3, 4). This hypothesis has been advanced on the basis of observations that
a) accumulation of Ca^{2+} in mitochondria interferes with their

capacity to generate ATP, b) increased cytosolic Ca^{2+},
levels waste energy sources by stimulation of ATPases, c)
increased Ca^{2+} levels are responsible for inducing protease
and phospholipase attack on cellular membranes and d) in the
presence of reduced ATP levels, excessive amounts of Ca^{2+}
induce contracture. The critical role for Ca^{2+} overload in
causing myocardial injury, by the Ca^{2+} paradox and a high
dose of catecholamines is obvious (6, 7). An unanswered
question remains: "Which factors within the myocardial cell
cause deregulation of Ca^{2+} homeostasis during ischaemia and
reperfusion"? A detailed knowledge of the sequence of derangements of Ca^{2+} occurring in ischaemic-reperfused myocardium
is required to answer this. This knowledge will also aid in
the development of interventions which aim to prevent, reduce
or delay myocardial injury.

Deregulation of cellular Ca^{2+} balance during ischaemia.

During myocardial ischaemia the fall of ATP content
leads to a reduction of Ca^{2+} pumping activity of the sarcolemma and the sarcoplasmic reticulum. A reduction of Na^+
pumping activity of the sarcolemma may also be expected
which attenuates indirectly the rate of Ca^{2+} efflux via the
Na^+/Ca^{2+} exchanger. Partial depolarization of the sarcolemma
by the increasing extracellular K^+ concentration and the
increasing adrenergic activity lead to partial opening of
Ca^{2+} channels through which Ca^{2+} enters the myocytes.
However, an opposed action of accumulated H^+ ions on Ca^{2+}
channels is expected. Ca^{2+} entry via the Na^+/Ca^{2+} exchange
occurs when the reduction of the sarcolemmal Na^+ gradient
and the increased depolarization of the sarcolemma reach
certain levels. A third possible route of Ca^{2+} entry is via
nonspecific pores or disrupted parts of the sarcolemma due
to the damaging actions of H^+ and Ca^{2+}-dependent protease or
phospholipase activities. The interaction of accumulated
lipid intermediates (free fatty acids, long-chain fatty
acylcarnitines and lysophospholipids) with membrane constituents might contribute also. These amphiphilic compounds
cause membrane expansion, displacement of Ca^{2+} and destruction of the lipid annulus surrounding the transport and

channel proteins. Whether the concentrations of these substances in vivo rise high enough during early ischaemia is
still unanswered (8, 9).

Deregulation of cellular Ca^{2+} balance during reperfusion.

The same factors, which play a role in deregulation of
Ca^{2+} balance during ischaemia, are also relevant during
reperfusion, although tissue accumulation of H^+ ions is less
by the increased washout and the ATP level may recover.
Their contributions to the Ca^{2+} deregulation will therefore
become less. However, the reavailability of extracellular
Ca^{2+}, the regenerated action potentials, the reoxygenation
of the mitochondria, inducing active Ca^{2+} influx, and the
impaired Ca^{2+} extrusion transport systems are additional
factors which may explain the excessive gain of Ca^{2+} during
reperfusion (10). It is difficult to differentiate between
the damaging effects of ischaemia and reperfusion since the
latter is required to obtain recovery of heart function,
biochemical and ultrastructural parameters. Besides Ca^{2+}
overload several other factors have been implicated as the
cause for reperfusion injury: the no-reflow phenomenon, the
sudden swelling of cells due to an elevated osmotic pressure
as a consequence of the increased tissue levels of lactic
acid and phosphate. Also the reoxygenation and the accumulated xanthine results in the formation of superoxide and
hydroxyl radicals inducing peroxidative damage to membranes
(11, 12). These free radical reactions and cell swelling may
indirectly affect Ca^{2+} homeostasis (13, 14). Because so many
other factors with no direct relation to the development of
Ca^{2+} overload contribute in causing reperfusion injury, Ca^{2+}
entry blockers are expected to be less effective in cardioprotection during reperfusion phase.

Role of Ca^{2+} entry blockers in myocardial ischemia-reperfusion.

Several groups explored the use of Ca^{2+} channel blockers
(e.g. verapamil, nifedipine, diltiazem) for myocardial protection during ischaemia and reperfusion (1, 2, 4, 15, 16).
It is questioned, however, if prevention of the development
of Ca^{2+} overload is their primary mechanism of protection.

Some studies suggest that Ca^{2+} entry blockers are only effective when administered prior to the induction of ischaemia (17, 18). Ca^{2+} entry into the myocardial cells is blocked during the action potential, intracellular Ca^{2+} stores will be depleted, and less Ca^{2+} released with each excitation-contraction cycle causing a negative inotropic action. The resulting reduction in the metabolic rate confers a protective effect since ATP depletes slower during the subsequent ischaemia. Other reports have shown that concentrations of diltiazem, verapamil or nifedipine which did not decrease cardiac output, afforded protection against global ischaemia in rat hearts (19). Protection by Ca^{2+} entry blockers might also be expected from enhanced blood-flow to the ischaemic region, the decrease in cardiac after-load (due to systemic vasodilation) and for some drugs from a negative chronotropic effect. However, in studies employing global ischaemia, coronary ligation of hearts without an extensive collateral circulation or animals on cardio-pulmonary bypass, these mechanisms can be excluded.

Since Ca^{2+} entry blockers exert their protective action also by reducing deregulation of the myocyte Ca^{2+} balance, one wonders what the membrane targets of the drugs are. In this context it is of interest that the anti-calmodulin drugs chlorpromazine, phenothiazines and W-7 protect myocardium against ischaemia-reperfusion damage as well (19, 20). Some Ca^{2+} entry blockers - felodipine, prenylamine and bepridil - inhibit effectively Ca^{2+} activation of the calmodulin-dependent enzymes cyclic nucleotide phosphodiesterase, myosin light chain kinase and sarcolemmal Ca^{2+} pumping ATPase (21, 22). The calmodulin subunit, required for full activation of the Ca^{2+} slow channels in heart cells, could represent the site of action of the drugs (23, 24). All these observations point toward a key role for Ca^{2+}-calmodulin-activated enzyme and Ca^{2+} transport systems in the development of ischaemia-reperfusion damage. Another hypothesis is based on the poor solubility in aqueous solution and the hydrophobicity of Ca^{2+} entry blocking and

anti-calmodulin drugs. Because of these properties they
dissolve easily into the lipidphase of the sarcolemma and
thereby maintain sarcolemmal integrity during ischaemia and
reperfusion (17).

Improved short-time recovery of regional function of
reperfused porcine heart by nifedipine.

When nifedipine (1 µg.kg^{-1}.min^{-1}) was infused just prior
(10 min) to the release of a 30 min partial obstruction (flow
reduction to 20-25% of the base line) of the left anterior
descending coronary artery (LADCA) in anaesthetized pigs,
recovery of regional function was better (75%) than in the
untreated animals   (50%, Fig. 1).

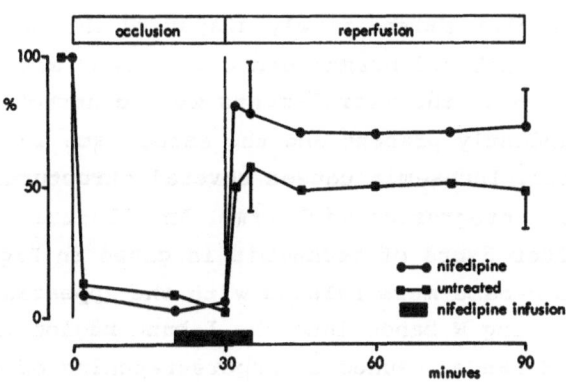

Fig. 1. Effect of administration of nifedipine before and
after release of subtotal obstruction on the recovery of
systolic wall thickening (%). Myocardial wall thickness was
monitored with an ultrasonic transducer sutured onto a part
of the epicardial surface perfused by the LADCA (26).

Since the flow in the ischaemic segment did not exceed 35%
of base line after nifedipine treatment, the lack of
improvement in function during ischaemia is not surprising,
because earlier observations in the same model showed that
when the flow is less than 40% of the base line an almost

complete loss of regional wall function results (25).
Despite this lack of effect of nifedipine during ischaemia,
an improved recovery of the systolic wall function during
the first 60 min of reperfusion was noticed (Fig. 1).
Ultrastructural changes in the ischaemic porcine heart:
effects of nifedipine treatment.

Ischaemia was induced by three successive ligations of
parts (or branches) of the LADCA at hourly intervals in the
anaesthetized pig. After 3 hrs, the heart was divided into
segments which had been ischaemic for 1, 2 and 3 hrs
(compare refs. 27 and 28). The non-ischaemic (0 h) tissue
sample was taken from a site nourished by the left circumflex coronary artery (LCXCA). Biopsies taken from the non-
ischaemic area revealed a normal ultrastructure (not
presented). The nuclei showed finely dispersed chromatin,
the mitochondria exhibited normal dense granules, matrix and
regular cristae, while the myofilaments were contracted.
Glycogen was abundantly present and the sarcolemma intact
and double-layered. Ischaemia caused several structural
alterations, which progressed with time. An illustration of
these changes after 3 hrs of ischaemia is given in Fig. 2 A.
The myofilaments became more relaxed with the appearance of
increasingly widening N bands into the I band region and
widening of the H bands, caused by superstretching of the
sarcomeres, after 2 hrs of ischaemia. At the same time
nuclear chromatin started to clump and marginate and glycogen
disappeared. In the 3 hrs ischaemic segments there was
marked intracellular edema (Fig. 2 A). The mitochondrial
matrix was more translucent, with disruption of the cristae
after 2 and 3 hrs of ischaemia. In 2 hrs ischaemic segments
electron-dense bodies appeared in many of the mitochondria.
This was more severe after 3 hrs ischaemia. The appearance
of these amorphous dense bodies has been ascribed to the
formation of insoluble proteins and lipids, with which at a
later stage of ischaemia and reperfusion, Ca^{2+} coprecipitates
(3). A number of pigs were treated with an intravenous
infusion of nifedipine with a dose (initially 0.75-1.0

$\mu g \cdot kg^{-1} \cdot min^{-1}$ and thereafter $0.2-0.5$ $\mu g \cdot kg^{-1} \cdot min^{-1}$) which lowered blood pressure by 20-25%. Infusion started 30 min before the first occlusion and lasted the entire experiment. In the nifedipine-treated animals changes were also found in mitochondria, nuclei and myofilaments but they developed more gradually in time (Fig. 2 B, see also refs. 29 and 30). In particular, the diminished occurrence of amorphous densities in the mitochondria suggests that the protective effects of nifedipine stem primarily from attenuation of excessive Ca^{2+} gain of myocardial cells (29-31).

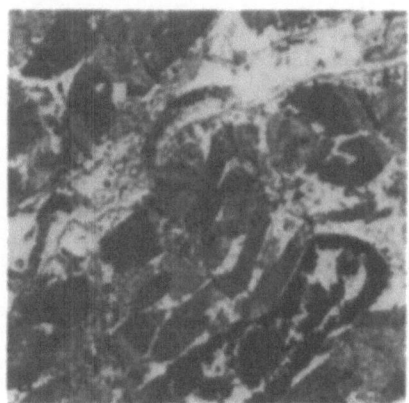 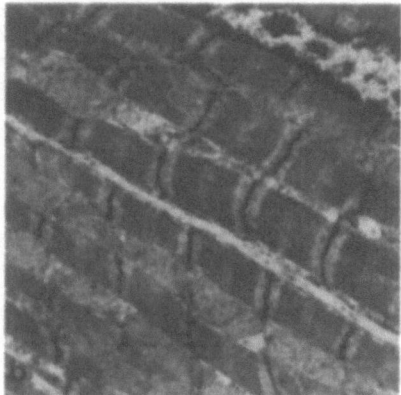

Fig. 2. Subepicardial myocardium 3 hrs after ligation of the LADCA (magnification 3000 x). Micrographs of myocardium are shown of untreated (a) and nifedipine-treated (b) animals (29, 30).

Functional integrity of sarcolemmal membranes isolated from ischaemic porcine heart: effects of nifedipine.

Biochemical functions in sarcolemmal vesicles isolated from ischaemic and non-ischaemic biopsies were also measured in the same LADCA ligation model. First, we ascertained that no significant differences in sarcolemmal protein yield (expressed as the percentage of total homogenate protein) or purification degree (expressed as the enrichment of the

sarcolemmal marker enzyme 5'-nucleotidase) existed between
any of the biopsies. Biochemical functions that were studied
in the sarcolemmal vesicles were: 1) cyclic AMP-dependent
phosphorylation of phospholamban-like protein; 2) AMPase; 3)
Na^+ gradient-induced Ca^{2+} uptake; 4) passive Ca^{2+} permeability (compare refs. 27-29). The most striking effect was the
time-dependent decrease of cyclic AMP-dependent ^{32}P
incorporation into phospholamban-like protein (Table 1).
Phosphorylated phospholamban plays a role in the second
messenger control of sarcolemmal and sarcoplasmic reticulum

Table 1.   AMPase and phosphorylation activities in sarcolemma
isolated from ischaemic myocardium.

Activity	Time (h) of ischaemia	Untreated		Nifedipine-treated	
		Contol	LADCA-ligated	Control	LADCA-ligated
P-incorp.	0	100	100	100	100
	1	101+7	61+8[a]	109	75+7[a]
	2	93+10	40+6[a]	110+14	51+3[a]
	3	104+12	32+5[a]	91+7	39+5[a]
AMPase	0	100	100	100	100
	1	98+6	86+6	89+13	105+13
	2	101+8	75+10[a]	98+12	87+10
	3	122+10	78+7[a]	90+14	114+20

The values are expressed as % ± S.E.M. of the non-ischaemic
area in the LADCA-ligated hearts or as % ± S.E.M. of the
corresponding area of non-ligated hearts. a indicates
significantly different (P < 0.05) from the % in the
corresponding biopsy from control hearts.

Ca^{2+} pumping ATPases (24, 28). The decreased in vitro
phosphorylation of the proteolipid component of the sarcolemma
from the ischaemic heart reflects a loss of functional
integrity of the sarcolemmal membrane. A detailed study of
the properties of phospholamban present in sarcolemma obtained
from ischaemic myocardium revealed, that the proteolipid is
either partially removed from the membrane or partially
degraded by Ca^{2+}-dependent protease (27, 28). Pretreatment

with nifedipine did not prevent the ischaemia-induced reduction in ^{32}P incorporation (Table 1). On the other hand, nifedipine prevented the reduction of 5'-nucleotidase activity observed in untreated animals after 2-3 hrs of ischaemia. This confirms earlier observations with nisoldipine (32) and verapamil (33). Thus, pretreatment with Ca^{2+} entry blockers protects against some sarcolemmal manifestation of ischaemic damage (29-31). The observed deficiency in phospholamban phosphorylation represents an independent factor (reduced rate of Ca^{2+} extrusion) which contributes to the production of cellular Ca^{2+} overload.

Effect of nifedipine on long-term recovery of myocardial function.

Murphy et al. demonstrated that in anaesthetized pigs no recovery of regional left ventricular function occurs during the first 2 hrs of reperfusion after 30 min and 60 min total coronary artery occlusion (34). We confirmed these observations in the same species. When, in another group of pigs, the chest was closed after 2 hrs of reperfusion, following 60 min of ischaemia, recovery of regional heart function (detected by two-dimensional echocardiography) was still absent after 14 days. However, in the animals subjected to 30 min of ischaemia, complete recovery of function had occurred (results not shown). Pretreatment with nifedipine did not affect long-term recovery in the animals subjected to 60 min of ischaemia.

Sarcolemmal integrity changes correlation with the long-term functional recovery of the heart.

^{32}P incorporation into phospholamban was measured in the sarcolemmal membranes isolated from biopsies taken after 2 hrs of reperfusion following 30 min or 60 min ischaemia. Table 2 not only shows a time-dependent reduction of in vitro ^{32}P incorporation but also the lack of any recovery during the first 2 hrs of reperfusion.

This suggests that the loss of second messenger control of the sarcolemmal Ca^{2+} pump is critical in ischaemia-reperfusion-induced Ca^{2+} overload which is related to long-

Table 2. ^{32}P incorporation into phospholamban-like protein of sarcolemma.

Duration (min) of		n^a	^{32}P incorporation (pmol.mg^{-1})	
ischemia	reperfusion		non-ligated area	ligated area
30	0	7	754+104	484+79^a
60	0	7	701∓ 69	287∓29^{b,c}
30	120	7	738∓ 76	528∓95^c
60	120	7	659∓ 68	212∓53^{b,c}

a = number of animals; b = P < 0.05 vs corresponding 30 min ligation value; c = P < 0.05 corresponding non-ligation value.

term (14 days) recovery of heart function. Pretreatment with nifedipine did not affect long-term outcome, although a short-term effect after a period of less severe ischaemia was demonstrated (Fig. 1).

Sarcolemmal destabilization and destruction correlates with long-term functional recovery of the heart.

Morphological studies have shown that clustering of sarcolemmal intramembranous particles takes place during global ischaemia of the Langendorff-perfused rabbit heart (35, 36). Applying fast-freezing techniques and thin-sectioning with lipid fixation, a disruption of the sarcolemma was observed in reperfused (90 min) ischaemic myocardium (36). This disruption was attended with the formation and extrusion of lipidic, liposomal structures. These phenomena are explained in terms of lateral phase separation of the lipids and destabilization of lipid in the sarcolemma, leading to structural blebbing-off of pure lipids (37). It is likely that both processes can be attributed to the presence of a low pH and high Ca^{2+} levels in cytosol during ischaemia and the initial phase of reperfusion. Freeze-fracturing studies confirmed this sarcolemmal breakdown, clearly showing the presence of multilamellar, particle-free particles and aggregation of intramembranous particles.

Sarcolemmal disruption was also present in hearts reperfused for 2 hrs after 60 min of LCXCA ligation (Figs. 3 and 4). These changes were, however, not observed when the LCXCA ligation lasted only 30 min. Thus some changes in

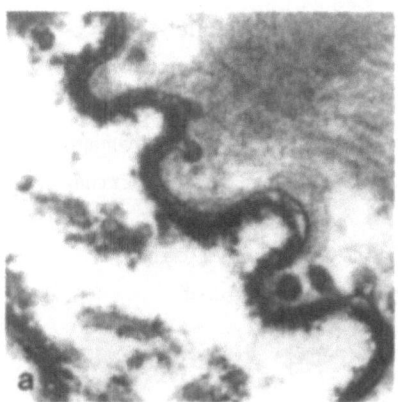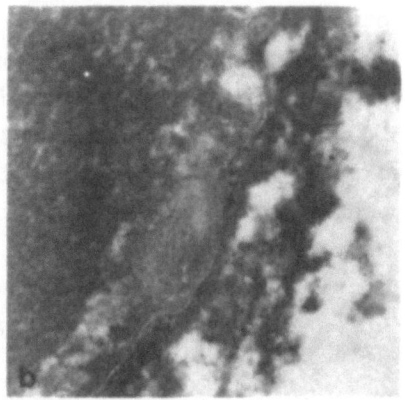

Fig. 3. Electonmicrographs of thin-sectioning of biopsies from 30 (a) or 60 min (b) occluded and 2 hrs reperfused myocardium. Magnifications: a) 61,000 x and b) 90,000 x.

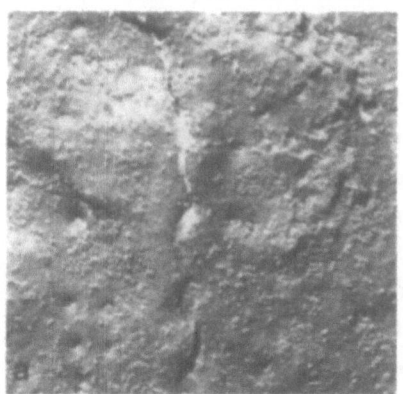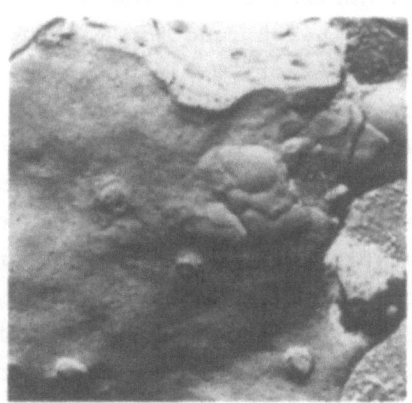

Fig. 4. Electron micrographs of freeze-fracturing of biopsies from 30 (a) or 60 min (b) occluded and 2 hrs reperfused myocardium. Magnifications: a) 65,000 x and b) 70,000 x.

sarcolemmal structure appear to correlate with long-term
recovery of regional function of the myocardium. Therefore
disruption of sarcolemma may be an indication of the transition from reversible to irreversible injury. Ca^{2+} entry
blockers and calmodulin antagonists are hydrophobic drugs
which dissolve easily into the lipidphase of the sarcolemma.
Protection against membrane destabilization may result from
drug penetration. In this context it is important that
hypothermia also protects the heart from ischaemic damage.
Hypothermia increases membrane microviscosity, which
stabilizes membrane bilayer configuration (38).

SUMMARY

Anaesthesized open-chest pigs were subjected to
different periods of ischaemia (30 min, 1, 2 or 3 hrs)
followed by either no, 2 hrs or 14 days of reperfusion.
Short (0-2 hrs)- and long (14 days)-term recovery of regional
wall thickening was estimated by echocardiography. When
infusion of the Ca^{2+} entry blocker nifedipine started 10 min
prior to release of a 30 min partial (to 25% of base-line
flow) obstruction of the LADCA, short-term recovery of
regional heart function was superior to that in untreated
animals. After 30 min of a total occlusion of the LCXCA,
recovery was absent after 2 hrs of reperfusion but complete
after 14 days. After a 60 min total LCXCA occlusion, recovery was still absent after 14 days. Pretreatment with
nifedipine did not affect this outcome. Biopsies showed
alterations in the ultrastructure, ^{32}P incorporation into
sarcolemmal phospholamban-like protein and 5'-nucleotidase
activity dependent on the duration of ischaemia (30 min, 1,
2 or 3 hrs). Nifedipine treatment prevented ultrastructural
and 5'-nucleotidase activity changes, but not the severe
reduction in phospholamban phosphorylation. The latter
process may be involved in the second messenger control of
the sarcolemmal Ca^{2+} pump, which participates in the
protection of myocardial cells against Ca^{2+} overload. The
reduced phosphorylation did not recover within 2 hrs of

reperfusion. Other signs of loss of sarcolemmal integrity were noticed by thin-sectioning and freeze-fracturing electron microscopy. After 60 min, but not after 30 min of ischaemia, clustering of intramembranous particles and membrane-blebbing were present during reperfusion. It is concluded that loss of sarcolemmal integrity correlates with long-term recovery of regional heart function. Cardioprotection by nifedipine was visible, when recovery was measured shortly (0-2 hrs) after partial occluson of the LADCA. Effects of the drug on long-term recovery may only become detectable when a partial restoration of regional heart function occurs.

ACKNOWLEDGEMENTS

The authors wish to thank Prof. Dr. W.C. Hülsmann for his critical reading of the manuscript and Miss A.C. Hanson and Miss M.I. Wieriks for aiding in the preparation of the final draft. This work was carried out with the aid of a Dutch Heart Foundation grant to Drs. J.A. Post.

REFERENCES

1. Fleckenstein, A. Circ. Res. 52. suppl. 1: 3-16, 1983.
2. Henry, P.D. Am. J. Cardiol. 46: 1047-1058, 1980.
3. Jennings, R.B. and Reimer, K.A. Am. J. Pathol. 102: 241-255, 1981.
4. Katz, A.M. Am. J. Cardiol. 44: 188-190, 1979.
5. Grinwald, P.M. and Nayler, W.G. J. Mol. Cell. Cardiol. 13: 867-880, 1981.
6. Rona, G. J. Mol. Cell. Cardiol. 17: 291-306, 1985.
7. Dhalla, N.S., Das, P.K. and Sharma, G.P. J. Mol. Cell. Cardiol. 10: 363-385, 1978.
8. Katz, A.M. and Messineo, F.C. Circ. Res. 48: 1-16, 1981.
9. Lamers, J.M.J., Stinis, J.T., Montfoort, A. and Hülsmann, W.C. Biochim. Biophys. Acta 774: 127-131, 1984.
10. Hearse, D.J. J. Mol. Cell. Cardiol. 9: 605-616, 1977
11. Schader, J. Bas. Res. Cardiol. 80, suppl. 2: 135-139, 1985.
12. Carmeliet, E. Circ. 70: 149-151, 1984.
13. Kako, K.J. Can. J. Cardiol. 2: 184-194, 1986.
14. Steenbergen, C., Hill, M.L. and Jennings, R.B. Circ. Res. 57: 864-875, 1985.
15. Weishaar, R.E. and Bing, R.J. J. Mol. Cell. Cardiol. 12: 993-1009, 1980.
16. Nayler, W.G., Ferrari, R., Williams, A. Am. J. Cardiol. 46: 242-248, 1980.
17. Drake-Holland, A.J. and Noble, M.I.M. Eur. Heart J. 4: 823-825, 1983.
18. Hugenholtz, P.G., Serruys, P.W., Fleckenstein, A. and Nayler, W.G. Eur. Heart J. 7: 270-278, 1986.

19. Higgins, A.J. and Blackburn, K.J. J. Mol. Cell. Cardiol. 16: 427-438, 1984.
20. Chien, K.R., Pfau, R.G. and Farber, J.L. Am. J. Pathol. 97: 505-530, 1979.
21. Shikano, K., Kusagawa, M., Itoh, H. and Hidaka, H. Cardiovasc. Res. 20: 364-368, 1986.
22. Lamers, J.M.J., Cysouw, K.J. and Verdouw, P.D. Biochem. Pharmacol. 34: 3837-3843, 1985.
23. Bkaily, G., Sperelakis, N. J. Cycl. Nucleot. Res. 11: 25-34, 1986.
24. Lamers, J.M.J. Gen. Physiol. Biophys. 4: 143-154, 1985.
25. Verdouw, P.D., Ten Cate, F.J. Schamhardt, H.C., Van der Hoek, T.M., Bastiaans, D.L. In: Quantification of Myocardial Ischemia (Eds. H. Kreuzer, W.W. Parmley, P. Rentrop and H.W. Heiss), Gerhard Witzstrock, New York, 1980, pp. 270-284.
26. Verdouw, P.D. Wolffenbuttel, B.H.R. and Ten Cate, F.J. Eur. Heart J. 4 suppl. C: 101-108, 1983.
27. Lamers, J.M.J., Stinis, J.T., Verdouw, P.D. and Hülsmann, W.C. In: Pathogenesis of Stress-induced Heart Disease (Eds. N.S. Dhalla, V. Panagia and R.E. Beamish) Martinus Nijhoff Publishing, Boston, 1985, pp. 132-146.
28. Lamers, J.M.J., De Jonge-Stinis, J.T., Hülsmann, W.C. and Verdouw, P.D. J. Mol. Cell. Cardiol. 18: 115-125, 1986.
29. Lamers, J.M.J., Essed, C.E., Pourquie, M.E.M., Hugenholtz, P.G. and Verdouw, P.D. Can. J. Cardiol., in press.
30. Verdouw, P.D., Essed, C.E., Hugenholtz, P.G., Lamers, J.M.J. In: Unstable angina. Current Concepts and Management (Eds. P.G. Hugenholtz and B.S. Goldman), Schattauer, New York, 1985, pp. 177-186.
31. Verdouw, P.D. and Lamers, J.M.J. In: Bepridil. A New Approach in the Management of Angina (Eds. P.A. van Zwieten, M. Kaltenbach, E. Schönbaum) Organon Int. B.V., Oss, 1986, pp. 17-31.
32. Takahashi, K. and Kako, K.J. Basic Res. Cardiol. 78: 326-337, 1983.
33. Daly, M.N., Elz, J.S. and Nayler, W.G. J. Mol. Cell. Cardiol. 17: 667-674, 1985.
34. Murphy, M.L., Peng, C.F., Kane, J.J. and Stranto, K.D. Am. J. Pathol. 50: 821-828, 1982.
35. Ashraf, M., Halverson, G.A. Am. J. Pathol. 88: 583-587, 1977.
36. Post, J.A., Leunissen-Bijvelt, J., Ruigrok, T.J.C. and Verkleij, A.J. Biochim. Biophys. Acta 845: 119-123, 1985.
37. Cullis, P.R., De Kruijff, B., Hope, M.J., Verkleij, A.J., Nayar, R., Farren, S.B., Tilcock, C., Madden, T.D. and Bally, M.B. In: Membrane Fluidity in Biology (Ed. R.C. Aloia), Acad. Press, New York, 1983, 1 pp. 39-81.
38. Fukunami, M. and Hearse, D.M. Cardiovasc. Res. 19: 95-103, 1985.

26

EFFECT OF NIFEDIPINE AND HYALURONIDASE ALONE AND IN COMBINATION ON
MYOCARDIAL PRESERVATION IN EXPERIMENTAL MYOCARDIAL INFARCTION - A
MORPHOLOGICAL AND BIOCHEMICAL PROFILE

M.P. GUPTA, S.D. SETH, S.C. MANCHANDA* AND UMA SINGH

Departments of Pharmacology and Cardiology*,
All-India Institute of Medical Sciences, New Delhi - 110 029, India.

INTRODUCTION

The extent of myocardial necrosis subsequent to coronary artery
occlusion is of utmost significance, because the patient's survival
depends largely on the extent of damage and the reversibility of
ischemic tissue. Though various pharmacological interventions have
been found to have some salutory effects on the ischemic myocardium,
nevertheless, no drug administered singly has been shown to be
totally effective in preventing further damage or to retrieve the
ischemic tissue. Hence the combinations of various cardioprotective
drugs, eg; calcium channel blockers, beta-blockers, nitroglycerine
etc. are being investigated for their synergistic effects (1-6).

Over the last two decades, it has been demonstrated that calcium
channel blockers protect ischemic myocardium. The protection is afforded
by preservation of mechanical function, tissue stores of ATP and mitochondrial function. Nifedipine (NFD) a potent anti-anginal agent is a
slow-channel blocker which increases myocardial oxygen supply by coronary
vasodilation and decreases myocardial oxygen demand by decreasing after
load. Unlike other vasodilator drugs, however, NFD also exerts a direct
negative inotropic effect on the myocardium consistent with its property
of selective inhibition of transmembrane flux of calcium in cardiac
muscle cells (7).

Hyaluronidase (HYL), a mucolytic enzyme which depolymerizes and
hydrolyzes hyaluronic acid has been employed to protect jeopardized
ischemic myocardium in clinical setting (8,9). HYL has been shown to
reduce ultimate infarct size in a number of experimental studies (10-15).
HYL increases substrate transport through the extravascular space by
depolymerizing mucopolysaccharides in the cardiac interstitium and
augmenting the cellular supply of glucose and other nutrients (16).

The present study was designed to investigate the efficacy of NFD and HYL administered alone and in combination on morphological and biochemical parameters in experimental myocardial infarction.

MATERIALS AND METHODS

Experimental protocol.

Twenty four adult healthy dogs of either sex, weighing 14-18 kg, kept under controlled conditions were anesthetised with sodium pentobarbitone (30 mg/kg i.v.). Dogs were intubated with a cuffed endotracheal tube and respiration was maintained by positive pressure ventilation with room air by INCO (India) volume respirator. A left lateral thoracotomy was performed through the fifth intercostal space. The pericardium was incised and the exposed heart was retained securely in a pericardial cradle. Immediately distal to the first large diagonal branch, the left anterior descending (LAD) coronary artery was isolated from the surrounding tissue and ligated in two stages according to the method of Harris(17).

The animals were divided into the following groups of six animals each :

Group I.   Control group

Group II. NFD treated group (10 μg/kg NFD i.v.).

Group III. HYL treated group (500 NF units HYL/kg i.v.).

Group IV. NFD + HYL treated group. (10 μg/kg NFD + 500 NF units/ kg HYL, i.v.).

Drugs were administered 20 min after coronary occlusion and the animals were killed 24 hours after occlusion. In the control group normal saline was infused intravenously (i.v.) equal to the volume of the drug infused, with a similar protocol.

Infarct size studies.

Ten minutes before the animals were killed, monastral blue dye (0.5 ml/kg was infused into the left atrium to delineate the in vivo area at risk (Ar). In vivo punch biopsies were taken rapidly from the three different zones of myocardium, the normal perfused zone (P), the ischemic zone (I) and the necrotic zone (N) after induction of ventricular fibrillation or standstill with an overdose of barbiturate. Thereafter, the heart was excised rapidly, the left ventricle was separated and 'bread-loafed' into 5 mm thick slices. The blue - stained normal perfused portion was separated from the unstained portion depicting the area at risk including area of necrosis (An) and weighed. To differentiate the infarcted tissue, both the portions, stained as well as unstained were incubated separately in buffered (1%) triphenyl tetrazolium chloride (TTC) solution for 20 min at 37°C. This differential staining method (18) discriminated necrotic area (pale yellow or white) from the normal perfused and reversibly injured tissue (viable tissue staining brick red) (19). Different regions of the myocardium are expressed in terms of per cent of left ventricular mass (LV mass) and the area at risk. Per cent reduction of Ar destined to necrosis was calculated as follows:

$$\left[1- \left(\frac{\text{An treated}}{\text{Ar treated}} \div \frac{\text{An control}}{\text{Ar control}} \right) \right] \times 100$$

Biochemical studies.

Tissue samples taken from clear-cut zones only were processed for biochemical investigations. Weight of these tissue samples was added to the weight of the respective zones of the ventricular mass.

Lactate was estimated by the method of Gutamann and Wahlefeld (20). Tissue samples for lactate estimation were immersed in pre-cooled perchloric acid (6%) and frozen immediately (in less than 10 seconds) in liquid nitrogen. Glycogen was estimated by the phenol-sulphuric acid method of Siulo et al (21). Samples of myocardial tissue were immediately immersed in hot 30% potassium hydroxide solution. For estimation of myocardial enzymes tissue samples taken from different zones of the ventricular myocardium were chilled on ice, weighed, minced with scissors and homogenized in 25 vol/g of 250 mM sucrose, 50 mM tris HCL, 4 mM neutralized ethylene diamine tetraacetic acid (EDTA), 30 mM potassium fluoride and 50 mM mercaptoethanol (pH 7.5) in polytron homogenizer for one minute. The homogenate was then centrifuged at 18,000 G for 10 min at 4°C. The supernatant was separated and centrifuged again at the same speed for 10 min. All procedures were carried out at 6-8°C in the cold room. The supernatant fluid of this homogenate was referred to as the fresh heart extract and used for the estimation of different myocardial enzymes. Phosphofructokinase (PFK) was estimated according to the method of Mansour (22), creatine phosphokinase (CPK) by the method of Foster et al (23) and lactate dehydrogenase (LDH) by the method of Bergmeyer and Bernt (24). The total amount of proteins were estimated in the supernatant fluid of the homogenate obtained for estimation of myocardial enzymes, by the method of Lowry et al (25). The estimation of the myo-cardial metabolites and enzymes was monitored in spectrophotometer (Spectroplus).

Statistical analysis.

Statistical analyses were performed using Student's t test or one way analysis of variance and the values are given herein. All data are expressed as means ± standard deviation (SD).

RESULTS

Infarct size studies.

Occlusion of the LAD coronary artery resulted in 33.79 ± 8.96% of left ventricular (LV) mass becoming ischemic area at risk (Ar) in the

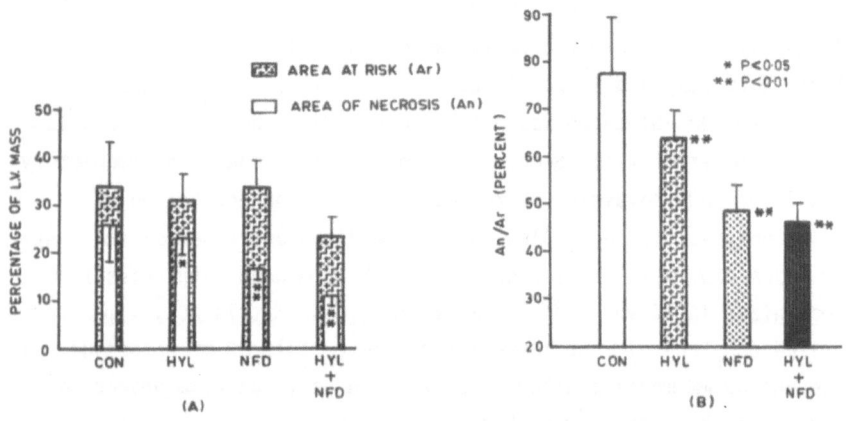

Fig. 1. (A) Area of necrosis (An) and viable tissue within area at risk (Ar) expressed as percentage of left ventricular mass (mean ± SD). In the drug-treated groups, infarct size (An) is significantly smaller as compared to control. (B) Comparison of the per cent of area of risk that evolved to infarction in the four experimental groups. Columns with bar represent mean ± SD. CON- control, HYL- hyaluronidase and NFD- nifedi-pine treated groups.

control animals. Ar per cent of LV mass was comparable in the NFD (33.72 ± 5.05) and HYL (30.91 ± 5.43) treated animals, but was significantly (P< 0.05) less in NFD + HYL (23.84 ± 4.12) treated group as compared to controls (Fig. 1 A). Area of necrosis (An) in control group was 77.43 ± 11.99% of Ar, whereas it was significantly (P< 0.01) reduced to 48.63 ± 5.11% of Ar in NFD, 64.16 ± 5.78% of Ar, in HYL and 45.76 ± 3.72% of Ar in NFD + HYL treated groups (Fig. 1 B).

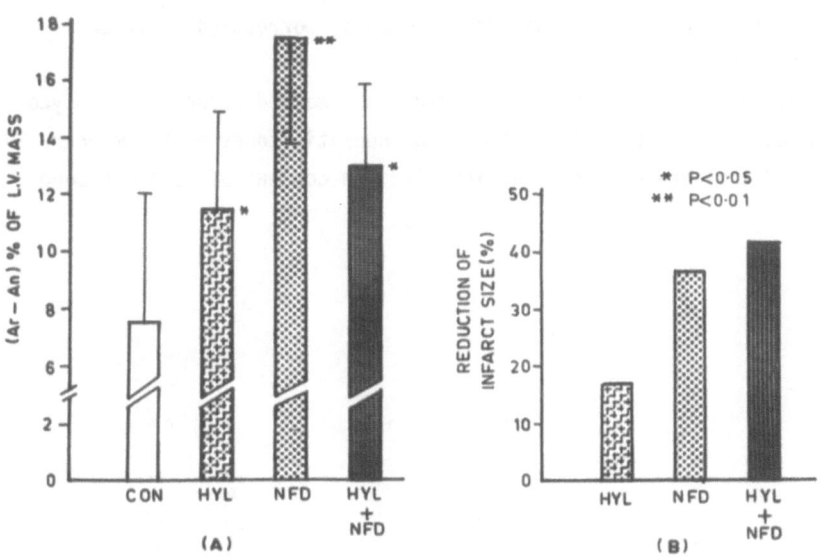

Fig. 2. (A) Comparison of the viable tissue (Ar-An) within the area at risk expressed as per cent of left ventricular mass in four experiment- al groups. Columns with bar represent mean ± SD. (B) Per cent reduction of area at risk destined to necrosis. CON- control, HYL- hyaluronidase and NFD - nifedipine treated groups.

The viable tissue expressed as per cent of LV mass was significantly (P< 0.01) increased only in NFD alone treated group (17.43 ± 3.70) as compared to the control group (7.43 ± 4.45). It was, however, comparable in HYL (11.56 ± 3.39) and NFD + HYL (13.01 ± 2.76) treated groups (Fig. 2 A). Viable tissue was 22.56 ± 11.99% of Ar in control group and

increased significantly (P< 0.01) in NFD (51.36 ± 5.11% of Ar), HYL
(35.83 ± 5.78% of Ar) and NFD + HYL (54.23 ± 3.72% of Ar) treated
groups. In HYL treated group, viable tissue within the area at risk
was mostly located in the subepicardial regions. These results demonstrate substantial per cent reduction of Ar destined to necrosis by the
different drug treatments viz. 36.36% with NFD, 16.88% with HYL and
41.53% with NFD + HYL (Fig. 2 B).

Biochemical Studies.

    Various anomalies in the biochemical parameters were manifested in
the different zones of the myocardium following coronary occlusion in
the control group. In the drug-treated groups, correction of these
anomalies was observed.

    Glycogen. Following coronary occlusion a marked reduction of glyco-
gen content was observed in ischemic and necrotic zones of the myocardium in control group (Fig. 3 A).The glycogen content of ischemic zone

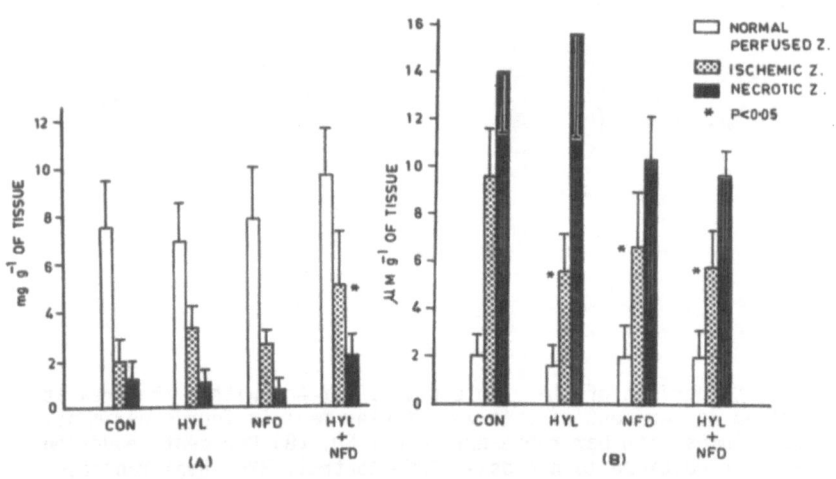

Fig. 3. Myocardial metabolite, glycogen (A) and lactate (B) concentrations in the different zones of myocardium in the four experimental
groups. Columns with bar represent mean ± SD. For statistical analysis
different zones of myocardium of drug-treated groups are compared with
the respective zone of the control animals. CON- control, HYL- hyaluronidase and NFD- nifedipine treated groups. Z - zone.

was less depressed and appreciably higher in NFD (37%) and HYL (74%) and significantly (P< 0.05) higher in NFD + HYL (168%) treated animals, than the same zone of the control animals.

Lactate. Coronary occlusion manifested a manyfold increase in the lactate content of ischemic and necrotic zones of the myocardium in the control animals. The lactate content of ischemic zone was significantly (P< 0.05) lower in drug treated animals (NFD 31%, HYL 40% and NFD + HYL 40%) than the same zone of control animals. Among the different groups, the lactate accumulation in necrotic zone was significantly (P< 0.05) reduced in NFD and NFD + HYL treated groups, when compared with HYL treated group (Fig. 3 B).

Phosphofructokinase (PFK). The activity of PFK enzyme under the influence of HYL rose significantly (P< 0.05) in normal perfused (81%)

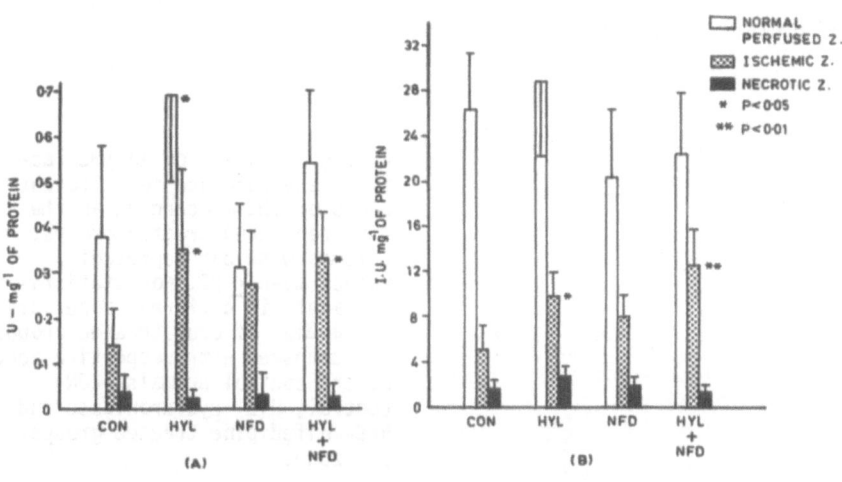

Fig. 4. Activity of the enzymes phosphofructokinase (A) and creatine phosphokinase (B) in different zones of the myocardium in the four experimental groups. Columns with the bar represent values mean ± SD. For statistical analysis different zones of myocardium of drug-treated groups are compared with the respective zone of the control animals. CON- control, HYL- hyaluronidase and NFD- nifedipine treated groups. Z - zone.

and ischemic (150%) zones of the myocardium when compared to controls. This rise of PFK activity was more apparent in NFD + HYL treated animals (Fig. 4 A). Activity of PFK in the necrotic zone of the myocardium of the four experimental groups was not significantly different from each other.

Creatine phosphokinase (CPK). No difference was observed in the CPK enzyme activity of the normal zones of the myocardium in different groups. However, in individual groups, it was moderately reduced in ischemic zone (P< 0.01) and greatly diminished in necrotic zone (P< 0.005) thus picturising the situation of a massive central infarct. CPK activity of ischemic zone in the intervention groups was significantly higher in HYL (P< 0.05) and NFD + HYL (P< 0.01) treated animals, than the control group (Fig. 4 B). On the other hand, no significant change was observed in NFD treated group. A linear relationship was found between the CPK activity of ischemic myocardium and the area at risk that evolved to infarction (An/Ar). It, therefore, suggests that viable tissue within the area at risk is closely related to the CPK activity, expressed per mg of protein of that particular zone.

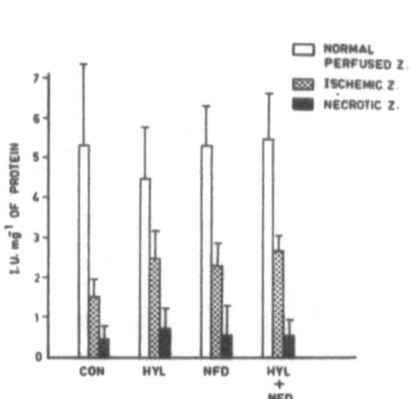

Fig. 5. Activity of enzyme lactate dehydrogenase in different zones of the myocardium in the different drug-treated groups. Columns with bar represent values mean + SD. For statistical analysis different zones of myocardium of drug-treated groups are compared with respective zone of the control animals. CON- control, HYL- hyaluronidase and NFD- nifedipine treated groups. Z - zone.

Lactate dehydrogenase (LDH). In the respective groups, LDH enzyme activity in ischemic and necrotic zones was depressed moderately as compared to the normal myocardium, whereas in ischemic zones of

different groups, LDH activity receded to less depressed in HYL (56%) and
NFD (53%) and rose moderately in NFD + HYL (80%) treated groups, when
compared with the same zone of controls (Fig. 5).

DISCUSSION

Coronary artery occlusion results in myocardial ischemia and the
preferential metabolic substrate free fatty acid in normoxic myocardium
shifts to glucose metabolism to meet the energy demands of the ischemic
myocardium (26). Prolongation of coronary occlusion beyond 20 min duration in anesthetised dogs is associated with evolution of myocardial
infarction evidenced by the development of tissue necrosis (27).

Data available from the present study demonstrates that NFD can
improve indices of myocardial ischemia by causing diminished breakdown
of glucose, enhancing glycolysis through PFK and decreasing tissue
levels of lactate which would in turn reduce acidosis. Furthermore, NFD
effectively increased the activity of enzyme PFK alongwith restoration
of the normal activity of myocardial CPK and LDH. This membrane stabili-
zing activity of NFD is of particular interest as it protects myocardial
structural integrity, restores partially damaged cells to full metabolic
function and prevents further tissue damage (28-30). NFD has been found
to lessen the effects of ischemia in several ways causing increased
coronary circulation (31), decreased myocardial oxygen requirements (32)
and suppressed Ca^{2+} overload of the myocardial cell (33-35).

The beneficial effects of NFD were found to be more pronounced when
combined with HYL. Several mechanisms may contribute to explain this
synergistic effect. HYL has been shown to salvage ischemic myocardium
effectively in experimental models (9-14) as well as in clinical setting
(7,8). In the present study the percentage of the area at risk that
evolved to infarction was markedly reduced in combination therapy group
of NFD + HYL treated animals in comparison to the NFD and HYL alone
treated groups. HYL in combination with NFD was effective enough to
increase significantly (P< 0.05) the glycogen content and decrease the
lactate content of the ischemic zone. In the present study an unexpected
rise of PFK enzyme activity was observed with HYL administration in the
normal perfused zone. Since PFK is a rate limiting step of the glycolytic
pathway, acceleration of this step accounts for faster rates of glycolysis, in the oxygen limited myocardium (36) facilitating improved ATP

synthesis, which is a major determinant of cellular survival and recovery
of jeopardized myocardium (37). In this regard our findings support the
earlier work (38,39) that the reduction of lactate accumulation (inhibitor of PFK) with HYL treatment is associated with higher levels of
energy rich phosphates (activitor of PFK). In the present study suppressed depletion of specific cardiac enzymes CPK and LDH was observed.
Reduced loss of myocardial creatine kinase by the administration of HYL
after coronary occlusion has been reported earlier (40). HYL functions
through its ability to depolymerize hyaluronic acid (41), to increase
capillary permeability (42), and thereby increased transport of energy
producing substrates from the blood stream through the interstitium to
the myocardial cells, referred to as the 'spreading factor'. Recent
studies (43) demonstrate diffusion of HYL into the centre of the distribution area of the occluded artery. This action would be important in
enhancing the delivery of substrates and increasing washout of harmful
metabolites such as lactate, through extravascular pathways. This may
also facilitate increased glucose entry into the myocardial cells (9)
also seen in the present study. HYL improves collateral flow (16) more
effectively in the outerwall (44). This may be the explanation for the
subepicardial preservation of myocardium under the influence of HYL
observed in the present study.

Apart from salvage of injured tissue, the meticulous correction of
the biochemical anomalies by the combination therapy renders it more
efficacious, offering advantage over the single drug therapy to achieve
a better prognosis in acute myocardial infarction.

SUMMARY

Intravenous administration of nifedipine (NFD) singly and in
combination with hyaluronidase (HYL) markedly reduced the myocardial
area of necrosis (An) from $77.43 \pm 11.99\%$ to $48.63 \pm 5.11\%$ (NFD) and
$45.76 \pm 3.72\%$ (NFD + HYL) of area at risk (Ar) in LAD coronary artery
ligated dogs. There was, however, less significant effect of HYL
administered singly on the infarct size with a reduction of $64.16 \pm$
5.78% of Ar. Combination therapy improved the glycogen content of
ischemic zone of the myocardium. The lactate level of the ischemic zone
was significantly decreased by the above mentioned drugs. HYL enhanced
the activity of enzyme phosphofructokinase (PFK) at least by two folds.

This rise in PFK activity also resulted with administration of NFD +
HYL. Creatine phosphokinase and lactate dehydrogenase activity
shifted towards normal with these pharmacological interventions. These
findings indicate that NFD and HYL administered singly and in combination
were effective enough to reduce infarct size and correct the biochemical
abnormalities resulting from ischemic insult of the myocardium. Combination therapy was, however, found more effective.

ACKNOWLEDGEMENTS

This work was financially supported by the Department of Science and
Technology, Government of India, New Delhi. The authors gratefully
acknowledge the gift of nifedipine from Bayer AG Leverkusen, Germany.

REFERENCES

1. Hammermeister, K.E., DeRouen, T.A. and Dodge, H.T. Circulation.59:
   421 - 429, 1979.
2. Saini, R.K., Fulmor, I.E. and Antonaccio, M.J. J.Cardiovasc.
   Pharmacol. 4 : 770 - 776, 1982.
3. Johnston, D.L., Lesoway, R., Humen, D.P. and Kostuk, W.J. Am. J.
   Cardiol 55 : 680 - 687, 1985.
4. Schanzenbacher P, Gottfert G, Lieubau G and Kochsie K.K. Am. J.
   Cardiol.55 : 33 - 36, 1985.
5. White, H.D., Polak, J.F., Wynne, J., Holman, B.L., Antman, E.M.
   and Nesto, R.W. Am. J. Cardiol. 55 : 1303 - 1307, 1985.
6. Fleckenstein, A. Annu. Rev. Pharmacol. Toxicol. 17 : 149 - 166,
   1977.
7. Maroko, P.R., Davidson, D.M., Libby, P., Hagen, A.D. and Braunwald,
   E. Ann. Intern. Med. 82 : 516 - 520, 1975.
8. Maroko, P.R., Hillis, L.D., Muller, J.E., Tarazzi, L., Heyndrick,
   G.R., Ray, M., Chiariello, M., Distante, A., Askenazi, T., Salerno,
   J., Carpentier, J., Reshetinaya, N.I., Radvani, P., Libby, P.,
   Raabe, D.S., Chazov, E.I., Bobba, P. and Braunwald, E. New Eng.
   J. Med. 296 : 898 - 903, 1977.
9. Kloner, R.A., Fishbein, M.C., maclean, D., Braunwald, E and Maroko,
   P.R. Am. J. Cardiol. 40 : 43 - 49, 1977.
10. Maclean, D., Fishbein, M.C., Maroko, P.R. and Braunwald E. Science.
    194 : 199 - 200, 1976.
11. Hillis, L.D., Fishbein, M.C., Braunwald, E and Maroko, P.R. Circ.
    Res. 41 : 26 - 31, 1977.
12. Wetstein, L., Simson, M.B., Haselgrove, J., Barlow, C.H. and
    Harken, A.H. Am. Heart. J. 104 : 529 - 536, 1982.
13. Nilsson, J.E., Sjogren, C and Sawe, U. Acta. Med. Scand. 216 :
    209 - 213, 1984.
14. Seth, S.D., Gupta, M.P., Gupta, M., Manchanda, S.C. and Srivastava,
    L.M. Ind. J. Pharmacol. 15 : 22 (abstr), 1983.
15. Maroko, P.R., Libby, P., Bloor, C.M., Sobel, B.E. and Braunwald, E.
    Circulation. 46 : 430 - 437, 1972.
16. Askenazi, J., Hillis, L.D., Diaz, P.E., Davis, M.A., Braunwald, E.

and Maroko, P.R. Circ. Res. <u>40</u> : 566 - 571, 1977.

17. Harris, A.S. Circulation. <u>1</u> : 1318 - 1328, 1950.
18. Darsee, J.R., Kloner, R.A. and Braunwald E. Circulation. <u>63</u> : 29 - 35, 1981.
19. Kloner, R.A., Darsee, J.R., DeBoer, L.W.V and Carlson, N. Arch. Path. Lab. Med. <u>105</u> : 403 - 406, 1981.
20. Gutamann, I and Wahlefeld, A.W. In : Methods of Enzymatic Analysis, (Ed. H.U. Bergmeyer) Verlag Chemie Weinheim, Academic Press Inc New York, San Francisco, London, 1974, Vol. 3, pp 1464 - 1468.
21. Siulo, Russel, J.C. and Taylor, A.W. J. Appl. Physiol. <u>28</u> : 234 - 236, 1970.
22. Mansour, T.E. In : Methods in Enzymology (Ed W.A. Wood) Academic Press New York, London, 1966, Vol. IX pp 430 - 436.
23. Foster, G., Brent, E. and Bergmeyer, U. In : Methods of Enzymatic Analysis. (Ed. H.U. Bergmeyer) Verlag Chemie Weinheim, Academic Press Inc. New York, San Francisco, London 1974, Vol. 2. pp 789 - 793.
24. Bergmeyer, H.U. and Bernt, E. In : Methods of Enzymatic analysis (Ed. H.U. Bergmeyer) Verlag Chemie Weinheim, Academic Press Inc. New York, San Francisco, London, 1974 Vol. 2, pp 574 - 579.
25. Lowry, O.H., Rosebrough, N.J. Farr, A.L. and Randall, R.J. J. Biol. Chem. <u>193</u> : 265 - 272, 1951.
26. Opie, L.H. Circ. Res. <u>38</u> : 1 - 52, 1976.
27. Reimex, K.A., Lowe, J.E., Rasmussen, M.M., and Jennings, R.B. Circulation. <u>56</u> : 786 - 794, 1977.
28. Seth, S.D., Ganguly, P.K., Srivastava, L.M. and Gupta, M.P. J. Mol. Cell. Cardiol. (Suppl) <u>12</u> : 149, 1980c.
29. Ganguly, P.K., Srivastava, L.M., Bora, P.S., Gupta, M.P. and Seth, S.D. Ind. J. Med. Res. <u>73</u> : 617 - 624, 1981.
30. Fleckenstein, A., Frey, M and von Witzleben, H. In : Proceedings of the 5th International Adalat Symposium (Eds. M. Kaltenbach and H.N. Neufeld) Excerpta Medica Amsterdam, Oxford, Princeton 1983 pp 36 -52.
31. Selwyn, A.P., Welman, E., Fox, K., Horlock, P. Pratt, T and Klein, M. Circ. Res. <u>44</u> : 16 - 23, 1979.
32. Vater, W., Kronberg, G., Hoffmeister, F., Kaller, H., Meng, K., Oberdorf, A., Puls, W., Schlossmann, K. and Stoepel, K. Arzneim - Forch. <u>22</u> : 1 - 14, 1972.
33. Clark, R.K., Christlieb, I.Y., Henry, P.D., Fischer, A.E., Nora, J.D., Williamson, J.R. and Sobel, B.E. Am. J. Cardiol. <u>44</u> : 825 - 831, 1979.
34. Fleckenstein, A. In : Proceedings of 3rd International Adalat Symposium (Eds. A.D. Jatene and P.R. Lichtlen) Excerpta Medica, Amsterdam, Oxford, 1976, pp 1 - 13.
35. Nayler, W.G., Ferrari, R. and Williams, A. Am. J. Cardiol <u>46</u> : 242 - 248, 1980.
36. Weishaar, R., Ashikawa, K. and Bing, R.J. Am. J. Cardiol. <u>43</u> : 1137 - 1143, 1979.
37. Hearse, D.J. and Chain, E.D. Biochem. J. <u>128</u> : 1125 - 1133, 1972.
38. Rovetto, M.J. Circ. Res. <u>41</u> : 373 - 379, 1977.
39. Seth, S.D., Gupta, M.P., Manchanda, S.C. and Srivastava, L.M. IUPHAR Int. Cong. Pharmacol. London p.51, 1984.
40. Ribeiro, L.G.T., Hillis, L.D., Lousie, E.K., Davis, M.A. Maroko, P.R. and Braunwald, E. Cardiovasc. Res. <u>12</u> : 334 - 340, 1978.
41. Meyer, K. Physiol. Rev. <u>27</u> : 335 - 359, 1947.

42. Szabo, G. and Magyar, S. Nature. 182 : 377 - 379, 1958.
43. Wolf, R.A., Chaung, L.H., Muller, J.E., Kloner, R.A. and Braunwald
    E. Circ. Res. 471 : 485 - 506, 1979.
44. Kloner, R.A., Braunwald, E. and Maroko, P.R., Circulation 58 :
    220 - 226, 1978.

27

ACTION OF CALCIUM ANTAGONISTS ON THE CONTRACTION OF ISOLATED
HUMAN CORONARY ARTERIES AND MYOCARDIUM

T. GODFRAIND

Laboratoire de Pharmacodynamie Générale et de Pharmacologie,
Université Catholique de Louvain, UCL 7350, avenue Emmanuel
Mounier 73, 1200 Bruxelles, Belgique.

INTRODUCTION

The concept of calcium antagonism has been pioneered
in Europe in the nineteen sixties in two different and
independent experimental approaches, one by Godfraind et al.
on vascular smooth muscles (1,2,3) the other by Fleckenstein
et al. (4) on cardiac muscle.

In the 1960s, Godfraind et al. analyzed the
pharmacological action of some drugs acting as polyvalent
antagonists on vascular smooth muscle, such drugs have the
property to inhibit, at the same concentration, the
vasoconstriction evoked by various agents including
norepinephrine, angiotensin, vasopressin and some other
spasmogens. Among those drugs were the diphenylpiperazines
cinnarizine and lidoflazine. Cinnarizine was used at that
time and still now as an anti-motion-sickness and
antiallergic drug and lidoflazine was used as an antianginal
drug. Because the active concentrations of each respective
antagonist were similar for the various agonists studied,
Godfraind et al. proposed that cinnarizine and lidoflazine
interfered with a common mechanism activated by various
agents to produce the smooth muscle contraction. A
hypothesis was that calcium entry was this common mechanism.

Godfraind and Polster (3) showed that the inhibitory
effect of cinnarizine, lidoflazine and chlorpromazine on the
contraction of several arteries, including pig coronary
arteries and human pulmonary arteries, evoked by KCl-rich
solutions, could be reversed by increasing the concentration

Table 1. Calcium Modulators

AGENTS AFFECTING Ca^{2+} MOVEMENTS (calcium antagonists and calcium agonists)

A. INHIBITORS: CALCIUM ANTAGONISTS
=================================

1. Agents acting at the plasma membrane

1.A Calcium entry blockers

    Group I : Specific calcium entry blockers

        Group I.A : Agents selective for slow calcium channels in myocardium (slow channel blockers)
          Phenylalkylamines : verapamil, gallopamil (D600); under investigation : anipamil, desmethoxyverapamil (D888), emopamil, falipamil (AQ-A-39), ronipamil
          Dihydropyridines : nifedipine, nicardipine, niludipine, nimodipine, nisoldipine, nitrendipine, ryosidine; under investigation : amlodipine, azodipine, dazodipine (PY 108-068), felodipine, flordipine, FR 34235, iodipine, isrodipine, mesudipine, ni(l)vadipine, oxodipine, PN 200-110, riodipine
          Benzothiazepines : diltiazem; under investigation : fostedil (KB-944)

        Group I.B : Agents inactive on slow calcium channels in myocardium
          Diphenylpiperazines : cinnarizine and flunarizine

    Group II : Non-specific calcium entry blockers

        Group II.A : Agents acting at similar concentrations on calcium channels and fast sodium channels
          Bencyclane, bepridil, caroverine, etafenone, fendiline, lidoflazine, perhexiline, prenylamine, SKF 525A, terodiline, tiapamil

        Group II.B : Agents interacting with calcium channels while having another primary site of action
          They include, among others : agents acting on sodium channels (local anesthetics, phenytoin); on catecholamine receptors (benextramine, nicergoline, phenoxybenzamine, phenothiazines, pimozide, propranolol, WB-4101, yohimbine derivatives); on benzodiazepine receptors (diazepam, flurazepam); on opiate receptors (loperamide, fluperamide); on cyclic nucleotide phosphodiesterases (amrinone, cromoglycate, papaverine); barbiturates; cyproheptadine; indomethacin; reserpine.

1.B <u>Sodium-calcium exchange inhibitors</u>

      Amiloride and derivatives

2. Agents acting within the cell

2.A <u>Acting on sarcoplasmic reticulum</u>

      Dantrolene, TMB-8

2.B <u>Acting on mitochondria</u>

      Ruthenium red

2.C <u>Calmodulin antagonists</u>

      Phenothiazines : trifluoperazine, chlorpromazine
      Naphtalene derivatives : W7
      Local anesthetics : dibucaine
      Dopamine antagonists : pimozide, haloperidol
      Calmidazolium (R 24571)

B. FACILITATORS
=============

1. Agents acting at the plasma membrane

  <u>Calcium agonists</u>

      Dihydropyridines : BAY K 8644, CGP 28392, YC 170

2. Agents acting on sarcoplasmic reticulum

      Inositol 1,4,5-triphosphate
      Caffeine

3. Ionophore

      A 23187, ionomycin

of calcium in the perfusate. To characterize the diphenylpiperazines, they used the term "antagoniste du calcium" (calcium antagonist), a term used co-incidently by Fleckenstein and his Colleagues to describe the effect of verapamil and prenylamine on cardiac tissue.

Several chemical families have been added to the first generation of compounds characterized on a pure phenomenological basis as calcium antagonists, in addition other drugs have been claimed to belong to this group (Table 1). The purpose of this paper is to examine some pharmacological properties of these drugs in human coronary artery and human myocardium in vitro in order to serve for the understanding of their clinical use in angina pectoris.

RESULTS AND DISCUSSION

The pharmacotherapeutic cascade

The pharmacological actions of any drug may be studied at various levels which illustrate the five steps of a cascade from the molecular to the clinical level (Table 2). Because the main target for the therapeutic action of calcium antagonists appears to be the arterial smooth muscle, this cascade may be studied in arteries.

The simplest experimental procedure to assess the relation between calcium entry and the development of smooth muscle contraction is to preincubate the preparation in Ca-free physiological solution, to depolarize it with Ca-free KCl-rich solution and gradually increase the calcium concentration in the bathing solution. This will result in an increase in tension dependent on Ca^{2+} concentration (1). When an agonist is used to stimulate the tissue, the calcium dependency of the response may also be examined. It should be pointed out that the response of a vessel to vasoconstrictors depends upon the interaction of the agent with specific receptors but that it may be modulated by factors extrinsic to the muscle cell. Some of those factors are derived from the endothelium. When endothelium has been

Table 2. The pharmacotherapeutic cascade of a drug.

Level of pharmacological action	Qualitative effect	Quantitative parameter
1. Molecule	Binding to Ca^{2+} channel	K_D, K_i
2. Cell	Changes in Ca^{2+} fluxes and action potentials	I_{50}
3. Tissue (in vitro)	Cardiac negative inotropic and chronotropic effects, smooth muscle relaxation	IC_{50}, pA_2
4. Organ (in vivo)	Hemodynamic modifications, (ECG, cardiac output, blood pressure)	Plasma levels
5. Clinical disorder	Anti-anginal and anti-hypertensive effects	Plasma levels

Table 3. Quantitative parameters of the pharmacotherapeutic cascade of nifedipine in angina pectoris.

Level of action	Quantitative parameter	Value (nM) in	
		Rat aorta	Human coronary
1	K_i	4[*]	
2	I_{50}	2[†]	
3	IC_{50}	2[†]	3; 30[‡]
5	Therapeutic free drug plasma level		7-20

[*] K_i value for displacement of (^3H)-nitrendipine by nifedipine.

[†] Concentration of nifedipine producing 50 % inhibition of ^{45}Ca influx (I_{50}) or contraction (IC_{50}) evoked by K^+-depolarization.

[‡] Inhibition of contractions evoked by K^+-depolarization (IC_{50} 3 nM) or serotonin (IC_{50} 30 nM).

(For references, see 8).

330

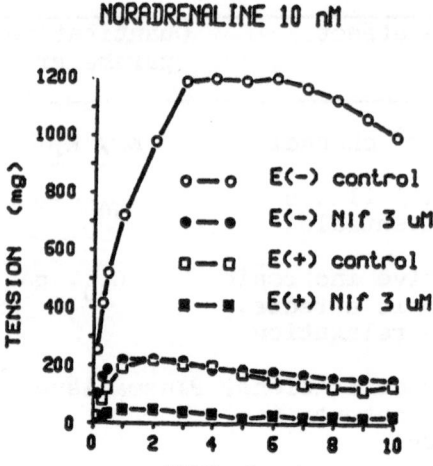

NORADRENALINE 10 nM

o — o E(-) control
● — ● E(-) Nif 3 uM
□ — □ E(+) control
■ — ■ E(+) Nif 3 uM

TENSION (mg)

TIME (min)

Fig. 1. : Response of rat aorta to noradrenaline 10 nM, with (E+) and without (E-) endothelium; inhibition by nifedipine 3 uM (8).

removed, there is an amplification of vasoconstrictive responses that was initially reported with clonidine and other adrenergic agents in rat aorta (Fig. 1) (5). This effect of endothelium in contractile responses may explain changes in vasomotor tone observed in some cardiovascular diseases associated with endothelial damages. Therefore in pharmacological experiments on vessels, it is mandatory to compare results obtained with and without endothelium when vasoactive agents, but not KCl-depolarization, are studied. Studies with human coronary arteries have not yet fully considered this question.

Calcium dose-effect curves have been established in the absence and the presence of various concentrations of dihydropyridines and of diphenylpiperazines. The results were similar except that the potency was different between these compounds. A shift to the right of the calcium dose-effect curve and a dose-dependent depression of the maximum response are usually observed. This graphical expression of the experimental results explains the use of the term "calcium antagonist" to characterize those drugs.

Another protocol of study has consisted in the analysis of the relaxing action of diphenylpiperazines and dihydropyridines on the contraction evoked by a K-depolarizing solution. Relaxation is dose-dependent (6) and the contraction can be completely abolished. In such experiments, differences between drugs were not only related

to active concentrations but also to the rate at which
relaxation was achieved.

Using isopycnic density gradient centrifugation,
Godfraind and Wibo (7) have shown that nitrendipine specific
binding sites are associated with the plasma membrane. They
have compared estimates, measured by various approaches, of
the apparent dissociation constants of dihydropyridines :
inhibition of smooth muscle contraction, (IC_{50}), of calcium
entry (I_{50}) and displacement of H^3-nitrendipine from its
binding sites in microsomes (Ki). As far as vasoconstrictor
agonists were concerned, for each dihydropyridine so far
examined, these three estimates were relatively close (8).

Such data therefore indicate that the effect of the
dihydropyridines on vascular smooth muscle contraction are
related to their binding to calcium channels resulting in
blockade of their opening by vasospastic stimuli. However,
although the basic mechanism of action appears identical for
all dihydropyridines, differences among them are found
considering their mode of interaction with potential
operated channels (giving or not use-dependence) (8).

Human coronary arteries in vitro

Experimental studies on the pharmacology of human
coronary arteries become of major interest due to the recent
evolution of concepts regarding the determinants of anginal
attack and of the initiation of myocardial infarct (9).

Human isolated coronary arteries display various types
of spontaneous rhythmic activity. As reported by Godfraind
and Miller (6), this activity is only noted in some arterial
segments and has not been found in arteries from 29-year-old
or younger hearts. In nonactive segments, rhythmic activity
could sometimes be induced by several agonists. When it was

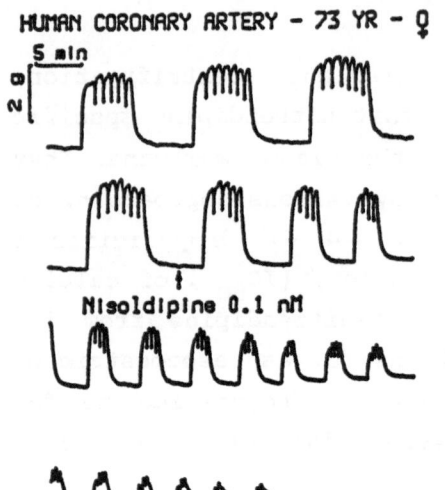

HUMAN CORONARY ARTERY - 73 YR - ♀

5 min

2 g

Nisoldipine 0.1 nM

Fig. 2. : Spontaneous contractile activity in human isolated coronary artery and its abolition by nisoldipine (8).

present, this activity appeared to be extremely sensitive to dihydropyridines such as nifedipine or nisoldipine (Fig. 2). The spontaneous fluctuations in tone may be attributed to fluctuations in calcium concentration in the myoplasm. When human coronary arteries are examined in vitro, K-rich solutions, known to depolarize smooth muscle membrane, evoke a sustained contraction that can be attenuated by drugs such as nifedipine, nisoldipine, lidoflazine.

Although potassium released from myocytes during cardiac anoxia could act as a vasoconstrictor, it is unlikely that it could initiate vasospastic angina, therefore it is worth to examine the action of various agonists. Several endogenous vasoconstrictors initiate the contractile activity of human coronary arteries in vitro. There are some variations in responsiveness to some agonists when the results from different laboratories are compared (6,10,11,12,13,14). We may identify at least two factors responsible for this heterogeneity : the age of the heart and the existence or absence of a cardiovascular disease responsible or not of the death. The main difference between reports occurs with noradrenaline.

In man, alpha-adrenergic mediated vasoconstriction may contribute significantly to myocardial ischemia in patients with coronary artery disease (15). Ginsburg et al. (10) and Toda (14) have reported that noradrenaline contracts coronary arteries. We could only elicit noradrenaline contractions in human coronary arteries in the presence of propranolol. However, the presence of functional sympathetic nerve endings is obvious from the potentiation of the response after blockade of neuronal uptake by cocaine. In the preparations that we studied, it appears that the beta-adrenergic responsiveness was more important than the alpha-adrenergic one. Indeed, precontracted coronary arteries were relaxed by isoprenaline concentrations down to 10^{-7} M, the maximum effect was reached with 10^{-5} M. This effect was blocked by propranolol. This relaxation appears to depend upon the age of the heart. Preparations taken from older hearts (60-70 years) failed to relax in the presence of isoproterenol. This loss of responsiveness is in accordance with observations done in animal vessels showing a reduction of isoproterenol-evoked relaxation with aging (6).

Serotonin and PGF_{2alpha} are the most potent vaso-constrictors. They usually increase the basal tone of the vessel and increase the rhythmicity.

Human coronary arteries contain both H_1 and H_2 receptors (6). H_1 receptors are responsible for the contraction evoked by histamine. Ginsburg et al. (11) have reported that atherosclerotic coronary segments are supersensitive to histamine. H_2 receptors appear to control relaxation of precontracted arteries. Godfraind and Miller (6) have reported that this effect is reduced or absent in older hearts.

Godfraind et al. (12) have reported that nifedipine is a powerful inhibitor of both the spontaneous activity and the activity evoked by spasmogens. The same is true for nisoldipine which appears to be a highly potent inhibitor of the rhythmic contractions in human coronaries (Fig. 1). The action of nifedipine on coronary spasm is dose-dependent. On human coronary artery contracted by serotonin, the abolition of the rhythmic activity was observed for concentrations $(10^{-8}$ M) that were found in the blood after a therapeutic dose of nifedipine. Higher doses completely relaxed the artery.

An analysis of the pharmacotherapeutic cascade is possible for the action of nifedipine in angina pectoris. As shown in Table 3 where the quantitative parameters of the cascade are reported, there is sufficient agreement between the various values obtained on isolated preparations to conclude that the effect observed is related to the molecular interaction with calcium channels.

The problem of selectivity

One of the most important questions related both to the mode of action and to the clinical use of calcium antagonists is : does tissue selectivity exist, and if so, to what properties of the antagonists and tissues is it due ?

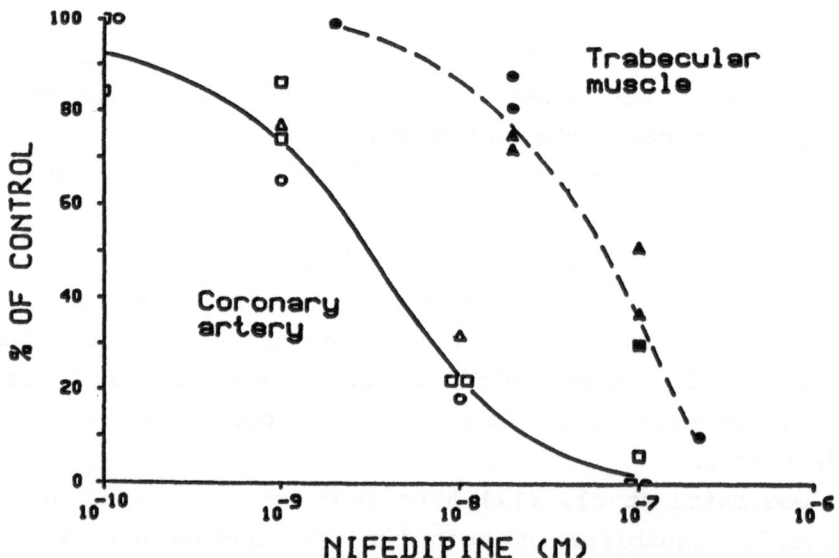

Fig. 3. : Concentration-effect curves of nifedipine in human isolated coronary artery segments contracted by depolarization (solid line and open symbols) and electrically stimulated trabecular muscle (broken line and solid symbols) taken from the same hearts aged 45 (O), 43 (□) and 15 (△) years. The ordinate represents the contractile effect as percentage of that in control tissues. Each point represents a single observation (12 modified).

As far as the cardiovascular system is concerned, agents that depress cardiac contractility are not generally sought after by clinicians and a primary concern is the relative selectivity of the antagonists for vascular tissue over cardiac tissue. Figure 3 illustrates the inhibition by nifedipine of the contraction of human trabecular muscle and of human coronary arteries taken from the same hearts and shows vascular specificity of the dihydropyridine.

Studies of the sensitivity of the human myocardium to the depressant action of nifedipine have shown that depression of the coronary contraction was achieved without significant change in the contractility of trabecular muscle (12). This indicates that at therapeutic concentration the action of nifedipine is only on the coronary spasm.

The selectivity of action, or lack of it, for several parts of the heart is an equally interesting possibility, offering the potential to alter specifically a particular function of the heart. In both rat and human cardiac preparations, it appears that the contractile force of atria is more depressed by nifedipine than the contractile force of ventricular preparations. Studies in rat heart with the calcium agonist Bay K 8644 (16) have shown that for a "physiological" concentration of calcium, the positive inotropic effect at maximal effective concentration was higher in ventricules than in atria. However the ED_{50} values of Bay K 8644 were not different in the two preparations. In addition, it was observed that pretreatment with nifedipine shifted to the right dose-effect curve of the calcium agonist allowing us to estimate the dissociation constant of nifedipine for the negative inotropic receptors. The value of this dissociation constant was much lower than the IC_{50} of nifedipine indicating that the negative inotropic effect of nifedipine depends of several factors and not only on the affinity of the receptors for dihydropyridines. Among those factors are the number of calcium channels per surface unit of the cardiac cell and the membrane potential. Membrane potential prevailing in vivo might be different from that existing in vitro. Factors such as affinity and calcium channels density might be different between species. This justifies the use of isolated human preparations for comparing different drugs of the same family and to define their specificity for a given tissue. For instance, we have observed that nisoldipine is 100 time more specific than nifedipine for human coronary arteries.

CONCLUDING REMARKS

There is an obvious need for quantitative information on the action of drugs in human beings. The use of human tissues, that is not limited by ethical considerations, may help for that purpose. It may furthermore provide an insight into the mechanism of action of the therapeutic effect of drugs in man that is not necessarily related to the mechanism of action of their pharmacological effect in animals. Analysis of the actions of Ca antagonists in human isolated coronary arteries and isolated cardiac preparations may serve as an illustration of such studies.

The pharmacological actions of any drug may be studied at various levels (molecule, cell, tissue in vitro, organ in vivo, clinical disorder) which illustrates in five steps a pharmacotherapeutic cascade from the molecular to the clinical level. In order to assume the existence of a link between the various steps, some consistency should exist in the order of magnitude of the quantitative parameters estimated for the various levels of action. An analysis of the pharmacotherapeutic cascade is possible for the action of nifedipine in angina pectoris.

When attempting to relate the therapeutic effects of drugs to their pharmacological properties, it is important to remember that the tissular conditions prevailing in pathological states may profoundly affect the drug activity. For instance, in ischaemic or anoxic conditions, there is an increase of extracellular K^+ which will modify the membrane potential and the function of calcium channels and thereby their interaction with calcium entry blockers.

SUMMARY

The action of Ca antagonist dihydropyridines has been studied in vitro on human coronary arteries and on human myocardium.

There is evidence that the effect observed at the tissue level is related to the molecular interaction with calcium channels. Nifedipine-evoked relaxation of depolarized human coronary arteries in vitro was observed at concentrations close to therapeutic plasma levels. IC_{50} values for the action of nifedipine on vascular and cardiac isolated preparations indicate that the effect on coronaries may be obtained without affecting cardiac contractility. This is still more marked for nisoldipine. However, IC_{50} values on intact cardiac tissue preparations are usually considerably higher than the dissociation constants measured on microsomal preparations. Such discrepancy may be attributed to the marked voltage-dependency of the interaction of dihydropyridines with their cardiac receptors.

REFERENCES
1. Godfraind, T. and Kaba, A. Br. J. Pharmacol. 36:549-560, 1969.
2. Godfraind, T., Kaba, A. and Polster, P. Arch. Int. Pharmacodyn. Ther. 172:235-239, 1968.
3. Godfraind, T. and Polster, P. Thérapie 23:1209-1220, 1968.
4. Fleckenstein, A., Tritthart, H., Fleckenstein, B., Herbst, A. and Grun G. Pflügers Arch. 307:R25, 1969.
5. Godfraind, T., Eglème, C. and Alosachie, I. Clin. Sci. 68:65s-71s, 1985.
6. Godfraind, T. and Miller, R.C. Circ. Res. 52:(suppl.) I81-I91, 1983.
7. Godfraind, T. and Wibo, M. Br. J. Pharmacol. 85:335-340, 1985.
8. Godfraind, T. Acta Pharmacol. Toxicol. 58(suppl.II):5-30, 1986.
9. Braunwald, E. N. Engl. J. Med. 307:1618-1627, 1982.
10. Ginsburg, R., Bristow, M.R., Harrisson, D.C. and Stinson, EB. Chest. 78:180-186(suppl.), 1980.

11. Ginsburg, R., Bristow, M.R., Davis, K., Dibiase, A. and Billingham, M.E. Circulation 69:430-440, 1984.
12. Godfraind, T., Finet, M., Socrates Lima, J. and Miller, R.C. J. Pharmacol. Exp. Ther. 230:514-518, 1984.
13. Godfraind, T. and Miller, R.C. In : Prostaglandins and Membrane Ion Transport (Eds. P. Braquet, S. Nicosia, J.C. Frohlich and R.P. Garay), Raven Press, New York, 1984, pp. 223-226.
14. Toda, N. Am. Physiol. Soc. H937-H941, 1983.
15. Mudge, G.H., Goldberg, S., Gunther, S., Mann, T. and Grossman, W. Circulation 59:544-550, 1979.
16. Finet, M., Godfraind, T. and Khoury, G. Br. J. Pharmacol. 86:27-32, 1985.

28

INHIBITORY EFFECTS OF ALLICIN (DIALLYL DISULFIDE-OXIDE, A CONSTITUENT OF GARLIC OIL) ON HUMAN PLATELET AND POLYMORPHONUCLEAR LEUKOCYTE FUNCTION

PHILIP R. MAYEUX, KRISHNA C. AGRAWAL, JEN-SIE H. TOU*, BARRY T. KING, ALBERT L. HYMAN, PHILIP J. KADOWITZ, AND DENNIS B. MCNAMARA

Departments of Pharmacology, Surgery and Biochemistry*, Tulane Medical School, New Orleans, LA.

INTRODUCTION

Garlic has had an important role in herbal medicine for thousands of years. It has been used to treat infections, heart diseases and respiratory ailments such as asthma. Ether extracts of garlic (<u>Allium stivum</u>) have been reported to inhibit human platelet aggregation <u>in vitro</u> (1). Partially purified distilled extracts of garlic have also been reported to inhibit human platelet aggregation <u>in vitro</u> but the effect on arachidonic acid (AA) metabolism in platelets is uncertain (2,3). It has been reported that garlic oil or garlic juice reduces serum cholesterol (4-6) and the severity of atherosclerosis (5,6) in rats and rabbits fed a high fat-high cholesterol diet. Allicin (diallyl disulfide-oxide), a known antibacterial agent in garlic (7) and the oil which gives garlic its characteristic odor, has also been reported to reduce serum and liver cholesterol levels in rats (8), but its effect on platelet aggregation and AA metabolism has not been studied.

Both thromboxane (TX) A_2 and prostaglandin (PG) I_2 are major cyclooxygenase products of AA and prostaglandin endoperoxide H_2 (PGH_2) metabolism in platelets and vascular tissue, respectively, and the TXA_2/PGI_2 ratio has been suggested to be important in maintaining normal platelet/vessel wall interactions (9), and alterations in metabolites of AA (e.g., PGI_2) are associated with progression of atherosclerotic disease (10).

The following study was undertaken to determine what effects allicin may have on human platelet aggregation <u>in vitro</u>, on AA and PGH_2 metabolism in the human platelet, and on PGH_2 metabolism in the bovine coronary artery and lung. We have also studied the effects of allicin on human polymorphonuclear leukocyte (PMN) lysosomal enzyme release since this process is an important mediator of the inflammatory process.

MATERIALS AND METHODS

Chemicals.

Arachidonic acid sodium, adenosine 5'-diphosphate sodium, papaverine hydrochloride, A23187, phenolphthalein β-glucuronide, phenolphthalein standard, and nordihydroguaiaretic acid were purchased from Sigma, St. Louis, Mo. (1-^{14}C)-Arachidonic acid (59.6 mCi/mmole) was purchased from Amersham, Arlington Heights, Il. U46619,(15S)-hydroxy-11α,9α-(epoxymethano) prosta 5Z,13E-dienoic acid), and prostaglandin standards were obtained from The Upjohn Co., Kalamazoo, Mich. Prostaglandin H synthetase was purchased from Oxford Biomedical Research, Inc., Oxford, Mi. Diallyl disulfide was purchased from Chemical Dynamics Corp., South Plainfield, N.J. All other chemicals were purchased from commercial chemical companies.

Synthesis of allicin.

Allicin was synthesized by a modified method of Stoll and Seebeck (11). To a solution of diallyl disulfide (3.24 g, 0.02 mole) in 15 ml of acetic acid, 30% hydrogen peroxide (5 ml) was added dropwise. During the addition, the reaction flask was kept in ice. The mixture was then stirred at room temperature for 1 hr followed by the addition of 50 ml of water. The solution was then reduced in volume to half under vacuum at 30°C. To the remaining solution an additional 50 ml of water was added and then extracted with ethyl ether (3 x 100 ml). The ether extracts were washed with a sodium bicarbonate solution (5%) and then with water. After drying over anhydrous $MgSO_4$, the ethyl ether was removed under vacuum. The oil was further purified by silica gel column chromatography, employing chloroform as the eluant. The UV absorbing fractions showing a single spot on TLC (silica gel) were collected. The solvent was then removed under vacuum to yield 1.85 g (51.4% yield) of pure allicin. The sample was analyzed for C, H, and N ($C_6H_{10}OS_2$). The spectral analysis (UV, IR, and NMR) of the oil was consistent with allicin. The oil was stored at -70°C. Solutions were made before the start of each experiment, kept on ice, and discarded after 2 hr.

Preparation of prostaglandin endoperoxide H_2.

(1-^{14}C)-PGH_2 was generated from 250 nmoles (1-^{14}C)-AA by incubation in 0.1 M phosphate buffer (pH 8.0) for 30 sec at 37°C with 150 units of prostaglandin H synthetase. The reaction was terminated by acidification with HCl to pH 2-3 and the reaction mixture was filtered under vacuum onto an ice-cold SPE Octadecylsilane (C18) 3 ml column (J.T. Baker,

Phillipsburg, N.J.). Greater than 98% of the radioactivity was extracted by the column. Stepwise elution with hexane:ether mixtures in the ratio 8:2, 6:4, 5:5, and 4:6 at 4°C yielded pure PGH_2 (>90%) in the 4:6 fractions. This methodology is a modification of the previously published method (12). Low specific activity $(1-^{14}C)-PGH_2$ was prepared from ram seminal vesicle microsomes using 3.3 μmoles AA plus 10 nmoles $(1-^{14}C)-AA$ (12) and purified in the same fashion. All PGH_2 was stored as a hexane:ether solution at -45°C.

Preparation of microsomes from bovine lung.

Bovine lungs were obtained from a local slaughterhouse where they were removed, kept on ice, and transported to the laboratory in a physiological salt solution (PSS), pH 7.4, consisting of (mM): NaCl, 118; KCl, 4.7; $CaCl_2$, 1.5; $NaHCO_3$, 25; $MgSO_4$, 1.1; KH_2PO_4, 1.2; and glucose, 5.6. The following procedures were done at 0-4°C. The tissue was minced and homogenized in 3 vol of 0.1 M phosphate buffer, pH 7.4, with a Polytron PT.20 homogenizer for 40 sec. The homogenate was centrifuged at 10,000 x g for 10 min. The supernatant was strained through cheesecloth and centrifuged at 100,000 x g for 1 hr. The microsomal pellet thus obtained was resuspended in phosphate buffer and stored at -45°C.

Preparation of microsomes from bovine coronary arteries.

Bovine hearts were obtained from a local slaughterhouse and transported on ice in PSS to the lab. The following procedures were done at 0-4°C. The circumflex and left anterior descending coronary arteries were dissected and cleaned. The tissue was homogenized in 10 vol phosphate buffer, pH 7.4. The microsomal fraction was isolated as described for the lung.

Preparation of homogenate from human platelet.

Platelet rich plasma (PRP) obtained from a local blood bank was centrifuged at 200 x g for 20 min to remove any residual red blood cells. The following procedure was carried out at 0-4°C. The PRP was then centrifuged at 1,200 x g for 15 min. The platelet pellet was resuspended in one-third original volume with 0.1 M phosphate buffer, pH 7.4, and disrupted using a Sonifier cell disruptor, model W-185. The resulting platelet homogenate was used immediately or frozen at -45°C and used the next day. Overnight storage of the platelet homogenate in this manner did not result in any loss in cyclooxygenase or TXA_2 synthetase activity (unpublished data).

Protein determination of the microsomal fractions from lung and coronary artery and of the homogenate from human platelet were made using the Bio-Rad protein assay kit (Richmond, Ca.).

Assay of arachidonic acid metabolism.

Platelet homogenate (1500 µg protein) was incubated in 100 µl of 5 mM tryptophan in 0.1 M phosphate buffer, pH 7.4, containing no other additions, 0.2% DMSO (dimethylsulfoxide) vehicle control, or various concentrations of allicin or other additions along with 20 µM AA, in duplicate. The reaction was initiated by addition of the reaction mixture (pre-incubated for 2.5 min at 37°C) to 2 nmole AA (266,400 cpm) dried at 0°C under a stream of N_2. Incubation with AA was for 1 hr in darkness at 37°C with constant stirring. The reaction was stopped and products extracted with addition of 400 µl ice-cold solution of ethyl acetate: methanol:0.2 M citric acid, pH 2.0 (15:2:1), vortexed and centrifuged. The upper organic layer was spotted for TLC on Analtech silica gel GHL plates along with authentic prostaglandin standards (6-keto-PGF$_{1\alpha}$, PGF$_{2\alpha}$, TXB$_2$, PGE$_2$, and PGD$_2$) and developed using the solvent system ethyl acetate:acetic acid:hexane:water (54:12:25:60, organic phase). The migration of prostaglandin standards was located by exposing the plates to iodine vapor and that of radiolabelled products by radiochromatogram scan on Packard 7201B or Technical Associates HY-35-4 scanners followed by computer analysis. Products were quantified based on percent conversion of substrate as described previously (12).

Assay of PGH$_2$ metabolism.

Microsomal fraction from bovine lung (200 µg protein) or bovine coronary artery (10 µg protein) or homogenate from human platelet (200 µg protein) was incubated in 100 µl of phosphate buffer, pH 7.4, containing no additions, 0.2% DMSO vehicle control, or various concentrations of allicin or other additions along with 10 µM PGH$_2$, in duplicate. The reaction was initiated by addition of the reaction mixture (pre-incubated for 2.5 min at 37°C) to 1 nmole PGH$_2$ (15,000 cpm) dried at 0°C under a stream of N_2. Incubation with PGH$_2$ was for 2 min at 37°C followed by addition of 400 µl of the stop solution. PGH$_2$ metabolites were extracted and quantified as described for products of AA.

Platelet aggregation study.

Blood from healthy donors, who had not ingested any aspirin or other nonsteroidal antiinflammatory drugs for at least two weeks, was collected by venopuncture into one-tenth vol of 3.8% trisodium citrate. Whole blood and PRP were in contact only with plastic or siliconized glass. PRP was prepared by centrifugation of whole blood at 200 x g for 20 min at room temperature. Platelet poor plasma (PPP) was prepared by centrifugation of PRP at 1,200 x g for 15 min.

Aggregation was monitored by continuous recording of light transmittance in a Chrono-log dual-channel aggregometer (Chrono-log Corp., Haverston, Pa.). A constant volume of PRP (0.45 ml) was used in all experiments. All drugs were prepared in 0.9% NaCl (saline) and kept on ice. Final volume in all experiments after addition of the aggregating agent was 0.5 ml. PRP was preincubated at 37°C for 3 min before addition of the aggregating agent. In experiments using allicin, the addition of allicin or the appropriate volume of saline was at 1 min of preincubation. Control aggregatory responses to AA, U46619, and ADP were 70-85% of PPP. In experiments using papaverine, allicin or saline was added at 1 min of preincubation of papaverine and PRP followed by addition of the aggregating agent at 3 min. The viability of the platelet preparation was evaluated every fifth experiment by repeating control aggregatory responses to 1.6 mM AA. If the percent maximum aggregation to AA differed more than 5% when compared to control aggregatory responses determined at the start of the experiments, no further experiments were performed and the previous four experiments were not used.

Determination of cyclic AMP levels.

The determination of cyclic AMP levels in PPP and PRP was performed in the following manner. Incubations of 0.45 ml of PPP or PRP, prepared from blood obtained from healthy donors, plus any additions (saline, allicin, or PGE_1 was added after 1 min to a final volume of 0.5 ml), were terminated after 3 min with 0.5 ml of 10% (w/v) trichloroacetic acid. Samples (1 ml) were sonicated and centrifuged for 1.5 min at 10,000 x g. The supernatant was extracted 4 times with 5 volumes of H_2O-saturated diethyl ether. The aqueous phase was dried in a 70°C water bath under a stream of air. The samples were reconstituted, acetylated (13,14), and cyclic AMP levels determined using a commercial cyclic AMP assay kit (Dupont, Boston, MA).

Preparation of human PMNs.

Human PMNs were prepared as previously described by Tou (15). Thirty ml portions of venous blood from normal donors were collected

into 4 ml of 0.15 M sodium citrate, pH 5.2, and 5 ml of 5% dextran T500
(Pharmacia Fine Chemicals, Pescataway, N.J.) in 0.15 M NaCl and allowed
to sediment at room temperature for 30 min. The supernatants containing
leukocyte-rich plasma were removed and centrifuged at 250 x g for 10 min
at 20°C. After hypotonic lysis of contaminating erythrocytes, leukocytes
were washed once and resuspended in Krebs-Ringer HEPES (N-2-hydroxyethyl-
poperazine-N-2-ethanesulfonic acid) buffer (16 mM, pH 7.4) modified to
contain 5 mM glucose at $1-2 \times 10^8$ cells/ml. Three ml cell suspensions
were layered on 3 ml Ficoll-Hypaque (Pharmacia Fine Chemicals, Pescataway,
N.J.) cushions and centrifuged at 400 x g for 20 min at 20°C to yield a
neutrophil pellet which was washed twice and suspended at a concentration
of 10^7 cells/ml in Krebs-Ringer HEPES buffer. Cell counts were made in
a hemocytometer, and cell viability was measured by trypan blue exclusion.
Cell preparations contained more than 95% neutrophils.

Assay for PMN β-glucuronidase release.

One ml of isolated PMNs was preincubated for 2 min at 37°C in a
Dubnoff shaker with 1 mM $CaCl_2$, allicin, or 0.1% DMSO vehicle. PMN
lysosomal release was stimulated by addition of the calcium ionophore
A23187 (5 μM final concentration). Incubation continued for 15 min
followed by centrifugation at 12,000 x g for 1 min using a desk top
Brinkmann centrifuge (Brinkmann Instruments, Westbury, N.Y.). The
supernatants were quickly aspirated and kept on ice until assaying for
β-glucuronidase activity (used as an index of β-glucuronidase release)
by the method of Talalay et al. (16). Briefly, a 200 μl sample was
incubated in duplicate with 600 μl 0.1 M sodium acetate buffer, pH 4.0,
and 0.01 M phenolphthalein glucuronide as substrate. Incubation was for
18 hr at 37°C with constant shaking. The reaction was terminated with
the addition of 2 ml 0.2 M glycine buffer, pH 10.4. The optical density
of each sample was determined at 550 nm and quantified against a
phenolphthalein standard curve prepared in the same assay buffers.
Percent inhibition of β-glucuronidase was based on the enzyme activity
of the supernatant from incubation with A23187 alone (taken as 100%)
compared with those from incubations pretreated with allicin prior to
the addition of A23187.

Statistical analysis.

The data were evaluated for differences over the concentration range
used and between control and vehicle control using a one-way analysis of

variance. Significant difference was indicated when p <.05 using the Scheffe aftertest. All data are expressed as mean ± SEM.

RESULTS

Typical tracings of the effect of allicin on human platelet aggregation induced by AA, U46619 (a stable analog of PGH_2), and ADP in vitro is summarized in Fig. 1. Allicin in the concentration range $1.3 \times 10^{-4}M$ to $1 \times 10^{-3}M$ preincubated with PRP for 2 min produced concentration-dependent inhibition of aggregation induced by 1.6 mM AA ($IC_{50} = 4.0 \times 10^{-4}M$), 2.8 µM U46619 ($IC_{50} = 3.4 \times 10^{-4}M$), and 10 µM ADP ($IC_{50} = 3.1 \times 10^{-4}M$) [data not presented]. Allicin alone induced no spontaneous aggregatory response from PRP over a 5 min period. The highest concentration of DMSO vehicle (0.2%) induced no spontaneous aggregation nor did it inhibit aggregation induced by AA, U46619, or ADP. Papaverine, an inhibitor of phosphodiesterase (17), was studied in combination with allicin on platelet aggregation. Illustrated in Fig. 2 are concentration-response curves comparing the inhibitory action of allicin alone and in the presence of 20 µM papaverine. The concentration

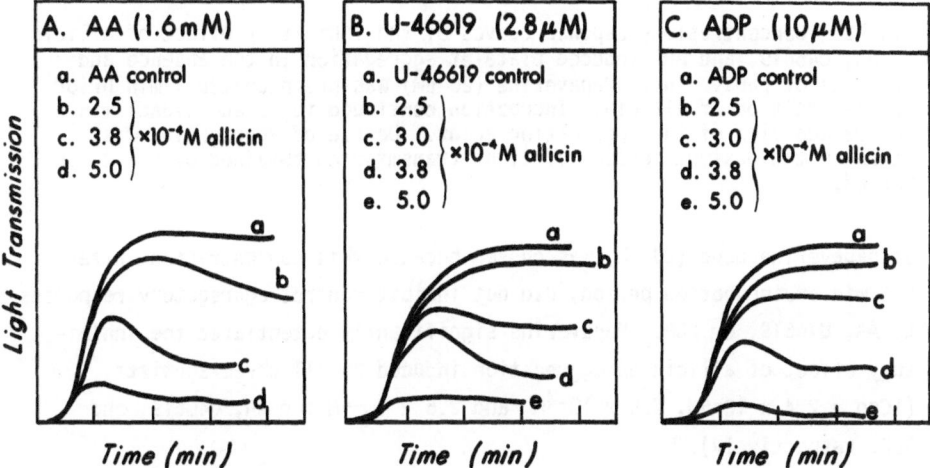

Fig. 1. Typical tracings of the inhibitory effect of allicin on platelet aggregation induced by AA, U46619, and ADP. Allicin at the concentrations indicated was incubated 2 min prior to the addition of the aggregating agent.

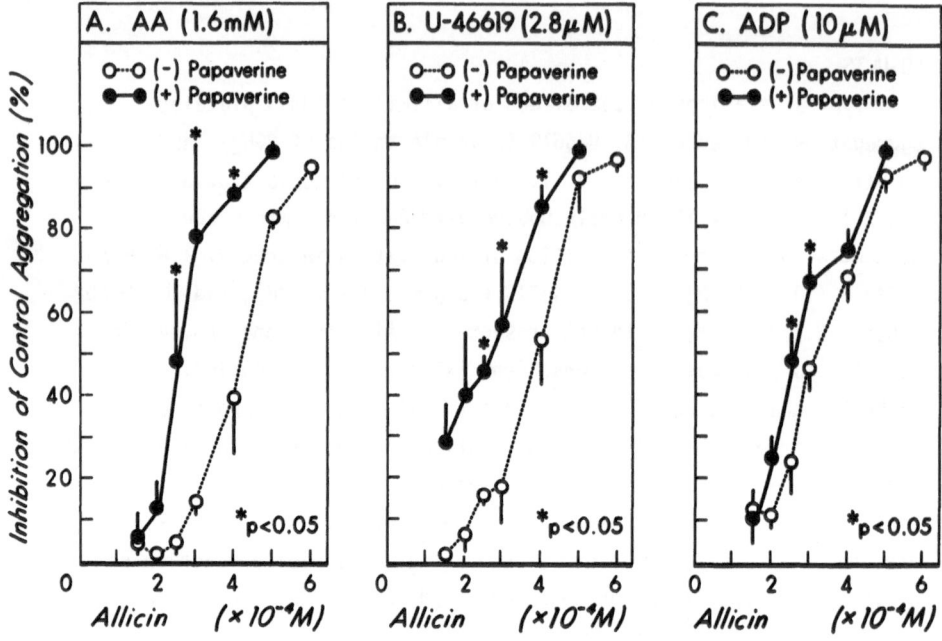

Fig. 2. Concentration-response curves of the inhibitory effect of allicin on AA, U46619, and ADP-induced platelet aggregation in the absence and presence of papaverine. Papaverine (20 μM) was preincubated 1 min prior to the addition of allicin. Incubation continued for 2 additional min before addition of the aggregating agent. Degree of aggregation was taken as the maximum percent of light transmission obtained over a 4 min period.

of papaverine used (20 μM) was chosen because this concentration, after a 3 min preincubation period, did not inhibit control aggregatory responses to AA, U46619, or ADP. Papaverine significantly potentiated the inhibitory effect of allicin on aggregation induced by all three agonists (IC_{50} = 2.4 x 10-4M, 2.5 x 10-4M, and 2.5 x 10-4M for AA, U46619, and ADP, respectively).

Allicin, at concentrations of 1.9 x 10-4M, 3.8 x 10-4M, and 5.0 x 10-4M preincubated 2 min with PRP, did not alter cyclic AMP levels within the platelets (Table 1). The combination of papaverine (20 μM, preincubated 1 min prior to the addition of allicin) and allicin (3.8 x 10-4M) induced no change in cyclic AMP levels either. PGE_1, at a concentration of $1.0 \times 10^{-6}M$ significantly increased cyclic AMP when preincubated 2 min with PRP.

Table 1. Effect of allicin on cyclic AMP levels in human platelets

	Allicin		
Control	$1.9 \times 10^{-4}M$	$3.8 \times 10^{-4}M$	$5 \times 10^{-4}M$
23 ± 5	27 ± 5	27 ± 7	32 ± 7

Papaverine 20 µM		PGE_1
	+Allicin	$1 \times 10^{-6}M*$
Control	$3.8 \times 10^{-4}M$	172 ± 65
31 ± 6	27 ± 8	

Values are expressed as pmoles of cyclic AMP per 1×10^9 platelets as measured by RIA. The cyclic AMP level in PPP was subtracted from each PRP determination in order to express the cyclic AMP level as that generated by the platelets.

*Significantly different from control, $p < .05$; n=7.

Results of experiments with human platelet homogenates are presented in Table 2. Allicin at concentrations of $10^{-6}M$ to $10^{-3}M$, incubated with 1500 µg homogenate protein and 20 µM AA or 200 µg protein and 10 µM PGH_2, induced no change in the formation of TXB_2, the stable breakdown product of TXA_2. However, the cyclooxygenase inhibitor, indomethacin, inhibited AA conversion to TXB_2 in a concentration-dependent manner ($IC_{50} = 7.0 \times 10^{-7}M$, data not presented). The AA incubations were performed with 1500 µg of platelet homogenate protein when it was determined that the average platelet protein content of each aggregation determination was 1466 ± 182 µg (n=5 individuals).

Results of experiments with microsomes prepared from bovine coronary artery are presented in Table 3. Allicin at concentrations of $10^{-6}M$ to $10^{-3}M$ incubated with 10 µg protein and 10 µM PGH_2 induced no change in the formation of 6-keto-$PGF_{1\alpha}$, the stable breakdown product of PGI_2. Results of experiments with microsomes prepared from bovine lung are presented in Table 4. Allicin at concentrations of $10^{-7}M$ to $10^{-3}M$ incubated with 200 µg microsomal protein and 10 µM PGH_2 induced no change in 6-keto-$PGF_{1\alpha}$ or TXB_2 formation. The TXA_2 synthetase inhibitor, dazoxiben,

Table 2. Effect of allicin on human platelet TXB_2 formation.

	TXB_2	
	Arachidonic acid	PGH_2
Control	537 ± 50	285 ± 10
Vehicle	539 ± 34	278 ± 9
Allicin		
$10^{-6}M$	670 ± 60	289 ± 18
$10^{-5}M$	536 ± 35	271 ± 15
$10^{-4}M$	537 ± 18	283 ± 16
$10^{-3}M$	540 ± 52	252 ± 7

The data are expressed as pmoles (mean ± SEM) of product formed per 60 min incubation with 1500 µg homogenate protein and 20 µM AA or 2 min with 200 µg homogenate protein and 10 µM PGH_2. Vehicle control was incubation in 0.2% DMSO. Allicin induced no significant change in product formation at any of the concentrations studied. n=5

Table 3. Effect of allicin on 6-keto-$PGF_{1\alpha}$ formation in the bovine coronary artery.

	6-keto-$PGF_{1\alpha}$
Control	158 ± 39
Vehicle	169 ± 41
Allicin	
$10^{-6}M$	174 ± 44
$10^{-5}M$	168 ± 38
$10^{-4}M$	165 ± 34
$10^{-3}M$	165 ± 39

The data are expressed as pmoles (mean ± SEM) of product formed per 2 min incubation with 10 µg microsomal protein and 10 µM PGH_2. Vehicle control was incubation in 0.2% DMSO. Allicin induced no significant change in product formation at any of the concentrations studied. n=3

selectively inhibited TXB_2 formation in a concentration-dependent manner (IC_{50} = 1.4 x $10^{-7}M$, data not presented). These results indicate that allicin, at the concentrations used, does not affect PGI_2 synthetase activity in microsomes from bovine coronary artery nor does allicin affect PGI_2 synthetase activity or TXA_2 synthetase activity in microsomes from bovine lung.

Table 4. Effect of allicin on TXB_2 and 6-keto-$PGF_{1\alpha}$ formation in the bovine lung.

	TXB_2	6-Keto-$PGF_{1\alpha}$
Control	295 ± 14	89 ± 13
Vehicle	298 ± 11	84 ± 15
Allicin		
10^{-7}M	265 ± 17	82 ± 12
10^{-6}M	282 ± 19	94 ± 17
10^{-5}M	283 ± 15	97 ± 16
10^{-4}M	295 ± 18	109 ± 12
10^{-3}M	259 ± 8	112 ± 13

The data are expressed as pmoles (mean ± SEM) of product formed per 2 min incubation with 200 μg microsomal protein and 10 μM PGH_2. Vehicle control was incubation in 0.2% DMSO. Allicin induced no significant change in product formation at any of the concentrations studied. n=4

Allicin produced concentration-dependent inhibition of A23187-stimulated lysosomal enzyme release from human PMN (Table 5). A 15 min exposure to A23187 (5 μM) stimulated PMN lysosomal enzyme release (as measured by released β-glucuronidase) which was inhibited by a 2 min preincubation with allicin in the concentration range of 10^{-7}M to 10^{-4}M (IC_{50} = 5 x 10^{-6}M). A23187 stimulated release of 20 ± 5% of the releasable β-glucuronidase as determined by hypotonic lysis (data not presented). UV spectral analysis confirmed the absence of chemical interaction between allicin and A23187. In addition, β-glucuronidase activity was not affected by addition of allicin (100 μM) and incubation for 17 min prior to assaying (data not presented). These controls indicate that the inhibition of A23187-stimulated lysosomal enzyme release by human PMN is due to the action of allicin on the PMN and not artifactual due to chemical interactions with A23187 or β-glucuronidase.

DISCUSSION

We report here that allicin inhibits human platelet aggregation in vitro induced by AA, U46619, and ADP. The inhibition of aggregation induced by U46619 was potentiated by the phosphodiesterase inhibitor papaverine, yet neither allicin nor the combination of allicin plus papaverine significantly raised the level of cyclic AMP within the

Table 5. Effect of allicin on β-glucuronidase release from human PMN stimulated with A23187.

Allicin	$10^{-8}M$	$10^{-7}M$	$10^{-6}M$	$10^{-5}M$	$10^{-4}M$
% Inhibition of release	2 ± 2	22 ± 10	43 ± 8	58 ± 20	67 ± 9

One ml of PMN (10^7 cells) was incubated 15 min with 5 M A23187 with or without a 2 min preincubation with allicin. Data are expressed as percent inhibition (mean $\pm$ SEM) of A23187 stimulated release β-glucuronidase using β-glucuronidase activity as an index of enzyme release. n=3-4

platelet. We have shown that allicin does not affect AA or PGH_2 metabolism in homogenates of human platelets nor is metabolism of PGH_2 affected in microsomes prepared from bovine coronary artery and bovine lung. Allicin does inhibit PMN lysosomal enzyme release stimulated by the calcium ionophore A23187.

Steam distilled extracts of garlic and partially purified methanolic extracts of garlic have been reported to inhibit human platelet aggregation in vitro (2,3). Allicin is formed naturally through the action of the enzyme allicinase on the parent compound alliin when the tissue of the garlic bulb is disrupted (18). Due to the labile nature of allicin, steam distilled extracts as prepared by Vanderhoek et al. (2) should not have contained allicin. In their study, steam distilled extracts of garlic were shown to inhibit human platelet aggregation induced by ADP as well as to inhibit AA metabolism by cyclooxygenase and lipoxygenase. The methanolic extract prepared by Apitz-Castro et al. (3) may have contained allicin although they did not specifically report its presence. Their study indicated that methanolic extracts did inhibit platelet aggregation yet left cyclooxygenase and lipoxygenase activities unaffected. These two studies suggest that there are different components of garlic that may have inhibitory activity on platelet aggregation. The present data demonstrate that pure allicin can inhibit human platelet aggregation in vitro induced by agonists which initiate the aggregating process through different mechanisms. AA-induced aggregation is initiated through metabolism of AA to TXA_2, a potent stimulus of aggregation (19). Initiation of aggregation by a substance like U46619 is, therefore, not dependent on cyclooxygenase or TXA_2 synthetase activity or on the availability of

AA (21). ADP is believed to initiate aggregation through inducing shape changes in the platelet followed by stimulation of endogenous AA metabolism (22). The IC_{50} of allicin for the three agonists is not significantly different. This suggests a mechanism of inhibition of aggregation that is equally effective against each of the three agonists. This would not be the case if inhibition were through inhibition of AA or PGH_2 metabolism. Inhibition of aggregation induced by U46619 suggests a mechanism that is not associated with AA metabolism or release. Further evidence to support a non-AA mediated mechanism for inhibition of platelet aggregation comes from the present observation of the absence of any effect on TXA_2 formation using AA or PGH_2 as substrate in homogenates of human platelet.

The potentiation of the inhibitory action of allicin by papaverine against all three aggregating agents suggests a cyclic nucleotide mechanism. Agents which increase or maintain the level of cyclic AMP are known to inhibit platelet function, irrespective of the initiating event (22). Although papaverine potentiates the anti-aggregatory action of allicin, the lack of any detectable rise in cyclic AMP indicates that this potentiation is not mediated through a change in cyclic AMP levels. The concentrationof papaverine used may have been too low to produce a detectable rise in cyclic AMP (17). At the concentration used in the present study, papaverine has been reported to dilate the dog basilar artery mainly through inhibition of the voltage-dependent influx of calcium and also through inhibition of the receptor-activated release of intracellular calcium stores in a manner thought not to be causally related to an increase in cyclic AMP (23). It has also been suggested that at a papaverine concentration as low as 50 μM, the inhibitory action of papaverine on rat ileal smooth muscle results from blockade of the calcium influx (24). It may be that papaverine potentiates the anti-aggregatory action of allicin through inhibition of calcium mobilization. A rise in the level of cyclic GMP within the platelet has been associated with inhibition of platelet aggregation (25). It is not known what effect, if any, allicin has on cyclic GMP.

The inhibition by allicin of calcium-dependent lysosomal enzyme release by A23187 suggests that allicin may alter PMN functions requiring calcium movements. A23187 increases the free calcium concentration within the PMN which could directly induce lysosomal enzyme release or

352

stimulate a variety of calcium-dependent enzyme systems such as phospholipase (PL) A$_2$, PLC, or lipoxygenase which may contribute to lysosomal enzyme release (26). In our system, inhibition of cyclooxygenase activity by indomethacin (10 μM) does not inhibit A23187-stimulated lysosomal enzyme release whereas nordihydroguaiaretic acid (10 μM), an inhibitor of cyclooxygenase and lipoxygenase, does inhibit A23187-stimulated release (unpublished data). The effect of allicin on lipoxygenase activity is unknown.

Although inhibition of lipoxygenase may inhibit PMN lysosomal enzyme release, lipoxygenase inhibition in the platelet would not inhibit aggregation and might even be expected to promote aggregation in response to AA (27). Inhibition of platelet aggregation and inhibition of PMN lysosomal enzyme release can both be accomplished through inhibition of calcium mobilization. Although no direct measurements have yet been made, if allicin were to inhibit calcium mobilization such as that triggered by TXA$_2$ in the platelet or A23187 in the PMN, this could be a common mechanism through which allicin inhibits platelet aggregation and PMN lysosomal enzyme release. Further studies are indicated to test the hypothesis that allicin exerts its effects on platelet and PMN function by inhibition of calcium mobilization or channel function.

SUMMARY

Allicin inhibits platelet aggregation and PMN lysosomal enzyme release. Since allicin has no effect on cyclic AMP levels in the platelet and no effect on AA or PGH$_2$ metabolism, the data suggest that allicin may be exerting its effects through inhibition of calcium mobilization. Garlic is still used today as a folk remedy for ailments such as infections, hypertension, heart disease, pneumonia, and asthma. Garlic oil is comprised of many compounds. One such compound is allicin, the oil which gives garlic its characteristic odor. Our studies indicate that allicin has pharmacologic activities in vitro which may lend credence to its usefulness as an herbal medicine.

REFERENCES

1. Bordia, A. Atherosclerosis 30:355-360, 1978.
2. Vanderhoek, J.Y., Makhefa, A.N. and Bailey, J.M. Biochem. Pharmacol. 29:3169-3173, 1980.

3. Apitz-Castro, R., Cabrera, S., Cruz, M.R., Ledezma, E. and Jain, M.K. Thromb. Res. 32:155-169, 1983.
4. Sodimu, O., Joseph, P.K. and Augusti, K.T. Experientia 40:78-80, 1984.
5. Bordia, A., Verma, S.K., Vyas, A.K., Khabya, B.L., Rathore, A.S., Bhu, N. and Bedi, H.K. Atherosclerosis 26:379-386, 1977.
6. Sainani, G.S., Desai, D.B., Natu, M.N., Katrodia, K.M., Valame, V.P. and Sainani, P.G. Jap. Heart J. 20:351-357, 1979.
7. Cavallito, C.J. and Bailey, J.H. J. Am. Chem. Soc. 66:1950-1951, 1944.
8. Augusti, K.T. and Mathew, P.T. Experientia 30:468-470, 1974.
9. Sinzinger, H., Feigl, W. and Silberbauer, K. Lancet 2:469, 1979.
10. Gryglewski, R.J., Dembinska-Kiec, A., Zmuda, A. and Gryglewska, T. Atherosclerosis 31:383-394, 1978.
11. Stoll, A. and Seebeck, E. Hel. Chim. Acta 31:189-210, 1948.
12. She, H.S., McNamara, D.B., Spannhake, E.W., Hyman, A.L. and Kadowitz, P.J. Prostaglandins 21:531-541, 1981.
13. Harper, J.F. and Brooker, G.J. Cyclic Nucleotide Res. 4:207-218, 1975.
14. Frandsen, E.K. and Krishna, G. Life Sci. 18:529-541, 1976.
15. Tou, J-S. Lipids 21:324-327, 1986.
16. Talalay, P., Fishman, W.H. and Huggins, C. J. Biol. Chem. 166: 757-772, 1946.
17. Mills, D.C.B. and Smith, J.B. Biochem. J. 121:185-196, 1971.
18. Cavallito, C.J., Bailey, J.H. and Buck, J.S. J. Am. Chem. Soc. 67: 1032, 1945.
19. Parise, C.V., Venton, D.L. and LeBreton, G.C. J. Pharmacol. Exp. Ther. 228:240-244, 1984.
20. Coleman, R.A., Humphrey, P.P.A., Kennedy, I., Levy, G.P. and Lumley, P. Br. J. Pharmacol. 73:773-778, 1981.
21. Brace, L.D., Venton, D.L. and LeBreton, G.C. Am. J. Physiol. 249: H1-H7, 1985.
22. De Gaetano, G. Clinics in Haematol. 10:297-336, 1981.
23. Fujioka, M. Br. J. Pharmacol. 83:113-124, 1984.
24. Huddart, H. and Saad, K.H.M. J. Exp. Biol. 86:99-114, 1980.
25. Mellion, B.T., Ignarro, L.J., Ohlstein, E.H., Pontecorvo, E.G., Hyman, A.L. and Kadowitz, P.J. Blood 57:946-955, 1981.
26. Goldstein, I.M. In: Contemporary Topics in Immunobiology (Ed. R. Snyderman), Plenum Press, N.Y., Vol. 14, 1984, pp. 189-219.
27. Aharony, D., Smith, J.B. and Silver, M.J. Biochim. Biophys. Acta 718:193-200, 1982.

ACKNOWLEDGMENTS

The authors wish to thank Ms. Janice Ignarro for her expert help in the preparation of the manuscript. This investigation was supported in part by National Institutes of Health grants HL29456, HL15580, HL11802, and HL18070 and a grant from the American Heart Association-Louisiana, Inc.